# Psychotic Disorders: Conceptualization and Treatment

# Psychotic Disorders: Conceptualization and Treatment

Editor: Paul Walker

MURPHY & MOORE
www.murphy-moorepublishing.com

www.murphy-moorepublishing.com

MURPHY & MOORE

**Cataloging-in-Publication Data**

Psychotic disorders : conceptualization and treatment / edited by Paul Walker.
p. cm.
Includes bibliographical references and index.
ISBN 978-1-63987-466-8
1. Psychoses. 2. Psychoses--Treatment. 3. Psychology, Pathological. I. Walker, Paul.
RC512 .P79 2022
616.89--dc23



Murphy & Moore Publishing,
1 Rockefeller Plaza,
New York City, NY 10020, USA

ISBN 978-1-63987-466-8 (Hardback)

# Contents

# Preface

Psychotic disorders refer to a group of severe ailments which impact the mind. They can affect a person's ability to think clearly, communicate effectively, make sound judgments and comprehend reality. A few types of psychotic disorders are schizophrenia, schizophreniform disorder, schizoaffective disorder, delusional disorder and shared psychotic disorder. Schizophrenia causes hallucinations or delusions in the patients, along with changing their behavior. Schizophreniform disorder displays schizophrenic symptoms but for a duration shorter than 6 months. Schizoaffective disorder involves the symptoms of both schizophrenia and mood disorder. Psychotic disorders can be treated through antipsychotic medications and therapies such as individual talk therapy, cognitive behavioral therapy and psychoanalytic therapy. This book attempts to understand the multiple disorders that fall under the psychotic disorders and how they can be treated. It will provide comprehensive knowledge to the readers. This book will serve as a valuable source of reference for graduate and post graduate students.

This book is a result of research of several months to collate the most relevant data in the field.

When I was approached with the idea of this book and the proposal to edit it, I was overwhelmed. It gave me an opportunity to reach out to all those who share a common interest with me in this field. I had 3 main parameters for editing this text:

1. Accuracy - The data and information provided in this book should be up-to-date and valuable to the readers.

2. Structure - The data must be presented in a structured format for easy understanding and better grasping of the readers.

3. Universal Approach - This book not only targets students but also experts and innovators in the field, thus my aim was to present topics which are of use to all.

Thus, it took me a couple of months to finish the editing of this book.

I would like to make a special mention of my publisher who considered me worthy of this opportunity and also supported me throughout the editing process. I would also like to thank the editing team at the back-end who extended their help whenever required.

**Editor**

1

# Negative Symptoms of Schizophrenia: Constructs, Burden, and Management

Agota Barabassy, Balázs Szatmári,
István Laszlovszky and György Németh

**Abstract**

The aim of the chapter is to raise awareness about recent constructs of negative symptoms, their burden on patients, caregivers and society, and about their management. Schizophrenia consists of positive, negative, and cognitive symptoms. However, treating physicians are not necessarily aware about recent constructs of negative symptoms, their presence at prodromal stage, and the distinction among primary, secondary, persistent, prominent, or predominant negative symptoms. Negative symptoms have a substantial impact on the day-to-day functioning of patients with schizophrenia and contribute more to impaired quality of life and poor functioning than positive symptoms do. Additionally, they are associated with high costs for society and a substantial burden for caregivers. Negative symptoms are not adequately treated by available antipsychotic therapies. Publications have shown that no antipsychotic has a beneficial effect when compared to another. Cariprazine is the only antipsychotic that has proven superiority over another antipsychotic (risperidone) in one clinical study.

**Keywords:** primary, secondary, prominent, predominant, negative symptoms, deficit syndrome, alogia, affect blunted, avolition, anhedonia, asociality, antipsychotic treatment

## 1. Introduction

It is well known and established in the scientific community that schizophrenia symptoms can be categorized as positive, negative, and cognitive. While positive symptoms are easy to recognize, negative symptoms are often more difficult to distinguish, as they can be mistaken for depressive symptoms [1, 2]. For the treatment of schizophrenia symptoms, several antipsychotics were discovered, developed, and registered from the 1950s. These drugs are efficiently improving the positive symptoms of schizophrenia but have slight or no effect on the negative and cognitive symptoms. Since no real treatment was available for negative symptoms, little focus has been laid on this particular field of the disease so far. With very recent development approaches and the new potential treatments on the horizon, discussions on how to define, distinguish, and treat negative symptoms are increasing day by day.

Negative symptoms are a key element of schizophrenia including symptoms such as blunt affect, lack of motivation, asociality, and impoverished speech. They are associated with disruptions and/or lack of normal emotions and behavior [1, 3]. These symptoms may occur with or without positive symptoms and can, at times, be difficult to recognize as part of the disorder.

Recently, a consensus has been reached on how to describe negative symptoms [4]:

Five constructs (the 5 "A") were identified as negative symptoms namely affect (blunted), alogia, anhedonia, asociality, and avolition and were clustered into two factors: one including blunted affect and alogia and the other consisting of anhedonia, avolition, and asociality (**Table 1**). For each construct, symptoms due to identifiable factors, such as medication effects,

**Blunted affect and alogia cluster**

Affect blunted/flat affect

Blunted affect refers to a decrease in emotions and expressions. Patients may appear immobile, lifeless, and have a wooden expression [5]. They may make little to no eye contact and speak in a dull monotone voice [1]. Absence of emotions is called flat affect [3]

Alogia

Patients with schizophrenia often have reduced speech and may give short answers to questions. Many questions may be required in order to receive sufficiently detailed information from the patient [3, 6]

**Anhedonia, avolition and asociality cluster**

Avolition

Avolition refers to lack of motivation, sense of purpose, or ability to follow through on plans. For example, the patient may have a desire or interest to grow a garden but never act on the plan [6]

Anhedonia

Anhedonia refers to lack of pleasure. Patients suffering from schizophrenia may not take interest in activities they previously enjoyed. For example, a patient who was an avid gardener before may have a complete lack of interest in gardening when suffering from schizophrenia [5]

Asociality/Social withdrawal

Patients with schizophrenia may exhibit social withdrawal, show diminished interest and pleasure in social interactions, and often neglect activities of daily living (such as personal hygiene) [1, 3]. Asociality should not be defined in purely behavioral terms (whether the subject has social interactions and close relationships), but mainly as a reduction in motivation for social contacts (whether the subject values and desires social interactions and close social bonds) [7, 8]

**Table 1.** Characteristics of the most important negative symptoms.

| | |
|---|---|
| Primary | Considered a core symptom of schizophrenia which persist during clinical stability [9] |
| Secondary | A consequence of positive symptoms, neurological side effects, depressive symptoms, or environmental factors [10, 11] |
| Deficit syndrome | Presence of at least two out of the following six negative symptoms in patients meeting criteria for schizophrenia: 1. restricted affect (referring to observed behavior), 2. diminished emotional range (i.e., reduced range of the patient's subjective emotional experience), 3. poverty of speech, 4. curbing of interests, 5. diminished sense of purpose, 6. diminished social drive for at least 12 months including periods of clinical stability. The above symptoms are primary, i.e., not secondary to factors such as anxiety, drug effect, psychotic symptoms, intellectual disability or depression [12–14] |
| Prominent | Prominent negative symptoms were defined as: 1. Baseline score ≥4 on at least 3, or ≥5 on at least 2 negative PANSS subscale items; or 2. PANSS negative score >3 on item 1 and item 6 and at least one third item with a score >3 and a maximum of two items with a score >3 from the positive subscale [15, 16] |
| Predominant | Predominant negative symptoms were defined as: 1. Baseline score ≥4 on at least 3 or ≥5 on at least 2 of the 7 negative subscale items and a PANSS positive score of <19; 2. PANSS negative score ≥6 points over PANSS positive score; 3. PANSS negative score of at least 21 and at least 1 point greater than the PANSS positive score and 4. A common sense definition, negative subscale greater than positive subscale [15, 16] |
| Persistent | Persistent negative symptoms are defined as the presence of at least one negative symptom of moderate or higher severity, not confounded by depression or parkinsonism, at baseline and after 1 year of treatment [17] |
| Liemburg—core negative symptoms | Avolition, anhedonia<br>(Intensity of expected pleasure from activities diminished, asocial behavior) [18] |
| Liemburg—expressive deficit | Blunted affect, alogia<br>(Facial expression, expressive gestures, vocal expression, spontaneous elaboration, quantity of speech diminished) [18] |

**Table 2.** List and characteristics of frequently used negative symptom definitions.

psychotic symptoms or depression, should be distinguished from those regarded as core symptoms of the disease.

Besides this new adaptation, negative symptoms can also be characterized as primary, secondary, prominent, predominant or persistent, as deficit syndrome, or clustered as Liemburg "core negative symptoms" and "expressive deficit" clusters. **Table 2** gives an overview of frequently used negative symptom definitions.

## 2. Differential diagnosis

Negative symptoms can be part of various conditions/diseases and must be distinguished from those related to schizophrenia. The most important differentiation for clinical practice is between primary and secondary negative symptoms. While primary negative symptoms are considered a core symptom of schizophrenia, which persist during clinical stability [9], secondary negative symptoms are believed to be a consequence of other factors such as:

- positive symptoms (for example, social withdrawal because of paranoid ideas),
- neurological side effects of antipsychotic treatment (Parkinson like symptoms),
- depressive symptoms
- or environmental factors (social under stimulation due to hospitalization) [10, 11].

The importance of distinguishing primary from secondary negative symptoms lies in its therapeutic implication; while secondary negative symptoms can be improved by removing the underlying cause, primary negative symptoms are likely to persist despite treatment [9].

Additionally, negative symptoms, especially symptoms of **anhedonia, avolition, and asociality** can also occur in a number of other psychiatric diseases including depressive episodes, substance abuse, and internal or neurological disorders [19]. Schizoaffective disorder, depressive type (ICD-10 F25.1), and severe major depressive disorder with psychotic symptoms (ICD-10 F32.3) are two diseases that are particularly difficult to distinguish from schizophrenia with negative symptoms. Schizoaffective disorder, depressive type is "a disorder in which both schizophrenic and depressive symptoms are prominent, so that the episode of illness does not justify a diagnosis of either schizophrenia or depressive episode" [20]. The patient experiences a combination of schizophrenia symptoms, such as hallucinations or delusions, and mood symptoms, such as potentially anhedonia, avolition, and asociality. Severe major depressive disorder with psychotic symptoms is a disease where "the patient suffers from lowering of mood, reduction of energy, and decrease in activity. Capacity for enjoyment, interest, and concentration is reduced, and marked tiredness after even minimum effort is common. The lowered mood varies little from day to day, is unresponsive to circumstances, and may be accompanied by so-called 'somatic' symptoms, such as loss of interest and pleasurable feelings, marked psychomotor retardation, agitation, loss of appetite, weight loss, and loss of libido. Hallucinations, delusions, psychomotor retardation, or stupor so severe that ordinary social activities are impossible" might be present [20]. A correct diagnosis and distinction from schizophrenia with negative symptoms has a great impact on therapy in these diseases: while for schizoaffective disorder and major depressive disorder the therapy includes antidepressants next to antipsychotics [21], for negative symptoms of schizophrenia, this has not been shown as effective [22].

The differential diagnosis of **blunted affect** includes next to schizophrenia, post-traumatic stress disorder (PTSD). PTSD is a mental disorder that is triggered by a terrifying event (war, torture, sexual assault). Symptoms include flashbacks, nightmares, inability to feel positive emotions, dissociative symptoms, severe anxiety, and avoidance of triggers [19]. Blunted affect, anhedonia, and feelings of detachment are also core symptoms of PTSD, which cause diminished interest in activities that produce pleasure, and reduced tendency of emotional expressions [23].

**Alogia** is caused by a dysfunction in the fronto-striatal area of the brain and can therefore also occur in several neurological diseases (such as Huntington's and Parkinson's diseases, dementia, etc.) [24]. However, physical symptoms that accompany such diseases make the differentiation from schizophrenia not so difficult.

Overall, it can be concluded that while symptoms of anhedonia, avolition, and asociality also occur in the course of several other diseases (especially those with depressive episodes), blunted affect and alogia seem to be more inherent to schizophrenia with negative symptoms [25].

## 3. Course

Schizophrenia typically begins with a prodromal period, which precedes first episode psychosis and can last from a few days to around 18 months. The prodromal period and the very early phases of the disease are characterized by negative symptoms [26]. In contrast, early stages and acute exacerbations are more characterized by positive symptoms. Over time, the positive symptoms diminish due to treatment or due to the natural course of the illness and are replaced by more prominent negative symptoms. Finally, during the residual phase of the illness, negative symptoms are most prevalent [27]. **Figure 1** shows a typical course of the disease.

Although this is a common pattern for schizophrenia, the course can vary considerably. Some patients have psychotic episodes lasting weeks or months with full remission of their symptoms between each episode; others have a fluctuating course in which symptoms are continuous but rise and fall in intensity; yet others have relatively little variation in the symptoms of their illness over time.

In order to define clinically relevant course variants, a healthcare professional needs to be able to characterize both the current state as well as the longitudinal pattern of the illness in the individual patient [28]. For this, ICD-10 provides the following course specifiers [20] (**Table 3**).

At one end of the spectrum, the person has a single psychotic episode of schizophrenia followed by complete recovery; at the other end of the spectrum is a course in which the illness never abates and debilitating effects increase (**Figure 2**).

Negative symptoms are common in the prodromal phase of the disease, in between psychotic episodes and at the end of the disease in the residual phases. According to the ICD-10, which

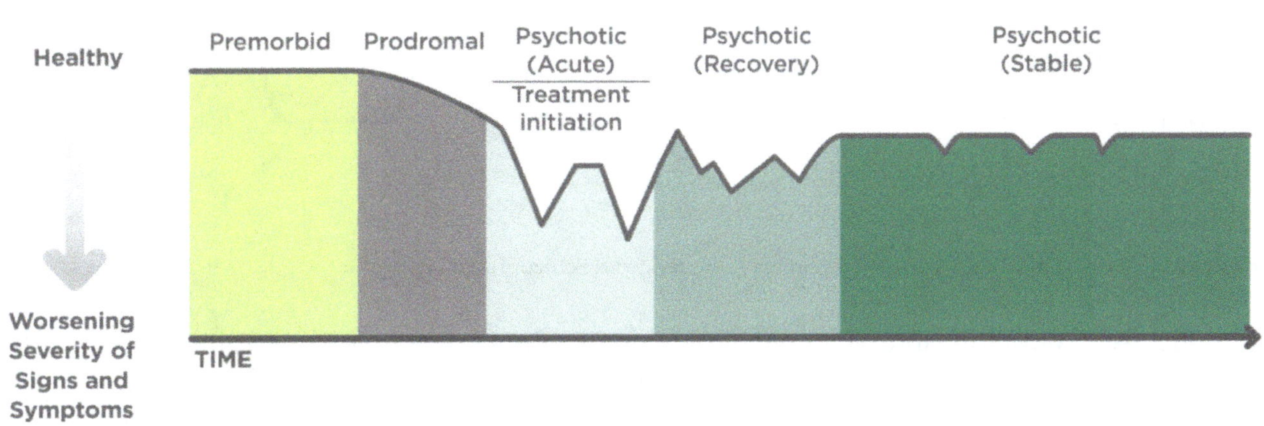


**Figure 1.** Individual clinical course of schizophrenia (adapted from American Psychiatric Association [32]).

| Class | Course |
|---|---|
| F20.x0 | Continuous; no remission of psychotic symptoms throughout the period of observation |
| F20.x1 | Episodic; with a progressive development of "negative" symptoms in the intervals between psychotic episodes |
| F20.x2 | Episodic; with persistent but nonprogressive "negative" symptoms in the intervals between psychotic episodes |
| F20.x3 | Episodic (remittent); with complete or virtually complete remissions between psychotic episodes |
| F20.x4 | Incomplete remission |
| F20.x5 | Complete or virtually complete remission |
| F20.x8 | Other pattern of course |
| F20.x9 | Course uncertain, period of observation too short |

**Table 3.** ICD-10 course specifiers.

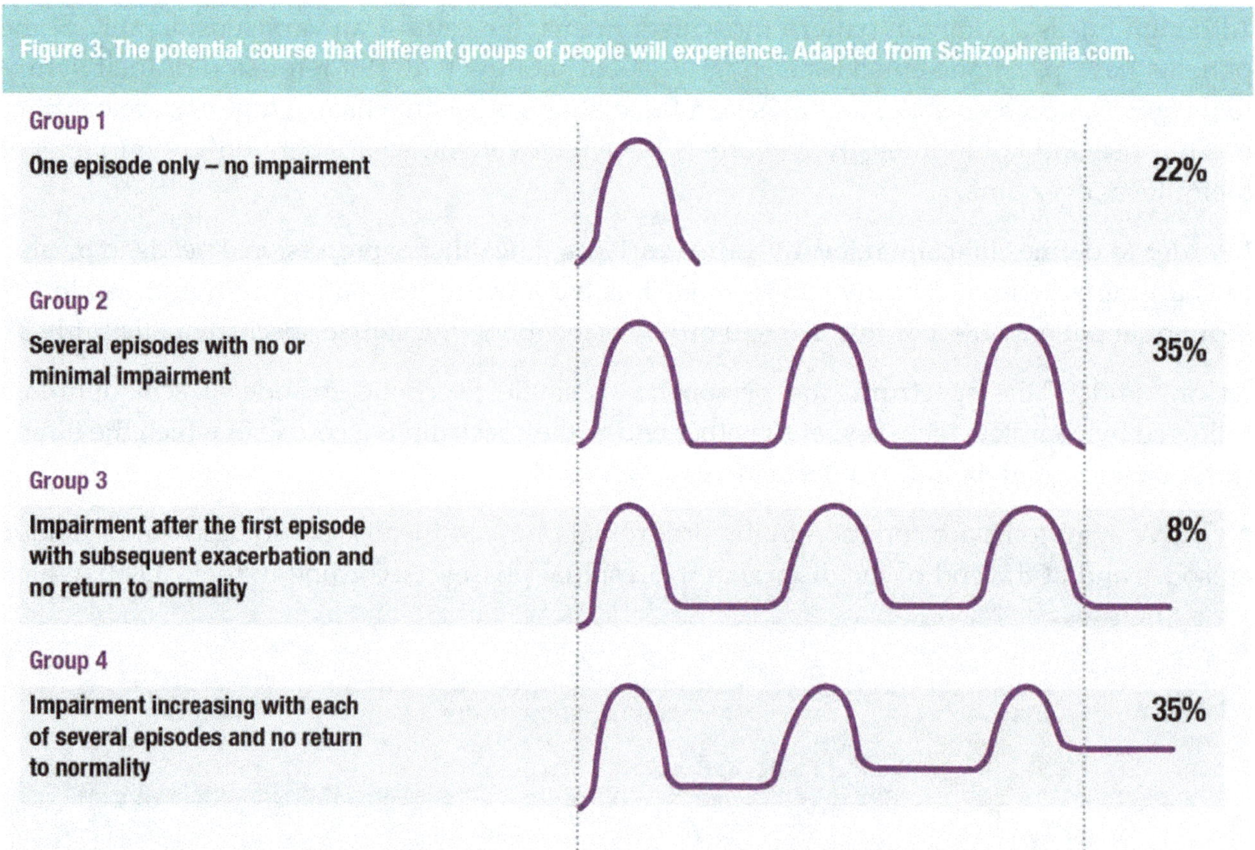


**Figure 2.** Overall clinical course of schizophrenia (adapted from Schizophrenia.com).

classifies schizophrenia into different subtypes (**Table 4**), negative symptoms prominently occur in hebephrenic, simple, and residual schizophrenia.

Hebephrenic schizophrenia is "a form of schizophrenia in which affective changes are prominent, delusions and hallucinations fleeting and fragmentary, behavior irresponsible and unpredictable,

| | |
|---|---|
| F20.0 | Paranoid schizophrenia |
| F20.1 | Hebephrenic schizophrenia |
| F20.2 | Catatonic schizophrenia |
| F20.3 | Undifferentiated schizophrenia |
| F20.4 | Post-schizophrenic depression |
| F20.5 | Residual schizophrenia |
| F20.6 | Simple schizophrenia |
| F20.8 | Other schizophrenia |
| F20.9 | Schizophrenia, unspecified |

**Table 4.** Subtypes of schizophrenia according to ICD-10.

and mannerisms common. The mood is shallow and inappropriate, thought is disorganized, and speech is incoherent. There is a tendency to social isolation. Usually, the prognosis is poor because of the rapid development of 'negative' symptoms, particularly flattening of affect and loss of volition. Hebephrenia should normally be diagnosed only in adolescents or young adults" [20].

"Simple schizophrenia is a disorder in which there is an insidious but progressive development of oddities of conduct, inability to meet the demands of society, and decline in total performance. The characteristic negative features of residual schizophrenia (e.g., blunting of affect and loss of volition) develop without being preceded by any overt psychotic symptoms" [20].

"Residual schizophrenia is a chronic stage in the development of a schizophrenic illness in which there has been a clear progression from an early stage to a later stage characterized by long-term, though not necessarily irreversible, 'negative' symptoms, e.g., psychomotor slowing; underactivity; blunting of affect; passivity and lack of initiative; poverty of quantity or content of speech; poor nonverbal communication by facial expression, eye contact, voice modulation and posture; poor self-care and social performance" [20].

In summary, negative symptoms constitute a core element of the disease. They dominate the clinical picture at the beginning and at the end of the disease but are also found in between psychotic episodes.

## 4. Epidemiology

Historically, applying different diagnostic criteria for patients with negative symptoms has affected the incidence and prevalence numbers of such patients. Depending on the diagnostic criteria applied, negative symptoms may comprise 5–60% of patients with schizophrenia, as shown by Rabinowitz et al., who found that in a large sample of negative symptom patients, 8.1–62.3% met criteria for prominent negative symptoms and 10.2–50.2% met criteria for predominant negative symptoms [16]. Bobes reported that approximately 60% of individuals with schizophrenia-spectrum disorders experience one or more negative symptoms [29] and about 13% of the schizophrenic patients could be described as having primary negative symptoms [29]. Buchanan claimed 15–20% experience enduring negative symptoms that are primary to the disorder [27]. In a further study by Sicras-Mainar, it was reported that 52% of the patients presented one or more negative symptoms, the most common being passive/apathetic social withdrawal and emotional withdrawal [30, 31]. Furthermore, the prevalence of negative (deficit) states has been estimated to be 15% in first episode patients, 25–30% in clinical samples and 14–17% in population studies [9].

In conclusion, it is evident that negative symptoms are highly prevalent in the schizophrenic population.

## 5. Risk factors

Brain imaging, electrophysiological, and oculomotor data, showing either less or different abnormalities in negative symptom patients (here defined as deficit syndrome), suggest that deficit syndrome represents a separate disease entity with respect to other forms of schizophrenia, and not just the extreme end of a severity continuum. This is further supported by evidence that deficit syndrome has different risk factors than general schizophrenia [9].

These are

- male gender—while in general schizophrenia, there is no difference in gender [9, 32]
- summer births, compared to a winter birth in general schizophrenia [9]
- serum antibodies to cytomegalovirus [9]
- low serum folate concentration [9]
- higher genetic contribution in negative symptoms than to positive symptoms [27]
- obstetric complications [33]
- structural abnormalities, such as enlarged ventricles [33]
- dysfunctional beliefs about performance (increased defeatist performance beliefs), acceptance, likelihood of success, and resources, which reduce motivation [33]

## 6. Burden

Negative symptoms account for much of the long-term morbidity, poor functional outcomes, and high rates of disability in patients with schizophrenia [14, 34, 35]. They have a substantial impact on the day-to-day functioning of patients affecting the ability to live independently, to perform activities of daily living, to be socially active, to maintain personal relationships, and to work and study [16, 36–40]. Research evidence suggests that the negative symptoms of schizophrenia contribute more to impaired quality of life and poor functioning than positive symptoms do [35, 38, 41] and that their severity is associated with a lower quality of life [42].

The three major challenges of schizophrenia's negative symptoms are their modest therapeutic response, pervasiveness, and diminution of patients' quality of life and functioning [43].

Evidence suggests that even after significant improvements in psychotic symptoms, patients with schizophrenia continue to experience poor quality of life due to residual negative symptoms, depression/anxiety, or cognitive impairment [44].

Mohr et al. (using their own definition of disease states based on the PANSS, as described above) found that patients who began therapy in disease state four (high negative symptoms but low to moderate other symptoms) seemed relatively intractable to treatment, with lower odds ratios than patients starting in disease states five (cognitive impairment predominant) and seven (positive predominant) [45].

Negative symptoms are major contributors to low function levels and deterioration in most patients with schizophrenia, because poorly motivated patients cannot function at school or work, cannot maintain relationships with family and friends in the face of unresponsive affect, and do not develop personal interests when experiencing anhedonia, apathy, and inattention [43].

One longitudinal study showed that negative symptoms predicted long-term impairment in global psychosocial functioning and work performance, with negative symptom severity being a significant individual predictor of the degree of impairment in relationships [34]. Additionally, the degree of impairment in participation and enjoyment of recreational activities was significantly correlated with the severity of negative symptoms [34].

Negative symptoms affect patients' ability to cope with daily activities and have a negative impact on their quality of life. Negative symptoms are relatively common and account for much of the long-term morbidity and poor functional outcome of patients with schizophrenia.

Patients with schizophrenia have severe problems with personal and social relations, which affect their quality of life (QoL) [46]. Negative symptoms, in particular, are often enduring and lead to poor functional outcomes in individuals with schizophrenia [47]. Increased risk of suicide, an unhealthy lifestyle, poor physical health, and CV disease (which is a leading cause of death) are main reasons associated with excess early mortality in schizophrenia [31].

Negative symptoms are recognized by both the Food and Drug Administration (FDA) and European Medicines Association (EMA) as features of schizophrenia that are not adequately treated by available antipsychotic therapies and are considered a valid target for drug development [16]. Negative symptoms can often persist despite psychosocial treatments and antipsychotic medication [47, 48].

As previously discussed, increased costs are positively correlated with lower functioning and negative symptoms are the major contributor to low function levels in patients with schizophrenia. Patients with negative symptoms have been shown to use more healthcare resources (including primary care, emergency care, and specialized care visits, laboratory tests, radiology tests, and pharmaceutical prescriptions), especially with regard to primary care visits [30]. The highest direct costs are due to a high frequency of hospital admissions in negative symptom patients [49]. In addition to this direct cost, negative symptoms represent a burden for patients, caregivers, and society and therefore constitute a relevant economic burden [30].

## 7. Treatment

With the development of second-generation antipsychotics, there was initially hope within the medical community of targeting the negative and cognitive symptoms, as well as the positive symptoms of schizophrenia. Indeed, various therapeutic guidelines suggest second-generation antipsychotics (SGAs) over first-generation antipsychotics (FGAs); however, this suggestion is controversial.

The second-generation antipsychotics demonstrated efficacy in treating positive symptoms with less motor side effects than first-generation antipsychotics (with accompanied improvement in secondary negative symptoms), but the treatment goal of also improving the primary, negative, and cognitive symptoms was not achieved with these medications [22].

To explore any differential efficacy against negative symptoms, Leucht et al. [50] conducted a meta-analysis of 150 RCTs that directly compared an FGA with an SGA and included data from more than 21,000 patients. They found that four SGAs (clozapine, olanzapine, amisulpride, and risperidone) were most effective overall, but also specifically with respect to negative symptoms, when compared to FGAs. The magnitude of this difference, however, was small, with the largest effect size reported being 0.32 for olanzapine. With respect to EPS side effects, these four drugs were better than high dose FGAs but not when compared to low doses. The findings of pragmatic studies comparing the clinical effectiveness of SGAs and FGAs in schizophrenia [51, 52] are consistent with the findings of Leucht et al. meta-analysis.

More recent publications have shown that no drug has a beneficial effect on negative symptoms when compared to another [53–55]. In the only meta-analysis assessing available treatments for negative symptoms versus placebo, some statistically significant differences were found for various treatments (e.g., second-generation antipsychotics, antidepressants, glutamatergic agents, psychological interventions), but no effect reached the level of clinically significant improvement [55].

The results of the Cutlass1 study showed no advantage of second-generation drugs in terms of quality of life or symptoms over 1 year in patients with schizophrenia. In fact, those participants receiving a first-generation antipsychotic did rather better. In addition, there were no significant differences in rates of objectively assessed extrapyramidal side effects [51].

Amisulpride, the most widely studied antipsychotic in patients with negative symptoms, is indicated for negative symptoms in several European countries. However, most of the evidence showing efficacy is versus placebo and was obtained from clinical trials that were conducted in the 1990s (before the introduction of the current EMA recommendations) [56–59]. When amisulpride was evaluated in two recent studies conducted in patient populations specifically selected for predominant negative symptoms, the findings for amisulpride were equivocal [60]. A 6-month trial comparing olanzapine (5 or 20 mg/d) and amisulpride 150 mg/d with placebo only found significant improvement for low-dose olanzapine versus placebo, but not for amisulpride [61]. Additionally, in a 12-week double-blind trial comparing amisulpride and ziprasidone, equivalent improvement in negative symptoms was demonstrated for both drugs [62]. Improvement in patient functioning in conjunction with negative symptom improvement was not investigated in any of these studies [54], and pseudospecificity parameters were also not well controlled for.

Scant information is currently available to guide clinicians on the treatment of negative symptoms. This leads to

- **Treatment guidelines** rarely mentioning treatment of negative symptoms specifically, and if they do, they suggest second-generation antipsychotics. **Table 5** gives a few examples of treatment guideline suggestions. It is agreed that these antipsychotics are to be used for the treatment of negative symptoms, because so far no effective therapies were available. The scientific community agrees, however, that current antipsychotics do not adequately address negative symptoms. Therefore, it is to be shown, how therapeutic guidelines will change once an agent is available that shows better efficacy on negative symptoms than other antipsychotics.
- **Physicians prescribing** various medications including anxiolytics, antidepressants, and anticonvulsants, which sometimes add little value and create unnecessary polypharmacy [22]. Antidepressants are a common treatment choice given the overlap between predominant negative symptoms and depressive symptoms, but supporting evidence is limited [63].

In the light of these facts, it is paramount to find efficacious therapies for negative symptoms, as there is a huge unmet medical need. Extensive research is ongoing, and there are some promising agents in development that could potentially be used for negative symptom treatment later on [60, 64, 65]. However, at the moment, only one antipsychotic exists, which has shown superiority over another antipsychotic in the treatment of negative symptoms in a well-designed study examining treatment effects on primary, persistent negative symptoms and that agent is cariprazine [60].

Cariprazine is a new D3/D2 partial agonist antipsychotic with preferential binding to D3 receptors. Cariprazine differs from all available antipsychotics due to its higher affinity for D3 receptors, which is higher than that of any other antipsychotic or in fact than dopamine itself. Cariprazine can therefore affect a D3 receptor blockade [66] that no other antipsychotic can. Since the blockade of D3 receptors has been shown to be related to improvement of negative and cognitive symptoms [67], it is assumed that cariprazine's blockade of D3 receptors is responsible for its effects on negative symptoms.

This was demonstrated in a randomized, double-blind, risperidone-referenced clinical trial [60]. The study enrolled schizophrenic patients with persistent (at least 6 month), predominant (high level on negative symptoms low level of positive symptom), primary (extrapyramidal symptoms (EPS), high positive symptoms and depression were exclusionary) negative symptoms. After the 26 week treatment period, cariprazine-treated patients showed significant

| Organization | Terminology | Recommendation |
|---|---|---|
| World Federation of Societies of Biological Psychiatry (2012) | Negative symptoms | "For primary negative symptoms, treatment with certain SGAs (amisulpride, aripiprazole, clozapine, olanzapine, quetiapine, ziprasidone), but not with FGAs, is recommended with inconsistent evidence and with the need for more studies to prove the efficacy." |
| British Association for Psychopharmacology (2011) | Recommendations for the pharmacological management of negative symptoms | "Psychotic illness should be identified and treated as early as possible as this may offer some protection against the development of negative symptoms.<br>For any given patient, the antipsychotic that gives the best balance between overall efficacy and side effects should be used." |
| British Association for Psychopharmacology (2011) | Where negative symptoms persist beyond an acute episode of psychosis | "To ensure EPS (specifically bradykinesia) and depression are detected and treated if present, and consider the contribution of the environment to negative symptoms (e.g., institutionalization, lack of stimulation).<br>Consider augmentation of antipsychotic treatment with an antidepressant such as an SSRI, ensuring that choice is based on minimizing the potential for compounding side effects through pharmacokinetic or pharmacodynamic drug interactions.<br>If clozapine is prescribed, consider augmenting with lamotrigine or a suitable second antipsychotic." |
| American Psychiatric Association (2010) | Negative symptoms | "Treatment of negative symptoms begins with assessing the patient for syndromes that can cause the appearance of secondary negative symptoms. The treatment of such secondary negative symptoms consists of treating their causes, e.g., antipsychotics for primary positive symptoms, antidepressants for depression, anxiolytics for anxiety disorders, or antiparkinsonian agents or antipsychotic dose reduction for extrapyramidal side effects. If negative symptoms persist, they are presumed to be primary negative symptoms of the deficit state. There are no treatments with proven efficacy for primary negative symptoms." |

**Table 5.** Treatment guideline suggestions for negative symptoms treatment.

improvement in negative symptoms (measured by PANSS-Factor Score for Negative Symptoms /PANSS-FSNS/) and patient functionality (Personal and Social Performance /PSP/) alike compared to risperidone. Subanalyses of individual negative symptom items and PSP subdomains measuring day-to-day functioning showed that this effect was global and not only driven by selected items [60].

Responder analyses have a primary position in defining the clinical relevance of study results. In this study, these analyses with a 20 and 30% cut-off were both in favor of cariprazine over risperidone. One of the strongest methods to evaluate clinical relevance of PANSS results is the combined rate of CGI (improved/very much improved) with responder rates at 30 and 20% reduction level. Also here, cariprazine showed a clear, significant superiority of over risperidone.

The results are clinically relevant, especially bearing in mind that a significant difference over a comparator is much more difficult to achieve than over placebo, since the active comparator would be assumed to also have some activity [60].

Differences in PANSS total score, positive subscale score, general psychopathology, depression scale, or EPS scales were minimal and not statistically significant, substantiating that the change seen on negative symptoms was not due to improvement in secondary negative symptoms [60] but a true improvement on primary negative symptoms.

With no standard of care available for negative symptoms, the choice of risperidone in this study might be subject to potential criticism; however, it is the right choice considering the alternatives. Since the late 1990s, second-generation antipsychotics are the preferred treatment over first-generation antipsychotics. From the existing and available second-generation antipsychotics, only four are known to have somewhat better efficacy on negative symptoms, and these are clozapine, olanzapine, amisulpride, and risperidone [50]. Of these four:

- Clozapine is not considered a valid first-line treatment due to its severe side-effect profile. It is only a valid therapy if other antipsychotics have failed.
- Olanzapine is an effective antipsychotic medication and has, however, a completely different adverse event profile than cariprazine: its high weight gain and sedative properties would have unblinded the study. Therefore, it could not be used for this study. However, olanzapine was studied in a similarly designed negative symptom study and compared to asenapine. Olanzapine was not better in controlling negative symptoms of schizophrenia than asenapine [68], and its change from baseline to week 26 on the PANSS FSNS was lower (−7.1) than change from baseline to week 26 with cariprazine (−8.9).
- Amisulpride would have been a potential choice, since it is approved for the treatment of negative symptoms of schizophrenia in some European countries. However, which dose to choose is a challenging question: amisulpride is used in different doses for the treatment of positive symptoms (400–800 mg) and for the treatment of negative symptoms (50–300 mg) with no overlapping between the two dose ranges. Since the aim of the study was equally to improve negative symptoms and to keep positive symptoms well under control, no dose could be chosen as a well-established and empirically proven dose. Differences in equivalent doses and side-effect profiles further blurred the picture.
- Finally, risperidone was chosen, because it has a similar side-effect profile and a similar dose range to cariprazine. As no antipsychotic is considered truly better than another in the treatment of negative symptoms, risperidone is considered a valid choice and served as a representative for all antipsychotics. Risperidone kept the positive and depressive symptoms, as well as the level of EPS, well under control.

Other comparators for the study could have been placebo or aripiprazole. However,

- no empiric evidence is available for aripiprazole being an effective therapy for negative symptoms,
- and placebo would have been controversial from an ethical perspective (leaving patients untreated for 26 weeks). Moreover, such a study would have measured relapse rates instead of efficacy on negative symptoms and the results would have been difficult to interpret.

Additionally, cariprazine has demonstrated efficacy in the treatment of acute schizophrenic symptoms [44, 69, 70] as well as in relapse prevention and maintenance treatment [71]. It is generally safe and well tolerated and has a manageable safety profile. In a recent meta-analysis by Leucht et al. [72], several drugs were examined after 60 years of available antipsychotic treatment. Efficacy data on primary negative symptoms were not examined, but data on safety in the short-term acute schizophrenia trials were presented. Cariprazine showed a favorable safety profile concerning weight gain, QT prolongation, and prolactin increase [72] compared to the other antipsychotics.

## 8. Conclusions

Negative symptoms such as blunted affect, alogia, anhedonia, avolition, and asociality can be clustered into two main clusters: blunted affect and alogia cluster and anhedonia, avolition, and asociality cluster [4]. They can be further characterized as primary (key element of schizophrenia, and inherent to the disease) and secondary (due to external factors such as side effects, depression or positive symptoms). They affect patients' ability to cope with daily activities and have a negative impact on their quality of life.

Negative symptoms are relatively common (15–60%), and account for much of the long-term morbidity and poor functional outcome of patients with schizophrenia [16, 29–31, 68]. Despite the introduction of second-generation antipsychotics in the 1990s, the clinical management of these symptoms continued to be an unmet medical need [30]. Though these agents are very effective in managing positive symptoms of schizophrenia, they have relatively poor long-term efficacy for negative symptoms. Thus, many patients are left with negative symptoms after their positive symptoms have been partially or completely controlled [29].

Cariprazine is a new D3/D2 partial agonist antipsychotic with preferential binding, and subsequent blockade of D3 receptors [66]. Since the blockade of D3 receptors is assumed to be related to an improvement in negative and cognitive symptoms [67], cariprazine is assumed to be effective in the treatment of negative symptoms. This has been demonstrated in a well-designed clinical trial where cariprazine has shown a statistically significant improvement in negative symptoms and patient functioning compared to risperidone. Cariprazine has also shown to have an acceptable safety profile, with advantages in weight gain, QT prolongation and hyperprolactinemia compared to other antipsychotics [72].

In summary, with no antipsychotic therapies available for the treatment of primary negative symptoms, cariprazine is an exciting new potential. It could be the first-in-class compound and a game changer in the treatment of negative symptoms. With demonstrated efficacy on positive [44, 69–71] and negative symptoms [60], and a manageable safety profile, cariprazine monotherapy covers the full range of schizophrenic symptoms and could be a good long-term treatment choice for schizophrenia.

## Author details

Agota Barabassy*, Balázs Szatmári, István Laszlovszky and György Németh

*Address all correspondence to: barabassya@richter.hu

Gedeon Richter Plc., Budapest, Hungary

## References

[1] National Institute of Mental Health. Schizophrenia; 2017. https://www.nimh.nih.gov/health/publications/schizophrenia-booklet/index.shtml

[2] Fischer BA, Buchanan RW. Schizophrenia: Clinical Manifestations, Course, Assessment, and Diagnosis; 2017. www.up-to-date/schizophrenia

[3] Hales RE, Yudofsky SC. The American Psychiatric Publishing Textbook of Psychiatry. 5th ed. Washington DC, London: American Psychiatric Publishing; 2008

[4] Marder S, Galderisi S. The current conceptualization of negative symptoms in schizophrenia. World Psychiatry. 2017;**16**:14-24

[5] Merck Manual-Second Home Edition. Schizophrenia; 2017. http://www.merckmanuals.com/en-ca/home/mental-health-disorders/schizophrenia-and-delusional-disorder/schizophrenia

[6] American Psychiatric Association. Diagnostic and Statistical Manual of Mental Disorders (DSM-5). 5th ed. Arlington, VA: American Psychiatric Publishing; 2013

[7] Kirkpatrick B, Strauss GP, Nguyen L, Fischer BA, Daniel DG, Cienfuegos A, Marder SR. The brief negative symptom scale: Psychometric properties. Schizophr Bull. 2011 Mar;**37**(2): 300-305

[8] Kring AM, Gur RE, et al. The Clinical Assessment Interview for Negative Symptoms (CAINS): Final development and validation. American Journal of Psychiatry. 2013;**170**: 165-172

[9] Mucci A, Merlotti E, Üçok A, Aleman A, Galderisi S. Primary and persistent negative symptoms: Concepts, assessments and neurobiological bases. Schizophrenia Research. 2017 Aug;**186**:19-28

[10] Carpenter WT Jr, Heinrichs DW, Alphs LD. Treatment of negative symptoms. Schizophrenia Bulletin. 1985;**11**:440-452

[11] WFSBP Task Force on Treatment Guidelines for Schizophrenia. Hasan A, Falkai P, Wobrock T, Lieberman J, Glenthoj B, Gattaz WF, et al. World Federation of Societies of Biological Psychiatry (WFSBP) guidelines for biological treatment of schizophrenia, part 1: Update 2012 on the acute treatment of schizophrenia and the management of treatment resistance. The World Journal of Biological Psychiatry. 2012;**13**:318-378

[12] Carpenter WT Jr, Heinrichs DW, Wagman AM. Deficit and nondeficit forms of schizophrenia: The concept. The American Journal of Psychiatry. 1988 May;**145**(5):578-583

[13] Kirkpatrick B, Buchanan RW, McKenney PD, Alphs LD, Carpenter WT Jr. The schedule for the deficit syndrome: An instrument for research in schizophrenia. Psychiatry Research. 1989 Nov;**30**(2):119-123

[14] Kirkpatrick B, Buchanan RW, Ross DE, et al. A separate disease within the syndrome of schizophrenia. Archives of General Psychiatry. 2001;**58**:165-171

[15] European Medicines Agency. Guideline on Clinical Investigation of Medicinal Products, Including Depot Preparations in the Treatment of Schizophrenia. European Medicines Agency, Committee for Medicinal Products for Human Use (CHMP). London; 2012

[16] Rabinowitz J, Werbeloff N, Caers I, Mandel FS, Stauffer V, Menard F, Kinon BJ, Kapur S. Negative symptoms in schizophrenia – The remarkable impact of inclusion definitions in clinical trials and their consequences. Schizophrenia Research. 2013;**150**:334-338

[17] Galderisi S, Mucci A, Bitter I, Libiger J, Bucci P, Fleischhacker WW, Kahn RS; EUFEST Study Group. Persistent negative symptoms in first episode patients with schizophrenia: Results from the European First Episode Schizophrenia Trial. European Neuropsychopharmacology. 2013 Mar;**23**(3):196-204

[18] Liemburg E, Castelein S, Stewart R, van der Gaag M, Aleman A, Knegtering H; Genetic Risk and Outcome of Psychosis (GROUP) Investigators. Two subdomains of negative symptoms in psychotic disorders: Established and confirmed in two large cohorts. Journal of Psychiatric Research. 2013 Jun;**47**(6):718-725

[19] Fatemi SH, Clayton PJ. The Medical Basis of Psychiatry. 4th ed. New York: Springer; 2016. pp. 104-105

[20] World Health Organization. International Statistical Classification of Diseases. Online version; 2010. http://apps.who.int/classifications/icd10/browse/2016/en#/F20-F29

[21] Farahani A, Correll CU. Are antipsychotics or antidepressants needed for psychotic depression? A systematic review and meta-analysis of trials comparing antidepressant or antipsychotic monotherapy with combination treatment. The Journal of Clinical Psychiatry. 2012 Apr;**73**(4):486-496. DOI: 10.4088/JCP.11r07324

[22] van Os J, Kapur S. Schizophrenia. Lancet. 2009 Aug 22;**374**(9690):635-645

[23] Kashdan TB, Elhai JD, Christopher Frueh B. Anhedonia, emotional numbing, and symptom overreporting in male veterans with PTSD. Personality and Individual Differences. 2007 Sep;**43**(4):725-735. DOI: 10.1016/j.paid.2007.01.013

[24] Chen RY, Chen EY, Chan CK, Lam LC, Lieh-Mak F. Verbal fluency in schizophrenia: Reduction in semantic store. The Australian and New Zealand Journal of Psychiatry. 2000 Feb;**34**(1):43-48

[25] Chaturvedi SK, Prasad Rao G, John Mathai P, Sarmukaddam S, Gopinath PS. Negative symptoms in schizophrenia and depression. Indian Journal of Psychiatry. 1985 Jul-Sep; **27**(3):237-241

[26] Larson MK, Walker EF, Compton MT. Early signs, diagnosis and therapeutic of the prodromal phase of schizophrenia and related psychotic disorders. Expert Review of Neurotherapeutics. 2010;**10**:1347-1359

[27] Buchanan RW. Persistent negative symptoms in schizophrenia: An overview. Schizophrenia Bulletin. 2007;**33**:1013-1022

[28] Tandon R, Gaebel W, Barch DM, Bustillo J, Gur RE, Heckers S, et al. Definition and description of schizophrenia in the DSM-5. Schizophrenia Research. 2013 Oct;**150**(1):3-10

[29] Bobes J, Arango C, Garcia-Garcia M, Rejas J; CLAMORS Study Collaborative Group. Prevalence of negative symptoms in outpatients with schizophrenia spectrum disorders treated with antipsychotics in routine clinical practice: Findings from the CLAMORS study. The Journal of Clinical Psychiatry. 2010 Mar;**71**(3):280-286

[30] Sicras-Mainar et al. Impact of negative symptoms on healthcare resource utilization and associated costs in adult outpatients with schizophrenia: A population-based study. BMC Psychiatry. 2014;**14**:225

[31] Sicras-Mainar et al. Prevalence of metabolic syndrome according to the presence of negative symptoms in patients with schizophrenia. Neuropsychiatric Disease and Treatment. 2015;**11**:51-57

[32] American Psychiatric Association. Practice Guideline for the Treatment of Patients with Schizophrenia. 2nd ed. Arlington, VA: American Psychiatric Publishing; 2010

[33] Rector NA, Beck AT, Stolar N. The negative symptoms of schizophrenia: A cognitive perspective. Canadian Journal of Psychiatry. 2005;**50**:247-257

[34] Milev P, Ho B-C, Arndt S, Andreasen NC. Predictive values of neurocognition and negative symptoms on functional outcome in schizophrenia: A longitudinal first-episode study with 7-year follow-up. The American Journal of Psychiatry. 2005;**162**(3):495-506

[35] Kurtz MM, Moberg PJ, Ragland JD, Gur RC, Gur RE. Symptoms versus neurocognitive test performance as predictors of psychosocial status in schizophrenia: A 1- and 4-year prospective study. Schizophrenia Bulletin. 2005 Jan;**31**(1):167-174

[36] Alonso J, Croudace T, Brown J, Gasquet I, Knapp MR, Suárez D, Novick D. Health-related quality of life (HRQL) and continuous antipsychotic treatment: 3-year results from the Schizophrenia Health Outcomes (SOHO) study. Value in Health. 2009 Jun;**12**(4):536-543

[37] Harvey PD, Heaton RK, Carpenter WT Jr, Green MF, Gold JM, Schoenbaum M. Functional impairment in people with schizophrenia: Focus on employability and eligibility for disability compensation. Schizophrenia Research. 2012 Sep;**140**(1–3):1-8

[38] Rabinowitz J, Levine SZ, Garibaldi G, Bugarski-Kirola D, Berardo CG, Kapur S. Negative symptoms have greater impact on functioning than positive symptoms in schizophrenia: Analysis of CATIE data. Schizophrenia Research. 2012 May;**137**(1–3):147-150

[39] Kirkpatrick B, Buchanan RW. Anhedonia and the deficit syndrome of schizophrenia. Psychiatry Research. 1990 Jan;**31**(1):25-30

[40] Fenton WS, McGlashan TH. Natural history of schizophrenia subtypes. II. Positive and negative symptoms and long-term course. Archives of General Psychiatry. 1991 Nov;**48** (11):978-986

[41] Kirkpatrick B, Fenton WS, Carpenter WT Jr, Marder SR. The NIMH-MATRICS consensus statement on negative symptoms. Schizophrenia Bulletin. 2006;**32**(2):214-219

[42] Rudnick A, Kravetz S. The relation of social support-seeking to quality of life in schizophrenia. The Journal of Nervous and Mental Disease. 2001 Apr;**189**(4):258-262

[43] Tandon R, Jibson M. Negative symptoms of schizophrenia: How to treat them most effectively. Current Psychiatry. 2002;**1**(9):36-42

[44] Kane JM, Zukin S, Wang Y, Lu K, Ruth A, Nagy K, Laszlovszky I, Durgam S. Efficacy and safety of cariprazine in acute exacerbation of schizophrenia: Results from an international, phase III clinical trial. Journal of Clinical Psychopharmacology. 2015 Aug;**35**(4):367-373

[45] Mohr PE, Cheng CM, Claxton K, Conley RR, Feldman JJ, Hargreaves WA, Lehman AF, Lenert LA, Mahmoud R, Marder SR, Neumann PJ. The heterogeneity of schizophrenia in disease states. Schizophrenia Research. 2004 Nov 1;**71**(1):83-95

[46] Arsova S, Kopacheva Barsova G. Patients with schizophrenia and social contacts. Open Access Macedonian Journal of Medical Sciences. 2016 Sep 15;**4**(3):388-391

[47] Luther L, Fukui S, Firmin RL, McGuire AB, White DA, Minor KS, Salyers MP. Expectancies of success as a predictor of negative symptoms reduction over 18 months in individuals with schizophrenia. Psychiatry Research. 2015 Sep 30;**229**(1–2):505-510

[48] Tandon R, Nasrallah HA, Keshavan MS. Schizophrenia, "just the facts" 5. Treatment and prevention. Past, present, and future. Schizophrenia Research. 2010 Sep;**122**(1–3):1-23

[49] Millier A, Horváth M, Ma F, Kóczián K, Götze A, Toumi M. Healthcare resource use in schizophrenia, EuroSC findings. Journal of Market Access & Health Policy. 2017;**5**(1): 1372027. DOI: 10.1080/20016689.2017.1372027

[50] Leucht S, Corves C, Arbter D, Engel RR, Li C, Davis JM. Second-generation versus first-generation antipsychotic drugs for schizophrenia: A meta-analysis. Lancet. 2009 Jan 3; **373**(9657):31-41

[51] Jones PB, Barnes TR, Davies L, Dunn G, Lloyd H, Hayhurst KP, Murray RM, Markwick A, Lewis SW. Randomized controlled trial of the effect on Quality of Life of second- vs first-generation antipsychotic drugs in schizophrenia: Cost Utility of the Latest Antipsychotic Drugs in Schizophrenia Study (CUtLASS 1). Archives of General Psychiatry. 2006;**63**(10):1079-1087

[52] Lieberman JA, Stroup TS, McEvoy JP, Swartz MS, Rosenheck RA, Perkins DO, Keefe RS, Davis SM, Davis CE, Lebowitz BD, Severe J, Hsiao JK; Clinical Antipsychotic Trials of Intervention Effectiveness (CATIE) Investigators. Effectiveness of antipsychotic drugs in patients with chronic schizophrenia. The New England Journal of Medicine. 2005 Sep 22; **353**(12):1209-1223

[53] Millan MJ, Fone K, Steckler T, et al. Negative symptoms of schizophrenia: Clinical characteristics, pathophysiological substrates, experimental models and prospects for improved treatment. European Neuropsychopharmacology. 2014;**24**:645-692

[54] Arango C, Garibaldi G, Marder SR. Pharmacological approaches to treating negative symptoms: A review of clinical trials. Schizophrenia Research. 2013 Nov;**150**(2–3):346-352. DOI: 10.1016/j.schres.2013.07.026. Epub 2013 Aug 9

[55] Fusar-Poli P, Rocchetti M, Sardella A, Avila A, Brandizzi M, Caverzasi E, Politi P, Ruhrmann S, McGuire P. Disorder, not just state of risk: Meta-analysis of functioning and quality of life in people at high risk of psychosis. The British Journal of Psychiatry. 2015 Sep;**207**(3):198-206

[56] Danion JM, Rein W, Fleurot O. Improvement of schizophrenic patients with primary negative symptoms treated with amisulpride. Amisulpride Study Group. The American Journal of Psychiatry. 1999;**156**:610-616

[57] Loo H, Poirier-Littre MF, Theron M, Rein W, Fleurot O. Amisulpride versus placebo in the medium-term treatment of the negative symptoms of schizophrenia. The British Journal of Psychiatry. 1997;**170**:18-22

[58] Boyer P, Lecrubier Y, Puech AJ, Dewailly J, Aubin F. Treatment of negative symptoms in schizophrenia with amisulpride. The British Journal of Psychiatry. 1995;**166**:68-72

[59] Paillere-Martinot ML, Lecrubier Y, Martinot JL, Aubin F. Improvement of some schizophrenic deficit symptoms with low doses of amisulpride. The American Journal of Psychiatry. 1995;**152**:130-134

[60] Németh G, Laszlovszky I, Czobor P, Szalai E, Szatmári B, Harsányi J, Barabássy Á, Debelle M, Durgam S, Bitter I, Marder S, Fleischhacker WW. Cariprazine versus risperidone monotherapy for treatment of predominant negative symptoms in patients with schizophrenia: A randomised, double-blind, controlled trial. Lancet. 2017 Mar 18;**389**(10074): 1103-1113

[61] Lecrubier Y, Quintin P, Bouhassira M, Perrin E, Lancrenon S. The treatment of negative symptoms and deficit states of chronic schizophrenia: Olanzapine compared to amisulpride and placebo in a 6-month double-blind controlled clinical trial. Acta Psychiatrica Scandinavica. 2006;**114**:319-327

[62] Olie JP, Spina E, Murray S, Yang R. Ziprasidone and amisulpride effectively treat negative symptoms of schizophrenia: Results of a 12-week, double-blind study. International Clinical Psychopharmacology. 2006;**21**:143-151

[63] Möller HJ, Czobor P. Pharmacological treatment of negative symptoms in schizophrenia. European Archives of Psychiatry and Clinical Neuroscience. 2015 Oct;**265**(7):567-578

[64] Veerman SRT, Schulte PFJ, de Haan L. Treatment for negative symptoms in schizophrenia: A comprehensive review. Drugs. 2017 Sep;**77**(13):1423-1459

[65] Davidson M, Saoud J, Staner C, Noel N, Luthringer E, Werner S, Reilly J, Schaffhauser JY, Rabinowitz J, Weiser M, Luthringer R. Efficacy and safety of MIN-101: A 12-week randomized, double-blind, placebo-controlled trial of a new drug in development for the treatment of negative symptoms in schizophrenia. The American Journal of Psychiatry. 2017 Dec 1;**174**(12):1195-1202. DOI: 10.1176/appi.ajp.2017.17010122. Epub 2017 Jul 28

[66] Stahl SM. Mechanism of action of cariprazine. CNS Spectrums. 2016;**21**:123-127

[67] Maramai S, Gemma S, Brogi S, Campiani G, Butini S, Stark H, Brindisi M. Dopamine D3 receptor antagonists as potential therapeutics for the treatment of neurological diseases. Frontiers in Neuroscience. 2016;**10**:451

[68] Buchanan RW, Panagides J, Zhao J, Phiri P, den Hollander W, Ha X, Kouassi A, Alphs L, Schooler N, Szegedi A, Cazorla P. Asenapine versus olanzapine in people with persistent negative symptoms of schizophrenia. Journal of Clinical Psychopharmacology. 2012 Feb;**32**(1):36-45

[69] Durgam S, Starace A, Li D, Migliore R, Ruth A, Nemeth G, Laszlovszky I. An evaluation of the safety and efficacy of cariprazine in patients with acute exacerbation of schizophrenia: A phase II, randomized clinical trial. Schizophrenia Research. 2014;**152**:450-457

[70] Durgam S, Cutler AJ, Lu K, Migliore R, Ruth A, Laszlovszky I, Németh G, Meltzer HY. Cariprazine in acute exacerbation of schizophrenia: A fixed-dose, phase 3, randomized, double-blind, placebo- and active-controlled trial. The Journal of Clinical Psychiatry. 2015; **76**(12):1574-1582

[71] Durgam S, Earley W, Li R, Li D, Lu K, Laszlovszky I, Fleischhacker WW, Nasrallah HA. Long-term cariprazine treatment for the prevention of relapse in patients with schizophrenia: A randomized, double-blind, placebo-controlled trial. Schizophrenia Research. 2016 Oct;**176**(2–3):264-271

[72] Leucht S, Leucht C, Huhn M, Chaimani A, Mavridis D, Helfer B, Samara M, Rabaioli M, Bächer S, Cipriani A, Geddes JR, Salanti G, Davis JM. Sixty years of placebo-controlled antipsychotic drug trials in acute schizophrenia: Systematic review, Bayesian meta-analysis, and meta-regression of efficacy predictors. The American Journal of Psychiatry. 2017 Oct 1;**174**(10):927-942

# 2

# Cognitive-Behavioral Theory and Treatment of Antisocial Personality Disorder

Ahmet Emre Sargın, Kadir Özdel and
Mehmet Hakan Türkçapar

**Abstract**

Antisocial personality disorder (ASPD) has a distinct cognitive profile according to cognitive theory of personality disorders. Antisocial individuals' view of the world is personal rather than interpersonal. They cannot accept another's point of view over their own. As such, they cannot take on the role of another. Their actions are not based on choices in a social sense because of this cognitive limitation. Cognitive theory of personality disorders conceptualizes personality disorder including the ASPD, according to their basic beliefs or schemas. The content of beliefs can vary in different personality disorders. Antisocial patients view themselves as loners, autonomous, and strong. Some of them see themselves as having been abused and mistreated by society and therefore justify victimizing others because they believe that they have been victimized. Their view about other people is very negative; they see others as exploitative and thus deserving of being exploited in retaliation. In this chapter, after overviewing general features of ASPD, we aim to give an explanation how cognitive behavioral therapy (CBT) conceptualizes personality disorders in general and ASPD in particular and highlight the important implementations of CBT and schema therapy.

**Keywords:** antisocial personality disorder, cognitive behavioral theory

## 1. Introduction

Antisocial personality disorder (ASPD) is defined as a pervasive pattern of disregard and violation of the right of others [1]. Patients with ASPD often have problems with judiciary system like being arrested or imprisoned because they do not respect the right of others, they have tendency to violate the laws, anger problems, and alcohol/substance addiction [2].

During psychiatric interview they may seem inoffensive and even little bit charming but under this mask of sanity there is aggression, hostility, rage, and tension. They have defensiveness when replying the self-report scales [3]. During their lifetime, they repeatedly exhibit traits of impulsivity, low conscientiousness, which cause social and interpersonal problems. They may repeatedly perform illegal acts, lie or malinger people. They are manipulative in order to gain personal profit or pleasure. They disregard the feelings or wishes of others. Due to their impulsivity, they may change their jobs, accommodation or relationships all of a sudden without taking into consideration of the consequences. They are irresponsible as a partner and as a parent. They frequently have more than one sexual partner and hardly sustain monogamous relationships. Their children generally live in bad conditions such as lack of hygiene, malnutrition, or accommodation. All these disadvantages result in high rates of unemployment, bad housing, and being imprisoned and dying prematurely due to reckless behavior [4, 5].

The two main diagnostic systems, Diagnostic and Statistical Manual of Mental Disorders (DSM-5) and WHO's International Statistical Classification of Diseases and Related Health Problems, 10th edition (ICD-10), have similar criteria for antisocial personality construct.

According to the latest version of Diagnostic and Statistical Manual of Mental Disorders (DSM-5), ASPD is conceptualized through a criterion set which includes criminal behavior, lying, reckless and impulsive behavior, aggression and irresponsibility [4]. Although it defines a similar construct, the diagnostic label for antisocial personality has different name in ICD-10, as dissocial personality disorder. Dissocial personality disorder is defined in ICD-10 as characterized by disregard for social obligations, and callous unconcern for the feelings of others. There is gross disparity between behavior and the prevailing social norms. Behavior is not readily modifiable by adverse experience, including punishment. There is a low tolerance for frustrationand and a low threshold for discharge of aggression, including violence; there is a tendency to blame others or to offer plausible rationalizations for the behavior bringing the patient into conflict with society.

The two classifications are not identical but similar. The ICD-10 emphasizes the impairment in the interpersonal and the affective domain while DSM-5 focuses merely on the antisocial behaviour. (For instance there is a criteria of low tolerance for frustration, low threshold for aggression and violence in ICD-10 whereas DSM-5 focuses merely impulsivity, disregard for others, and irresponsible behaviors.) Also conduct disorder before the age of 15 is not necessary in ICD-10 criteria.

Antisocial personality like clinical entity is first defined as "moral insanity" in nineteenth century by Dr. J.C. Prichard in England. The moral insanity term is later replaced by another term psychopathy [6]. Psychopathy is first defined in "The mask of sanity" book of Cleckley and later conceptualized by Hare with the psychopathy checklist-revised (PCL-R) [7, 8]. Psychopathy is accepted as more severe than ASPD or dissocial personality disorder. It generally includes remorselessness, deceitfulness, egocentricity, superficial charm to others, depression and anxiety, and externalization of blame [9]. The psychopaths generally have lack of fear to aversive events and a deficit in processing affective information regardless of whether it is positive or negative [10]. There are studies suggesting that psychopaths have deficiency in empathy [11].

The prevalence of ASPD varies from depending on the instruments, methodology, and the country. It is between 1.3 and 6.8% for men and 0 and 0.8% for women [5, 12]. The prevalence is higher in populations that are affected by low socioeconomic factors. The ratio of men/women is 3. Approximately 50–80% of the criminals meet the diagnostic criteria of ASPD [13, 14]. Patients with ASPD may also have comorbid substance use disorders, anxiety disorders, depressive disorders, somatic symptoms and impulse control problems such as gambling disorder [5, 15, 16].

Like most of the psychiatric disorders, antisocial personality disorder is a heterogeneous diagnosis which has both biological and psychological etiology. From the adoption studies, it is seen that a child who has genetic vulnerability living in an adverse environment is prone to ASPD [17].

It was also asserted that psychopaths may have lack of cortical physiological responses that are associated with experiencing feelings, especially fear. Accordingly, some studies determined that psychopaths do not have autonomic hyperarousal when faced with a provoking stimulus unlike people without ASPD [18, 19].

On the other hand, according to cognitive behavioral theory it is assumed that there is developmental delay in the moral maturity and cognitive functioning of antisocial individuals which we will focus on the next chapter deeply [20].

## 2. Cognitive behavioral theory of antisocial personality disorder

### 2.1. Cognitive behavioral theory

When conceptualizing the human behaviour, cognitions and emotions, cognitive model views the cognition under two main titles: Automatic thoughts and schemas. Automatic thoughts are cognitions that accompany the distressful emotions and are specific to that situation/activating event. They are not the product of directed/driven thoughts that are created after a willing process. They rather pop up suddenly and the individuals mostly do not notice the automatic thought but the emotion resulting from it. They do not follow grammatical rules but rather they are set of meanings or images (i.e., "I am a bad mother," or having an image of himself/herself lying in bed in emergency service) flowing in the mind which are immediately accepted without evaluation by the individual and cause a distressful emotion [21, 22]. So when an activating event (A) occurs, this leads to a cognition, interpretation, evaluation, an automatic thought which is merely maladaptive/functional (B) and this leads to an emotion and a behaviour (C). Accordingly, the cognitive behavioral model emphasizes that it is not the event/situation that determines how the individual feels or behaves (**Figure 1**). It is the interpretation of that event/situation that determines the feelings and behaviors. This is why cognitive behavioral therapists suggest disputing these maladaptive/dysfunctional thoughts to modify emotions [23].

Schemas are divided into two domains: core beliefs and intermediate beliefs (underlying rules and assumptions). Although some authors like Padesky have used the term schema only to describe core beliefs; in general, core beliefs are included as a domain of schema along

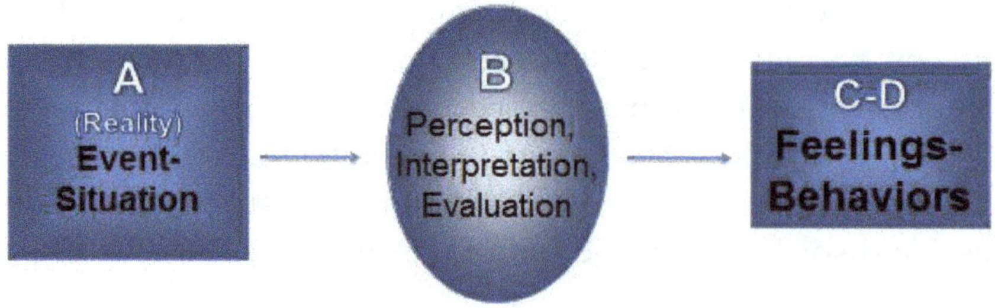


**Figure 1.** ABC model of cognitive behavioral therapy.

with intermediate beliefs [24]. Core beliefs are the cognitive constructs that determine how to regulate the information about himself/herself and his/her environment and include the essential assumptions about himself/herself, the others, and the world. After being developed as a result of early life experiences/memories and identifications with the important figures, core beliefs are reinforced with the similar experiences and learnings throughout the years [22, 25]. These beliefs about self and life constitute the emotional and behavioral traits of personality. These beliefs are so rigid, fundamental, and deep that even the individual himself/herself does not articulate them. The individual accepts these ideas as undisputable truths. Beck divides the core beliefs in three [25]:

(1) Unlovable core beliefs: "I am unlovable," "I am unattractive," "I am rejected," "I am not desired," "I am ugly," etc.

(2) Helpless core beliefs: "I am weak," "I am incompetent," "I am passive," "I am a loser," "I am coward," etc.

(3) Worthless core beliefs: "I am worthless," "I am bad," "I am disgusting," "I deserve to be punished," "I am guilty," etc.

Core beliefs exist in pairs in all the humans. For example, an individual has both "I am lovable" and "I am not lovable" core beliefs. A healthy person who does not have a psychiatric disorder or a personality disorder has the positive core belief as the effective trait ("I am lovable"). When the healthy individual experiences a negative event, the negative core belief gets activated. For example, when a healthy person breaks up from his/her partner, the core belief "I am not lovable" gets activated. This person may feel down for a while or he/she may have depression for a period. But when he/she gets rid of depression, the positive core belief becomes active. If the individual has chronic depression or a personality disorder, this means that the positive core belief is very weak. It is generally the negative core belief dominant in his/her life. As a result he/she is not able to get rid of what that core belief ("I am not lovable") is imposing. This kind of person only accepts the data confirming the negative core belief and discounts the data that does not fit into the schema. The negative core belief is like a broadcasting radio that never stops telling how much unlovable he/she is.

Underneath the superficial automatic thoughts, there lie the intermediate beliefs, rules, and assumptions. These rules, beliefs, and assumptions are the abstract regulators of the behaviour although they are not verbalized by the individual. They are settled rules, expectations, and attitudes about the individual himself/herself, the others or the world/experiences (i.e., "If I cry, it means that I am a weak person," "I must do everything perfect so that people would not understand I am actually incompetent"). Intermediate beliefs are the interconnections between the core beliefs and the automatic thoughts. Their functions are:

- Maintaining the core belief by bringing an explanation to the life experiences which are in contradiction with the core beliefs. For instance, an individual has a belief of "All human beings are bad." When this person comes across with someone who treats him/her in a good manner, he runs into a contradiction with his/her core belief. In order to overcome this contradiction, the individual comes up with the intermediate belief "If someone treats me well that means that he/she has an axe to grind."
- Having a life compatible with the core belief: If a person has a core belief of incompetency, he/she avoids taking any risks.
- Protecting the individual from the intense affect that arises from the activation of the core belief. For instance, if a person has a core belief of worthlessness, in order not to confront this core belief, the individual grabs to the intermediate belief: "If I become successful at work, I will be worthful."

Intermediate beliefs can be determined by determining the common and repeating themes in the automatic thoughts, by asking the meaning and the possible consequences of the automatic thought (downward arrow technique), or patient filling some scales (i.e., dysfunctional attitudes scale—DAS) [22].

To sum up, cognitive behavioral model assumes that we all have core beliefs that are rooted from genetic disposition and early childhood experiences. These core beliefs determine our intermediate beliefs (assumptions, rules, attitudes). Together these two are called schema. Schemas are kind of reservoir, which has explanations, assumptions, and strategies about the individual, others, and the world. When an activating event occurs, automatic thoughts are generated from this reservoir and shape feelings and behaviors (**Figure 2**). What cognitive

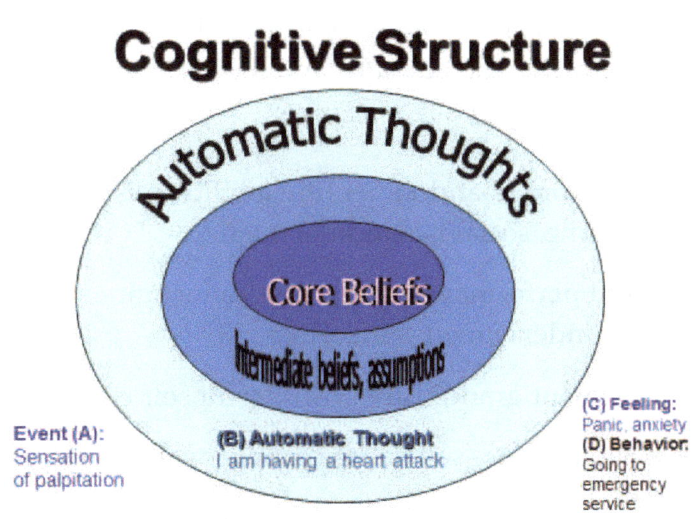


**Figure 2.** Cognitive structure.

behavioral therapy does, is to decrease the distressful emotions by disputing the maladaptive dysfunctional automatic thoughts first, and drying the reservoir (schemas) which from which these thoughts generate in the long run if the client frequently/chronically gets effected by these schemas. In cognitive behavioral therapy, cognitive processes can be integrated with the behavioral strategies to optimize the learning process.

Let us consider a person who has antisocial personality disorder and when this person gets across with new people he/she may have thoughts of cheating or giving harm. These thoughts may come from the intermediate beliefs of "I must be the one who hits first, otherwise I will be the loser," "Other people are nothing but wimps and they exist in life for being cheated/deceived," or "Laws are impediments for a satisfactory life and they are for weak people, if I obey the laws I will be exploited by other people." Of course these beliefs may be very well reflection of the core belief "I am weak and I may get hurt."

Today, with many schools focusing on the different components (i.e., schema therapy, dialectical behavioral therapy, acceptance, and commitment therapy, mindfulness based cognitive therapy) cognitive behavioral therapy (CBT)is found to be effective in numerous psychiatric disorders/psychological problems like depression, obsessive-compulsive disorder, panic disorder, generalized anxiety disorder, personality disorders, eating disorders, couple problems, family problems, and anger control problems [26–30].

### 2.2. Schema concept according to Young

Similar to cognitive behavioral therapy, Jeffrey Young stated that schemas develop in childhood in response to genetic predisposition and some environmental influences. Young viewed schema as resulting from unmet emotional needs in childhood [31]. To explain these unhelpful schemas, he introduced the concept of early maladaptive schemas (EMSs). According to Young, EMSs are unconditional and dysfunctional beliefs about the self. Like the adaptive schemas, EMSs develop from early experiences with the parents, caretakers, or peers during the childhood. A child who is not able to get his/her basic needs actualized; he/she develops schemas as the coping mechanisms to make sense of the experience and the world around him/her [32]. Young has delineated 18 schemas in five domains. These domains reflect the basic emotional needs of the child. The domains and the early maladaptive schemas are listed below [31]:

(a) **Disconnection and rejection:** Abandonment/instability, mistrust/abuse, emotional deprivation, defectiveness/shame, social isolation/alienation

(b) **Impaired autonomy and performance:** Dependence/incompetence, vulnerability to harm or illness, enmeshment/undeveloped self, failure

(c) **Impaired limits:** Entitlement/grandiosity, insufficient self-control/self-discipline

(d) **Other-directedness:** Subjugation, self-sacrifice, approval-seeking/recognition-seeking

(e) **Overvigilance and inhibition:** Negativity/pessimism, emotional inhibition, unrelenting standards/hypercriticalness, punitiveness

Because each schema has interpersonal, cognitive, and affective components, and it gives a perspective to the individual about the unmet needs that are experienced during early childhood; when EMSs are activated, high levels of affects show up causing significant distress and even psychiatric disorders. To overcome this distress, the individual may choose three options. Whichever option he/she chooses, he/she may decrease the intense affect, but the schema will be reinforced anyway. According to Young, these three options are [31]:

(1) **Schema maintenance:** Individuals, who have schema maintenance, accept the schema as completely true. Although they experience the negative emotions provoked by the schema, they keep on behaving in a way to confirm the schema. In their adulthood, they re-experience the similar traumas which created that schema. This type of behaviour is like taking the same action and hoping for a different outcome desperately.

(2) **Schema avoidance:** In this type of maladaptive coping mechanism, the individual completely tries to ignore the schema. They try not to think or feel anything that has a potential to trigger schema. In order to avoid the schema, they may spend their time to distract themselves like alcohol, etc. Similarly, they have a tendency to avoid therapy and to face these disturbing thoughts and feelings about their schema. It is not uncommon for these kinds of clients to engage in therapy interfering behaviors like being late or not doing the homework. This type of behaviour is like burying one's head in the sand like an ostrich.

(3) **Schema compensation**: Schema compensation means behaving in a way that the schema does not exist at all. At first glance, it may seem like a healthy mechanism but what the client does is merely an overcompensation effort to camouflage the schema beneath. This overcompensation effort may likely cause affective and interpersonal problems. Metaphorically speaking, this coping mechanism resembles a balloon being overinflated and blowing out ultimately. An example could be a person who has a schema of mistrust/abuse abusing others.

Having defined these concepts, Young developed schema therapy which has some adaptations cognitive behavioral therapy, psychodynamic therapy, and gestalt therapy. Because an individual always has more than one schema and there is always a shift from one schema to another in response to activating event, Young defined modes. A mode is a state of mind consisting of many schemas, coping behaviors in reaction to these schemas and the emotions. A mode can be maladaptive or healthy. An individual has many different modes and with result of the activating event, one of these modes get activated while others remain silent. As a new activating event occurs, another mode becomes active. To sum up, at any given time there is an active mode in an individual and due to the activating events there is always a shift from one mode to another.

Young defined the modes under four headings: child modes, coping modes, parent modes, and the healthy adult mode [31].

**Child modes:** There are four child modes. These are vulnerable child, angry child, impulsive/undisciplined child, and the contented child. Vulnerable child is characterized by the emotions of sadness, anguish, and shame. It includes subtypes of "lonely child," "abandoned and abused child," and "humiliated and inferior child" while angry child mode has subtypes of "stubborn child" and "enraged child". The last one "contended child" is the mode in which the basic needs of the child are met. Child modes are assumed to be universal and congenital [33].

**Maladaptive coping modes:** These modes are compliant surrenderer, detached protector, and overcompensator.

**Parent modes:** Because schemas come into existence because of the basic needs not implemented, or aversive experiences such as trauma, neglect, or abuse, parental modes usually derive from attachment figures which can be parents or anyone else (peers, social authority, etc.). While overwhelming emotions dominate the child modes, clients experience parental modes as negative thoughts. There are two parent modes: punitive parent and demanding parent.

**Healthy adult**: This is the aim of the schema therapy to accomplish ultimately. A healthy adult is able to set limits and/or accept and embrace the unhealthy maladaptive modes besides function in domains of social/family and occupational life.

The strategy in schema therapy is once modes are identified, the therapist and the client challenge the current maladaptive modes to deactivate it. After the deactivation, more adaptive and functional mode is introduced with some cognitive and experiential techniques which we will mention in the following chapters [33]. During this process, after identifying early maladaptive schemas, it is crucial to notice and validate the client's unmet emotional needs. Changing early maladaptive schemas to more adaptive and functional, adaptive schemas must be necessarily accompanied by changing maladaptive coping skills and replacing them with more appropriate ones.

Schema therapy has been investigated in many personality disorders but most of the studies were conducted about the efficacy in borderline personality disorder. Studies found that schema therapy was superior to treatment as usual and some other psychotherapy approaches with lower dropout rate and more cost effective [34–36]. In a study conducted by Bamelis et al., schema therapy was compared with clarification oriented psychotherapy (COP) and treatment as usual group in terms of clinical effectiveness and economical cost effectiveness-cost utility in six personality disorders (avoidant, dependent, obsessive-compulsive, paranoid, histrionic, and narcissistic). The study was conducted in 12 mental health institutes with 323 patients. It was found that schema therapy was more effective and had less dropout rates compared to treatment as usual or COP [37].

### 2.3. Cognitive behavioral theory of antisocial personality disorder

Although Young schema questionnaire (YSQ) scores are generally found to be higher in clients with personality disorders, there is still insufficient evidence to identify specific schemas for specific disorders. In the study that was conducted by Jovev and Jackson, it was aimed to examine which of the schema domains are specific in three personality disorders. For borderline personality disorder, high scores on dependence/incompetence, defectiveness/shame, and abandonment schema domains were detected while elevations on unrelenting standards and emotional inhibition schema domains were associated with obsessive-compulsive personality disorder and avoidant personality disorder, respectively [38]. While Nordahl et al. found that vulnerability to harm, emotional inhibition, and insufficient self-control were associated with narcissistic personality disorder [39], in their nonclinical sample, Reeves and Taylor found that men endorsed more symptoms of ASPD and higher levels of the core beliefs of emotional deprivation, social isolation, defectiveness/shame, and emotional inhibition [40].

The traditional view of ASPD is that these people have deficiency in internalizing the standards of the society [41]. Beck and Freeman suggest that there is evidence for developmental delay in moral maturity and cognitive functioning of antisocial individuals [20]. They have poor empathic ability and they are not able to perceive other people's point of view. They see themselves as loners, autonomous, and strong, and some of them may see themselves as abused and mistreated by society. They see others as either exploitative or weak and vulnerable [25].

According to Millon and Everly, antisocial individuals tend to be interpersonally aggressive, abusive, and cruel. They have learned to rely on themselves and to distrust others because they have a fear of being exploited and humiliated by others. They are secured only when they are in control of the situation and are independent of the will of others who may threaten their security (e.g., interpersonal control) [42].

When we look at the relation between the EMS and the aggressive behaviour, we see that Tremblay and Dozois found a relation between the domain of disconnection and rejection (abandonment, mistrust/abuse, social isolation) and domain of impaired limits (entitlement, insufficient self-control) and trait aggressiveness [43]. Gilbert and colleagues aimed to find out the prevalence of EMSs in offenders and they determined that entitlement, social isolation, dependence, insufficient self-control, and failure to achieve are associated with aggression [44]. Loper et al. investigated the relation between the schemas and the personality disorders in 116 incarcerated women who were convicted from robbery to assault. According to results, impaired limits presented with a sense of entitlement, poor impulse control, and lack of concern for others were correlated with cluster-B personality disorders including antisocial personality. This domain was also associated with hostility, institutional misconduct, self-reported violence, and victimization [45].

Polaschek and colleagues analyzed the interviews of the violent offenders and they identified implicit theories—a term which they define as structured interconnected belief network that guides behaviour and allows the individual to predict the result of a particular event [46]—instead of schema. From the transcript of the interview of the offenders, they uncovered four implicit theories: (1) beat or beaten, (2) I am the law, (3) violence is normal, and (4) I get out of control which corresponds to entitlement, mistrust/abuse, and insufficient self-control [47].

Ozdel et al. examined 38 patients diagnosed antisocial personality disorder selected from young soldiers most of whom were having substance abuse treatment in the army and 24 nonclinical volunteers. The purpose of the study was to identify core beliefs and early maladaptive schemas that characterize antisocial personality disorder. Diagnosis was made according to structured clinical interview for DSM-III-R personality disorders (SCID-II), Young schema questionnaire (YSQ), and the social comparison scale (SCS). SCS tries to identify judgments concerned with rank (inferior-superior) and determines how a person judges himself/herself as fitting in with or being similar to others. When the SCS scores of two groups were compared, it was found that there was a significant difference favoring the control group on these items: unlovable-lovable, lonely-not lonely, rejected-accepted, etc. In other words, control group subjects scored higher, meaning more positive social comparison perception. When the two groups were compared for YSQ, instead of simply comparing the means for specific schemas, the authors preferred to focus on schemas that showed significant differences and also had raw schema scores of 20 or more points. Using this procedure, significant findings were obtained for the specific schemas for emotional deprivation, entitlement/grandiosity, mistrust/abuse, vulnerability to harm, and social isolation. Three out of above five schemas-emotional deprivation, mistrust/abuse and social isolation fall into disconnection/rejection domain. Since this domain is conceptualized as stemming from a person's unmet needs for love, security, stability, and nurturance, it can be assumed that the current individual diagnosed with ASPD see himself/herself as unlovable, lonelier, and more rejected than the normal controls [48]. The results of SCS (the persons with ASPD tend to see themselves unlovable-lonely and rejected) supports the notion that antisocial persons may behave in order to compensate for a sense of victimization (ie., "I am weak so I must be the one who hits first."). Hence these findings may suggest that a conditional belief such as "I should hurt him before he hurts me" is behind the primary social strategies of attacking and exploiting used by individuals with ASPD [49]. This finding fits very well with the schema compensation strategy.

### 2.4. Treatment in antisocial personality disorder

When a therapist works with a client with antisocial personality disorder (ASPD) many challenges would be there from the beginning. First of all, most of the professionals believed that antisocial personality disorder is an untreatable condition. That's why they are reluctant to treat patients with ASPD. On the other side of the relationship antisocial patients that are coming for therapy are also very reluctant [50].

It is not common that an individual with ASPD goes to the therapist's office for getting help for the problems that are already considered so by the environment. They usually come to therapy when their conventional strategies have stopped working and have not been able to get what they wanted or the law or unofficial authority has threatened them. In these conditions, subjects of the admission are usually mood problems, behavioral problems, and alcohol and substance use problems. Another issue while working with ASPD is motivation. From the stages of change perspective, individuals with ASPD are usually at precontemplation or contemplation stages. This suggests that these people believe the source of the problem is from the outside; they are not the responsible one; or there is some kind of problem but they cannot do anything to solve it.

Above mentioned characteristics of the clinical picture of ASPD are also important guides to the therapist while working with them. This is all to say that the problem areas are mood problems including anger, anxiety, or depression; alcohol and substance use problems and the treatment strategy should consider teaching more functional attitudes and ways to get things wanted, and methods used in the treatment process must be motivational (i.e., pros and cons analysis).

Unfortunately, there is not any satisfactory evidence which therapeutic intervention is effective for antisocial personality disorder. In a meta-analysis searching for an effective therapy for ASPD concluded that although there are some interventions (i.e., contingency management with standard maintenance or CBT with standard maintenance, etc.) appeared to be effective for substance use problems, none of the psychological treatments were significantly effective [51].

Davidson et al. randomized 52 patients diagnosed with ASPD in two groups, one for CBT and one for treatment as usual. The CBT group received treatment either for 6 months or for 12 months. When the assessments made at baseline and at 12 months were compared, it was found that although 6 months of CBT decreased the problematic alcohol use and increased positive beliefs and social functioning more than the treatment as usual group, the difference was not significant [52].

From the cognitive behavioral point of view, treatment modalities are conventional CBT and schema therapy. Results of the studies used traditional CBT approaches are discouraging with nonsignificant behavioral changes and attitudes [53, 54]. However, a new cognitive behavioral model called the risk-need-responsivity (RNR) has become hope for the treatment of ASPD [55]. This approach assesses individuals with criminal and antisocial behavioral pattern based on their future risk of the criminal act, their needs, and environmental factors related to recidivism. In this approach, the aim is to reduce risk factors specifically connected lasting criminal behaviors since it is not usually used in untraditional mental health settings like prisons. The "risk" part of the model is about the intensity of the treatment because it is considered that the bigger the risk of future criminal behaviour, the more intense treatment is required. The "need" part of the model is about the goals of treatment. These goals are the ones that considered attempts of crimes mostly related to future. The "responsivity" part is about the consistency between the learning styles, ability, and motivational stages and interventions provided [56]. Since antisocial individuals have low motivation or learning abilities to change their somehow "working" strategies, completely individual treatment plan should be warranted. In this treatment plan, strategies pertaining to cognitive, behavioral, and social learning paradigms are used in order to construct an individual profile of learning. Andrew et al. proposed eight factors related to recidivism of the individuals with ASPD. In this risk-need-responsivity (RNR) model, risk factors are categorized under the two domains, which are static risk factors, such as previous crimes committed, and dynamic risk factors, such as current substance misuse. The main static risk factor is the history of antisocial behavior and the dynamic risk factors are disordered personality, criminal thinking (antisocial beliefs), antisocial associates, dysfunctional family or marital bonds, low levels of functioning and/or satisfaction in work/school, low levels of pro-social leisure activities, and substance abuse. Criminal thinking and disordered personality represent the focus for cognitive part of the therapeutic work. The other factors such as low family bond, unemployment, etc. represent the behavioral part of the therapy. Both cognitive and behavioral parts are sustained together. Antisocial personality beliefs can be assessed by an unstructured interview or some empirically supported tools such as personality belief questionnaire [57]. As for criminal thinking, there are various assessment tools for them. Once personality beliefs and criminal thinking aspects are found, cognitive interventions are implemented.

Cognitive interventions include introduction of conditional and unconditional beliefs; first cognitive restructuring of the intermediate beliefs in terms of rationality and functionality; positive schema log; and behavioral experiments.

Introduction of general CBT model and especially beliefs are of therapeutic effect. Attitudes, rules, and standards can be introduced as personal doctrines that can be hold or discharged according to their functionality and doctrine change would need time. Positive schema log is a cognitive technique in which client tries to detect concrete evidences contradicting to old core beliefs (these core beliefs can be about self or others). Behavioral experiments are well-designed individual experiments that try to test certain beliefs.

Behavioral interventions include functional analysis, self-monitoring, activity scheduling, and skills training (social skills training and assertiveness training).

Functional analysis is a work to examine triggers, behaviors, and the consequences of behaviors. These consequences are discussed in a short and long run. Intentions are not always in line with the consequences. This intervention has the individual focus on those consequences. Self-monitoring helps client to be able to stand back and observe him or herself. Activity scheduling helps clients to realize how they spend their times, which activities they usually engage in, and the effects of those activities. Skills training such as social skills training and assertiveness training should be better if added in treatment protocol when working with individuals with ASPD [58].

### 2.5. The basic concepts in schema therapy of antisocial personality disorder

As mentioned above, because antisocial personality disordered patients generally do not have enough motivation and referred to therapy for legal reasons, it is hard to keep them in therapy. Patients who have ASPD have very little concern about the consequences of their actions and how the others feel. They see themselves as lonely and victimized, so one of the most important things to move forward in therapy is to build a therapeutic rapport. Therapist uses two important strategies–limited reparenting and empathic confrontation–to build a relationship. ASPD patients have strong schemas due to their early childhood memories of unmet basic needs. Limited reparenting provides "corrective emotional experience" that feeds these unmet needs [59]. The responses, empathic attitude, and behaviors of the therapist construct the limited parenting in therapy sessions.

Empathic confrontation is another relational construct which is extremely useful during the change phase of the therapy. It is like a teeter–tooter. On one hand, the therapist accepts and shows the schema of the patient. He/she shows empathy about why the patient has that schema, what the utility of the schema was in the early childhood, and how it helped the patient to survive that traumatic period. On the other hand, the therapist confronts with the patient about the current consequences of the schema, how it destructs the patient's interpersonal relations, etc. Swinging between empathy and confrontation will lead the patient to be more open to alternative interpretations.

Cognitive strategies help the patient build a healthy adult mode, but before that the patient first has to realize his/her mode and then challenge it. It is very obvious that the patient will have difficulty in realizing his/her schema from many aspects; it is (was) a life-saving strategy for him/her. So cognitive strategies help the patient to step back and look at the picture from a distance. Cognitive strategies include [31]:

**Testing the validity of a schema:** It is like testing the validity of the automatic thoughts in CBT with the exception that, here the validity will be tested in considering the whole life rather than a particular situation. The therapist and the client search for the evidence for and against the schema.

**Reframing the evidence supporting the schema:** The therapist and the patient make a list of evidences supporting the schema, and then together generate alternative explanations to provide better understanding.

**Evaluating the advantages and disadvantages of the patient's coping responses:** The aim is to make patients notice that the schemas would have been once the key components for survival sometime during their lifetime but not anymore.

**Conducting dialogues between the "schema side" and the "healthy side":** Adapted from the "empty chair technique" of Gestalt therapy, the therapist guides the patient to produce healthy answers to the "schema side" and then they switch places and the client plays the "healthy side" or plays both the "healthy side" and the "schema side" and generates healthy answers to accusations of the schema.

**Schema flash cards:** Patients carry these coping cards when their schemas get activated.

**Schema diary:** Patients use these diaries again when their schemas are triggered. They identify the triggering event, emotions, thoughts, schema underneath, realistic and unrealistic concerns, and the healthy responses to these.

Following the cognitive strategies, experiential change strategies which include reparenting (imaginary dialogues between the vulnerable child, unhealthy adult, and the healthy adult) take place, letters to the parent and imagination for pattern-breaking [31].

Schema therapy of ASPD is a long journey with obstacles requiring the motivation of both the patient and the therapist. During the process, the therapist must prepare himself/herself for the therapy interfering behaviors/obstacles such as schema avoidance-detached protector mode, anger control problems, alcohol/substance abuse, and criminal behaviors/legal issues and keep his/her own schemas, avoidances, and overcompensations as well.

## 3. Conclusion

In conclusion, antisocial personality disorder has a great burden on the society in terms of both the financial expenses to treat the disorder and the juridical problems. Yet, there are no satisfactory results in the treatment of ASPD. Full (optimal) remission seems to be an unrealistic target for health professionals. The biggest obstacle is the demotivation of the client, which results in disengagement to the therapy or even not attending the sessions properly. It would not be surprising for the client to commit therapy interfering behaviors like cheating, lying, or even ridiculing the therapist. Cognitive behavioral-oriented therapies hypothesize that antisocial persons see themselves as unlovable, lonely, etc., which may be a compensation of victimization and suggest focusing on cognitive restructuring of the intermediate beliefs. Although there is not enough evidence of any psychotherapeutic interventions that are significantly effective, improvements in the symptoms like impulsivity, aggressive behaviour, or substance misuse will definitely have positive effects not only on the society in general (like reducing crime rates, etc.) but also on the interpersonal relations that the client have with the others.

## Author details

Ahmet Emre Sargın[1]*, Kadir Özdel[2] and Mehmet Hakan Türkçapar[3]

*Address all correspondence to: esargin79@yahoo.com

1 Department of Psychology, Uskudar University, Istanbul, Turkey

2 Dışkapı Yıldırım Beyazıt Training and Research Hospital, Ankara, Turkey

3 Department of Psychology, Hasan Kalyoncu University, Gaziantep, Turkey

## References

[1] American Psychiatric Association. Diagnostic and Statistical Manual of Mental Disorders. 4th ed. Washington, DC: American Psychiatric Publishing; 1994

[2] Dinwiddie SH, Daw EW. Temporal stability of antisocial personality disorder: Blind follow-up study at 8 years. Comprehensive Psychiatry. 1998;**39**(1):29-34

[3] De Ruiter C, Greeven PG. Personality disorders in a Dutch forensic psychiatric sample: Convergence of interview and self-report measures. Journal of Personality Disorders. 2000;(14):162-170

[4] American Psychiatric Association. Diagnostic and Statistical Manual for Mental Disorders. 5th ed. Washington, DC: American Psychiatric Publishing; 2013

[5] Swanson MC, Bland RC, Newman SC. Epidemiology of psychiatric disorders in Edmonton. Antisocial personality disorders. Acta Psychiatrica Scandinavica, Supplementum. 1994; **376**:63-70

[6] Ozarin L. Moral insanity: A brief history. Psychiatric News. 2001;**36**(10):21

[7] Cleckley H. The Mask of Sanity. 1st ed. St. Louis: Mosby; 1941

[8] Hare RD. The Hare Psychopathy Checklist-Revised (PCL-R). 2nd ed. Toronto, Canada: Multi-health Systems; 2003

[9] Lilienfeld S. Conceptual problems in the assessment of psychopathy. Clinical Psychology Review. 1994;**14**:17-38

[10] Herpertz SC, Werth U, Lukas G, Qunaibi M, Schuerkens A, Kunert H, Freese R, Flesch M, Mueller-Isberner A, Osterheider M, et al. Emotion in criminal offenders with psychopathy and borderline personality disorder. Archives of General Psychiatry. 2001;**58**:737-745

[11] Harpur TJ, Hakstian AR, Hare RD. Factor structure of the psychopathy checklist. Journal of Consulting and Clinical Psychology. 1988;**56**:741-747

[12] Torgensen S, Kringlen E, Cramer V. The prevalence of personality disorders in a community sample. Archives of General Psychiatry. 2001;**58**:590-596

[13] Hart SD, Hare RD. Psychopathy: Assessment and association with the criminal conduct. In: Stoff DM, Breiling J, Maser JD, editors. Handbook of Antisocial Behavior. 1st ed. New York, USA: Wiley; 1997. pp. 22-35

[14] Widiger TA, Corbitt EM. Comorbidity of antisocial personality disorder with other personality disorders. In: Stoff DM, Breiling JM, Maser JD, editors. Handbook of Antisocial Behaviors. 1st ed. New York, USA: Wiley; 1997. pp. 75-82

[15] Robins LN, Tipp J, Przybeck T. Antisocial personality. In: Robins LN, Legiar DA, editors. Psychiatric Disorders in America. 1st ed. New York: Free Press; 1991. pp. 258-290

[16] Lenzenweger MF, Lane MC, Loranger AW. DSM-IV personality disorders in the National Comorbidity Survey Replication. Biological Psychiatry. 2007;**15**:553-564

[17] Cadoret RJ, Yates WR, Troughton E, Woodworth G, Stewart MA. Genetic-environmental interaction in the genesis of agressively and conduct disorders. Archives of General Psychiatry. 1995;**52**(11):916-924

[18] Eysenck HJ, Gudjonsson GH. The Causes and Cures of Criminality. 1st ed. New York, USA: Plenum; 1989

[19] Hare RD. Electrodermal and cardiovascular correlates of psychopathy. In: Hare RD, Schalling D, editors. Psychopathic Behavior: Approaches to Research. 1st ed. New York, USA: Wiley; 1978. pp. 107-143

[20] Beck AT, Freeman A. Cognitive Theory of Personality Disorders. 1st ed. New York, USA: Guilford Press; 1990

[21] Beck AT, Rush AJ, Shaw BF, Emery G. Cognitive Therapy of Depression. New York, USA: Guilford Press; 1979

[22] Beck JS. Cognitive Behavior Therapy: Basics and Beyond. New York, USA: Guilford Press; 2011

[23] Ellis A. Reason and Emotion in Psychotherapy. New York, USA: Lyle Stuart; 1962

[24] Padesky CA. Schema change processes in cognitive therapy. Clinical Psychology Psychotherapy. 1994;**1**(5):267-278

[25] Beck AT, Davis DD, Freeman A. Cognitive Therapy of Personality Disorders. 3rd ed. New York, USA: Guilford Press; 2015

[26] Hofmann SG, Fang A. The efficacy of cognitive behavioral therapy: A review of meta-analyses. Cognitive Therapy and Research. 2012;**36**:427-440

[27] Butler AC, Chapman JE, Forman EM, Beck AT. The empirical status of cognitive-behavioral therapy: A review of meta-analyses. Clinical Psychology Review. 2006;**26**:17-31

[28] Clark DA, Beck AT, Alford BA. Scientific Foundations of Cognitive Theory and Therapy of Depression. Hoboken, NJ: Wiley; 1999

[29] Clark DA, Beck AT. Cognitive Therapy of Anxiety Disorders: Science and Practice. New York, USA: Guilford Press; 2010

[30] Shadish WR, Matt GR, Navarro AM, Phillips G. The effects of psychological therapies under clinically representative conditions: A meta-analysis. Psychological Bulletin. 2000;**126**:512-529

[31] Young JE, Klosko JS, Weishaar ME. Schema Therapy: A Practitioner's Guide. New York, USA: Guilford Press; 2003

[32] Young JE, Lindemann MD. An integrative schema-focused model for personality disorders. Journal of Cognitive Psychotherapy: An International Quarterly. 1992;**6**:11-23

[33] Dadomo H, Grecucci A, Giardini I, Ugolini E, Carmelita A, Panzeri M. Schema therapy for emotional dysregulation: Theoretical implication and clinical applications. Frontiers in Psychology. 2016;**7**:1987. DOI: 10.3389/fpsyg.2016.01987

[34] Giesen-Bloo J, van Dyck R, Spinhoven P, van Tilburg W, Dirksen C, van Asselt T, et al. Outpatient psychotherapy for borderline personality disorder, randomised trial of schema-focused therapy vs transference-focused psychotherapy. Archives of General Psychiatry. 2006;**63**:649-658

[35] Farrel JM, Shaw IA, Webber AA. A schema-focused approach to group psychotherapy for outpatients with borderline personality disorder: A randomized controlled trial. Behavior Therapy and Experimental Psychiatry. 2009;**40**:317-328

[36] Dickhaut V, Arnzt A. Combined group and individual schema therapy for borderline personality disorder: A pilot study. Journal of Behavior Therapy and Experimental Psychiatry. 2014;**45**(2):242-251

[37] Bamelis LL, Evers SM, Spinhoven P, Arntz A. Results of a multicenter randomized controlled trial of the clinical effectiveness of schema therapy for personality disorders. American Journal of Psychiatry. 2014;**171**(3):305-322

[38] Jovev M, Jackson H. Early maladaptive schemas in personality disordered individuals. Journal of Personality Disorders. 2004;**18**(5):467-478

[39] Nordahl HM, Holthe H, Haugum JA. Early maladaptive schemas in patients with or without personality disorders: Does schema modification predict symptomatic relief? Clinical Psychology & Psychotherapy. 2005;**12**(2):142-149

[40] Reeves M, Taylor J. Specific relationships between core beliefs and personality disorder symptoms in a non-clinical sample. Clinical Psychology and Psychotherapy. 2007; **14**:96-104

[41] Freeman A, Pretzer J, Fleming B, Simon KM. Clinical Applications of Cognitive Therapy. New York, USA: Plenum Press; 1990

[42] Millon T, Everly G. Personality and its Disorders: A Biosocial Learning Approach. New York: Wiley; 1985

[43] Tremblay PF, Dozois DJA. Another perspective on trait aggressiveness: Overlap with early maladaptive schemas. Personality and Individual Differences. 2009;**46**:569-574

[44] Gilbert F, Daffern M, Talevski D, Ogloff JR. The role of aggression-related cognition in the agressive behaviors of offenders: A general aggression model perspective. Criminal Justice and Behavior. 2013;**40**(2):119-138

[45] Loper AB. The relationship of maladaptive beliefs to personality and behavioral adjustment among incarcerated women. Journal of Cognitive Psychotherapy. 2003; **17**(3):253-266

[46] Ward T. Sexual offenders' cognitive distortions as implicit theories. Aggression and Violent Behavior. 2000;**5**:491-507

[47] Polaschek DL, Calvert SW, Gannon TA. Linking violent thinking: Implicit theory-based research with violent offenders. Journal of Interpersonal Violence. 2009;**24**:75-96

[48] Ozdel, K, Turkcapar MH, Guriz SO, Hamamci Z, Duy B, Taymur I, et al. Early maladaptive schemas and core beliefs in antisocial personality disorder. International Journal of Cognitive Therapy. 2015;**8**(4):306-317

[49] Beck AT, Freeman A, Davis DD. Cognitive Therapy of Personality Disorders. 2nd ed. New York: Guilford Press; 2004

[50] Meloy JR, Yakeley J. Antisocial personality disorder. In: Gabbard GO, editor. Gabbard's Treatment of Psychiatric Disorders. 5th ed. Arlington. APA Publishing; 2014

[51] Gibbon S, Duggan C, Stoffers J, Huband N, Völmm BA, Ferriter M et al. Psychological interventions for antisocial personality disorder. Cochrane Database of Systematic Reviews. 2010:CD 007668

[52] Davidson KM, Tyrer P, Tata P, Cooke D, Gumley A, Ford I, et al. Cognitive behavior therapy for violent man with antisocial personality disorder in the community: An exploratory randomized controlled trial. Psychological Medicine. 2009;**39**(4):569-577

[53] Matusiewicz AK, Hopwood CJ, Banducci AN, Lejuez CW. The effectiveness of cognitive behavioral therapy for personality disorders. Psychiatric Clinics of North America. 2010;**33**(3):657-685

[54] Hoffman SG, Asnaani A, Vonk IJ, Sawyer AT, Fang A. The efficacy of cognitive behavioral therapy: A review of meta-analyses. Cognitive Therapy and Research. 2012;**36**(5): 427-440

[55] Andrews Da, Bonta J. Psychology of Criminal Conduct. 5th ed. London and New York: Routledge; 2010

[56] Andrews DA, Bonta J, Wormith JS. The recent past and near future of risk and/or need assessment. Crime & Delinquency. 2006;**52**(1):7-27

[57] Butler AC, Beck AT, Cohen LH. The personality belief questionnaire-short form: Development and preliminary findings. Cognitive Therapy and Research. 2007;**31**(3):357-370

[58] Dobson D, Dobson KS. Evidence-based Practice of Cognitive-behavioral Therapy. 2nd ed. New York: Guilford Press; 2016

[59] Alexander F, French TM. Psychoanalytic Therapy: Principles and Applications. New York: Ronald Press; 1946

# 3

# Interdisciplinary Rehabilitation to Facilitate Recovery of People Living with Long-Term Schizophrenia in Developing Countries

Siew Yim Loh

**Abstract**

Schizophrenia is characterized by irregular, alternating episodes of exacerbation and remission of psychotic symptoms. The occupational care for people living with long-term schizophrenia (PLWS) after medical treatment, for re-engagement into work, leisure, and daily-living activities, still needs attention. Personalizing follow-up care of PLWS can improve the medical-psychosocial level of patient with differing medical, physical, and psychosocial effects from their treatment exposures. This chapter highlights the call for an individual care approach that is often lacking in resource-limited countries with additional burden from entrenched stigma. Patient categorization for PLWS may be a cost-effective step forward to overcome the less effective, one-size-fits-all approach. The need to address personalized assessment of risk exposure and to remediate its consequences on function, recovery, and quality of life calls for a better interdisciplinary-care approach, and a renewed investment to ensure occupational performance after recovery. Medicine is initial, but personalized rehabilitation is warranted for much improved functioning and better quality of life. Research is also needed to evaluate and document the effectiveness of various models of interdisciplinary care for PLWS that have been developed but may not be tested/evaluated and also on models tested effective but on other long-term nonphysical conditions.

**Keywords:** schizophrenia, work, leisure, daily-living activities, interdisciplinary, personalized, categorizing care, occupational therapy

## 1. Background

Schizophrenia is recognized as a severe brain disease, with 1% of any population predicted to develop schizophrenia during their lifetime [1]. The prevalence (i.e., the number of cases in a population at any one time point) and the incidence (i.e., the number of new cases annually) of schizophrenia is about 1% and about 1.5 per 10,000 people, with onset occurring typically during adolescence, at between 18 and 25 for men and between 25 and 35 for women [2]. The prevalence of schizophrenia in less developed countries was significantly lower than in the developed countries [3], but this difference could be due to underreporting [4]. This condition has been reported as highly unlikely to have a uniform etiology, because of the diversity of the aetiological factors involved, and the characteristically irregular and alternating episodes of exacerbation and remission of psychotic symptoms [5]. Therefore, it is considered the most disabling of all the major mental disorders and interferes with an individual's ability to think, feel and to receive, to understand sensory information, and/or how to behave appropriately.

The debilitating, public health burdens of schizophrenia also seem greater in less developed countries. About 85% of the world's population are in the 153 low- and middle-income countries [6], where 80% of people living with mental disorders reside. Mental illness accounts for 8.8% in low-income and 16.6% in lower-middle-income countries, of the total burden of disease [7, 8]. Living in a world distorted by hallucinations and delusions [9], people living with schizophrenia may feel frightened, anxious and confused, as they experience hearing voices (not heard by others), or believing that other people are reading their minds, controlling their thoughts or even trying to harm them. Their disorganized speech and behavior can be incomprehensible and may even be frightening to others. These encounters also worsen the entrenched stigma against people living with schizophrenia (PLWS), which increases the burden of care. This issue of PLWS experiencing stigma because of their illness is an ongoing battle in both developed and developing countries. They faced discrimination from many aspects of their lives including education, work, relationships and access to health-care services [10]. Studies on determinants of quality of life in schizophrenia found that gender, positive and disorganized symptoms of schizophrenia, and cognitive and physical impairments are the most important predictors of quality of life of a group of people with schizophrenia in Malaysia [11]. This issue calls for a better integrated care and a concerted public health de-stigmatization module to educate and reach more communities. It is therefore critical that medical treatment is provided with interdisciplinary rehabilitation care to address and impact these irregular, alternating episodes of exacerbation and remission and social stigma on their level of functioning in their daily living.

Occupational participation has a critical role in the recovery and functioning of people with schizophrenia. People living with schizophrenia look for treatments that relieve active symptoms and to improve their abilities to function at work, school and in their everyday lives. Research evidence suggests that occupational rehabilitative intervention can increase the likelihood of obtaining a competitive job with a positive impact on work hours, but it is often insufficient to enable optima work participation for people living with schizophrenia, and comprehensive, individualized treatments are necessary to address functional deficits which are a barrier for labor sustainability and their job performance [12]. The occupational rehabilitation for people living with long-term schizophrenia still needs attention and improvement to facilitate better social adjustment and reengagement into work, leisure and daily-living activities. However, the individual care approach is often lacking in resource-limited, developing countries where society's entrenched stigma on mental illness aggravates and complicates the recovery of PLWS. The need to address personalized assessment of risk exposure (from long-term treatment and psychosocial exposures) and to remediate its consequences on function, recovery and quality of life warrants a renewed investment to ensure performance beyond recovery. Patient categorization for PLWS may be a step forward to overcome the less effective, one-size-fits-all approach. Therefore, this chapter highlights the call for a need to categorize care towards personalizing follow-up rehabilitation care of PLWS to improve their specific medical and psychosocial needs for each individual patient who presents with differing side effects from their long-term treatment and the long-term exposures to their environments.

Medical treatment through the use of antipsychotic medication alone in long-term schizophrenia is often not enough for the characteristically irregular and alternating episodes of exacerbation and remission of illness in schizophrenia [5]. Improving and scaling up mental health services in developing countries requires flexible policies [13], to overcome limited resources, effective inter-professional communication and evidence-based training—both in numbers and in quality university-based training for the severe shortage of health professionals like occupational therapists.

A timely initiative for developing countries with low resources is towards the development of category patient-centered, rehabilitation services—beyond the initial phase of recovery from medical treatment. Categorization of care may be a focused way to address the complex range of needs from the individual's physical health, psychosocial, financial and occupational needs in people living with schizophrenia. It is universally accepted that the standard of care for people with schizophrenia should include the combination of antipsychotic medication and psychosocial interventions [14], but in many countries, this equation is neglected due to low manpower and resources. A more concerted plan to intervene by focusing on the category of needs of people living with schizophrenia may be more cost-effective than a "one-size-fit all" approach. Categorize care for PLWS is, in simpler term, about reappraising and re-addressing, and regrouping care needs to overcome the limitations from a "one-size-fit-all" approach. The principles are based on enabling PLWS to make informed choices, received personalized care, within a philosophy of recovery and well-being [14]. Categorizing these psychosocial-care interventions can be enhanced in context-appropriate ways to offer support to PLWS such as to (1) manage with negative/positive symptom and (2) deal with negative social reactions, including from family members and occupational needs [15]. Three principles of personalized care identified—(1) categorizing care, (2) early interdisciplinary intervention and (3) comprehensiveness of care—are important concepts when the therapists attempt to rehabilitate the client (as the expert patient), in line with the patient self-management approach for chronic disease [16].

## 2. Categorizing care to target better functioning and quality of life

Categorizing rehabilitation care for PLWS aims to ensure sustained recovery and improve their quality of living. With a target to increase the individual's level of functioning, the rehabilitation goal is to nurture the strengths and specific life skills, and to be able to live as independently as possible in the community [17]. The intervention targets at building up their strengths and reducing their deficits, and as such, the features of intervention program must be comprehensive, continuous, coordinated and all encompassing, to ensure better quality of living. With this, a need for more precision into the categorization of patient living with schizophrenia is warranted. This approach does require a paradigm shift in the culture of psychiatry interdisciplinary care, whereby health professionals collaborate closely towards implementing evidence-based findings (from epidemiologic knowledge and risk assessment tools) to develop a tailored, individual follow-up, and abandoning a generic approach for all people with schizophrenia. Medical and psychosocial care should eventually move into personalized precision approaches, as are recommended for all other chronic diseases too. Therefore, a care that intersect between evidence-based medicine and value-based medicine may prove to be more supportive of the patient's entitlement to autonomy, reflecting a truly commendable shift from focusing almost exclusively on a patient's clinical condition to considering him/her as a person [18]. It also sets the tone for a tailored, personalized and valued patient-centered care [19] that warrants careful identification of individual disorders, individual risk and functional needs. Studies are needed on what and how to categorize individual needs of PLWS across the spectrum of medical, psychosocial and occupational health status for a rehabilitation pathway to ensure multidimensional/comprehensive therapy where the occupational therapist can focus on value intervention to improve functional abilities and illness recovery [19]. Nevertheless, this chapter hopes to stimulate new discussions so that more studies are needed to evaluate what and how to categorize for personalized and valued care for better quality of life in people living with schizophrenia.

## 3. Early intervention interdisciplinary approach care

People living with schizophrenia may not present as a life-threatening condition, but early intervention should still be emphasized. Some people have only one such psychotic episode; others have many episodes during a lifetime, but even in the multi-episode group, they can lead relatively normal lives in between. Thus, any delay in medical treatment plays a significant role in the long-term outcome of these patients. The longer the duration of untreated illness, the more difficult it is to treat the patient and results in more permanent disabilities. Many have continuous or recurring pattern of illness and may not fully recover and typically requires long-term rehabilitation. Coping and self-management is needed with the symptoms of schizophrenia as they can be especially difficult for family members [16]. The numerous psychological, social and occupational dysfunctions experienced by people living with schizophrenia warrant greater comprehensive and an early therapy management, to facilitate their social functioning, and ensure a continuum of care from the hospital to their homes and community, or on the job. The occupational therapist, mental health counselors, social workers and working interdisciplinary with the psychiatrists treating these PLWS must be aware of the range of symptoms interfering with functions, so that evidence- and valued-based care can be considered for each individual.

## 4. Comprehensiveness of care

*Comprehensiveness* is defined by the institute of medicine in 1996 as "the provision of integrated, accessible health-care services by clinicians for addressing a large majority of personal health-care needs [20], but it is often refers to the bio-psychosocial or whole-person approach, that view patient as body and soul from a social context [21]". The increase in complexity of care, attending to co-morbidities and the evolution of interdisciplinary models of care calls for all health team to sustain such responsibilities and to provide better interdisciplinary care. In the comprehensive occupational therapy programs for people living with schizophrenia, the interventions planned are along the goal-directed use of time, energy and interest, with a comprehensive focus to foster adaptation, participation and performance by minimizing pathology and promoting the maintenance of health. However, in developing countries, there is a lopsided emphasis for medical personal over health-care professionals, and the low manpower of rehabilitation therapists is a significant issue for most developing countries. In Malaysia, a medical supremacy approach and an entrenched medical governance model for its health-care delivery system perpetuate the lingering issue of manpower shortages and low university-based program for training qualified occupational therapists.

## 5. Symptoms interfering with functions

People living with a diagnosis of schizophrenia encountered numerous dysfunctions from a serious mental illness with a very broad range of symptoms, which includes (1) "positive symptoms" (abnormal experiences), such as hallucinations (seeing, hearing, feeling something that is not actually there), delusions (false and usually strange beliefs) and paranoia (unrealistic fear); (2) "negative symptoms" (absence of normal behavior), such as emotional withdrawal and lack of motivation and enjoyment; and (3) cognitive dysfunction (problems with concentration, learning abilities and memory) [1, 2]. These symptoms also occurred with a disorganized and abnormal thinking, behavior and language. Often, they can become emotionally unresponsive or withdrawn, with the experience of progressive personality changes leading to a breakdown in their relationships with the outside world. Apart from stigma [15], the lack of insight of PLWS may be key factor contributing to the refusal of medical treatment and also medication non-adherence. At the Permai Hospital (a large mental institution in Malaysia), 54% of the patient with schizophrenia had poor insight [22], and a comparison study between patients with schizophrenia and other mood disorders psychosis found that schizophrenia patients had the worst insights—where the level of impairment of insight was associated with the functionality of patients [23]. Therefore, social isolation or withdrawal, along with the poor insights, unusual speech, thinking or behavior may precede, be seen along with or appear later on in the course of the illness. Some less obvious symptoms such as loss of interest, low energy, absence of warmth and care, and lack of humor are all dysfunctions that do not presently respond well to medications. These symptoms add to the distress for the schizophrenia sufferer and their families. In less-developed countries, the stigmatization phenomenon (from lack of awareness) aggravates the great distress to themselves and their families. Although the outlook for people living with schizophrenia has improved over the last 25 years, this is true only in developed countries. More research is needed as the current research has gradually led to new and safer medications and unraveling the mysteries behind the causes of the disease, but the occupational rehabilitation needed to enable people to live and function with a better quality of life is still needed.

## 6. Physical rehabilitation

Among people living with schizophrenia, physical fitness is a fundamental rehabilitation and self-management intervention, as it preserves a sense of physical wellness and mental well-being. The sufficient amounts of moderate daily exercise also form part of a healthier daily routine and facilitate sleep pattern. Research evidence has more often than not highlighted that physical health and mental health are intertwined [24]. As schizophrenics become withdrawn and unsociable, their desire to exercises wanes. Obesity and metabolic syndrome are among the major medical co-morbidities in schizophrenia, with evidences of relationship between weight gain or metabolic syndrome and antipsychotic medications [25–27]. A study on weight changes among first-episode schizophrenia 1 year after the initiation of antipsychotic medications reported that patients treated with olanzapine had the largest mean weight gain (14+ 10 kg) with treatment [28]. Patients treated with the antipsychotics trifluoroperazine, flupenthixol decanoate and clozapine are to be associated with the highest prevalence of metabolic syndrome [29, 30]. In addition, even the normal weight people with schizophrenia have higher visceral fats compared with normal weight healthy control subjects [31], and physical activity such as simple regular walking is important and beneficial to the body composition and quality of life of PLWS [32].

## 7. Psychosocial rehabilitation

People with schizophrenia become ill during the critical career-forming years of life (18–35 years old), which makes them, less likely, as a group of young adults to be able to complete their certification degrees or vocational training needed for skilled work. Many have difficulty with communication, motivation, self-care and relationships with others. Together with the antipsychotic medicines to treat the symptoms of the illness, counseling and social support from family, friends and health-care services is also a vital part of therapy. Thus, many of them not only faced dysfunction from thinking and emotional difficulties but they have dysfunctions from a lack of social and work skills and experience as well. With social rehabilitation, PLWS can be very much focussed on internal processes that his/her external social world collapses [24], with a loss of self-esteem [33]. Social engagement is a longitudinal predictor of objective and subjective health [34]. In fact, evidence points to the fact that any person who is socially incompetent due to mental illness is unable to function smoothly in society because of feelings of low self-esteem, isolation and anger [35].

## 8. Cognitive rehabilitation

All domains of cognition are affected in schizophrenia, with verbal and visuospatial memory, attention, executive function and speed of processing most profoundly being affected [36–38]. Verbal memory represents one of the most affected cognitive domains in schizophrenia, and the impairments are the most profound [39]. Of the three symptoms domain, on positive, negative and disorganization symptom, cognition is the strongest predictor of functional outcome [40]. Cognitive deficits are closely linked to activities of daily living (ADL) and have been shown to interfere with daily functioning including activities of daily living [41], employment and quality of life [42–44]. Green et al. [45, 46] pointed out that four specific neurocognitive domains were significantly associated with functional outcomes: executive functioning, immediate verbal memory, secondary verbal memory and vigilance. Dysfunctions in activities of daily living (ADL) have been predictive of future cognitive impairment, independent of current cognitive status or depression [47, 48]. Among all ADLs, bathing impairment may have the highest risk of future institutionalization [49]. With the acknowledgement that some ADL dysfunctions are more predictive of long-term institutionalization, policymakers can plan ahead of the resources to target these declines with occupational therapy and nursing services that has implication for future program spending on long-term-care services. Functional impairment leads to an acceleration of cognitive decline [41, 48]. Therefore, any strategy to increase or maintain cognitive functioning can enable people to remain functionally independent in medical management (which is important for people living with schizophrenia) and ensure independence in their daily living [48].

## 9. Daily-living performance

Activities of daily living (ADL) are a part of everyday self-care activities that are important for health maintenance and independent living [41, 48, 49]. A major goal of occupational therapy rehabilitation is to enable people to develop independent living skills—for personal daily care of oneself and independent community living. ADL dependence is correlated with increased health-care costs, an increased risk of mortality, poorer quality of life and institutionalization [50–52]. Self-care including oral health has often been neglected—a cohort study on 543 people with schizophrenia found that the mean decayed-missing-filled teeth was at a high 20.5, almost double as that of the general population which was only 11.7 [53]. Wey et al. also found that higher decayed-missing-filled teeth scores were significantly associated with both older age ($p < 0.001$) and longer illness duration ($p \leq 0.048$) [53]. Leisure time is another key area of rehabilitation focus for people living with schizophrenia, who are often limited in their financial capabilities and may find it hard to know what to do with the spare time on their hands. Initial assessment must be made to determine what new skills are needed, and then from there, a program could be developed and individualized for that client [54]. Lalonde [16] reported that the leisure desires and needs of schizophrenics determine the range of activity and how they use time effectively. PLWS should be encouraged to begin/continue participating in meaningful social recreational/community activities because social engagement can help slow down the onset of ADL disability [55]. However, it is also timely for clinicians to attend to the underlying factors that worsen ADL performance (but can be treated early such as depression, resistance to care and pain), because ADL impairment has significant ramifications for patients and leads to institutionalization and caregiver burnout.

## 10. Work rehabilitation

Worldwide, psychiatry disorders comprise about one-third of the burden of illness in young adulthood [56], because about 75% of adult mental health problems manifest around early adulthood [57]. Untreated mental health problems and disorders in adolescents and young adults are strong predictors of poor vocational achievements, problematic interpersonal and family functioning. Most schizophrenia rehabilitation programs need a vocational component. Financial stability is a crucial part of the rehabilitation of these young adults—and having some money in one's pocket is a potent source of self-esteem [58]. Work (paid or volunteer tasks) can become monotonous and unchallenging, but for people with schizophrenia, work can provide a social or an occupational environment/routine that is familiar and safe. A study on the quality of life of community-based chronic schizophrenia patients in Penang (Malaysia) found that people with schizophrenia experienced discrimination, social isolation and workplace exploitations [59]. A large study across 26 countries reported that 64% of PLWS (n = 469) who apply for work, training or education were discriminated [59–61]. Employment (and a task-orientated-coping style) has been found to be positively correlated with a better quality of life [62], whereby social relationship was the most impaired aspects of well-being [63] in this group where social functioning is often at risk [10]. Importantly, employment has been showed to be positively correlated with a better quality of life [64]. In short, work as a medium of rehabilitation can build up their work skills and good work habits [54], providing them with a sense of belonging, finance, meaning and purpose in life. Supported employment, a type of psychosocial therapy that offers job training, integrated together with work-related social skills training, has been used to enhance vocational and non-vocational outcomes for people with schizophrenia in mainland China [65]. Supported employment has been reported to be effective in various international settings and has a beneficial impact on competitive employment rates for about 2 years irrespective of economic conditions [66].

## 11. Interdisciplinary rehabilitation for schizophrenia

In the past, rehabilitation for people living with schizophrenia (PLWS) in developing countries with low resources has focus primarily on a one-size-fits-all approach, with integration of psychosocial interventions to enable these persons to engage in their highest possible level of independent functioning. Schizophrenia has been commonly associated with impairments in social and occupational functioning due to a combination of positive (hallucinations or delusions, disorganized speech) and negative symptoms (such as a flat affect or poverty of speech) and impairments in cognition (e.g., attention, memory and executive functions) [9]. In recent decades, the introduction of better, newer, more well-tolerated antipsychotic medications has opened up possibilities for more patients to participate in psychiatric rehabilitation programs including overall patient-self-management and supported employment. The rehabilitation goals have shifted towards a better level of symptom control and management, and a greater level of subjective life satisfaction and quality of life. Therefore, an early interdisciplinary approach to plan personalized- and categorized-care intervention is based on categorizing users into smaller clusters according to their needs in line with a need-based approach to recovery [15, 18]. The therapists need to establish the level of concerns for the particular intervention—and decides with the other health-care practitioners and with clients' inter-discipline. Specific occupational therapy intervention is needed and calls for greater research as well as clinical implementation to help define the category of care packages according to the needs of occupational therapy service users and the adapted OT intervention in mental health—a preliminary framework presented in **Table 1** [63, 67]. More work and research are needed

| The OT service category | Definition | Level of concerns<br>(low, mid, high) |
|---|---|---|
| 1. Patient self-efficacy—to engage in basic self-care, work and leisure | Adapting activities to match current abilities and thus support engagement, Focus on personal assets and resources rather than deficits only | [__] [__] [__] |
| 2. Behavioral activation (re-motivation process) | Building enjoyment in activity engagement to make spontaneous choices to participate in self-care, leisure and work. | [__] [__] [__] |
| 3. Self-management education to activate patients in symptom management | Increase understanding of managing the condition, and monitoring symptoms and managing changing emotions while developing coping skills | [__] [__] [__] |
| 4. Lifestyle adjustment | An intervention that is focused on developing/establishing daily routines, roles and responsibilities in a graded pattern of intervention, leading to a structured daily routine of self-care, productivity (work) and leisure which support the delivery of life roles | [__] [__] [__] |
| 5. Lifestyle management | Interventions focus on promoting health and prevention of ill health. Health promotion topics, that is, smoking cessation, healthier eating, mental well-being, increased physical activity addressed as part of enhancing the quality of life. | [__] [__] [__] |
| 5. Environmental modification and assistive technology to support engagement in activity | Support with environmental modification and assistive technology and establishing a sense of purpose/direction and satisfaction in functioning in new and unfamiliar physical and social environments | [__] [__] [__] |
| 6. Developing social relationships and networks | Building supportive social relationship at home and social engagement at the community | [__] [__] [__] |
| 7. Enablement: back to work/meaningful occupation | Sheltered employment and into supportive employment and open employment | [__] [__] [__] |

PLWS, people living with schizophrenia.

**Table 1.** Clustering of category of occupational therapy care progressing at a different level for PLWS.

to ensure outcome-based recovery approach. Psychosocial category of care that includes more community-based interventions must include home-based component, psychoeducation and family involvement, and some of cognitive retraining have been recommended as feasible in low-middle-income countries and self-management intervention skills training [15, 68]. In people living with schizophrenia, further category of care such as the supported employment for those who are trained with social skill has been found to be helpful in providing sustainable employment [69, 70]. The goal of interdisciplinary rehabilitation is aiming towards recovery, by facilitating and optimizing people living with long-term schizophrenia experienced by themselves as they become empowered to manage their lives. This is the rehabilitation pathway that allows them to achieve a meaningful life and one that contributes to a positive sense of belonging in the community—one that allows them to live independently, not just to exist. It calls for experts in the area of rehabilitation—in particular, the occupational therapists, psychologist and psychiatrists to collaborate directly with the "client" or the expert patient.

## 12. Summary

Indeed, medication is an initial must for every individual afflicted with schizophrenia, but it is by no means a cure and warrants customized rehabilitation to improve quality of life. Patient categorization for people living with long-term schizophrenia is a step forward to overcome the less-effective, one-size-fits-all approach. With more occupational therapist and psychiatrists now compared to decades ago, the rehabilitative care for PLWS needs more attention and should be improved. Occupational practice guidelines target at outcome-focused-care and interdisciplinary-care planning. It is a practice guided by the Model of Human Occupation to craft a framework that enables people to move forward—by addressing practical daily issues and gaining the needed confidence as goals are planned and achieved, and benefit from. Occupation-focused practice can transform people living with schizophrenia's daily experience of their situation, both as a patient in recovery and as a holistic human being, gradually establishing themselves as valued members of the community. Personalizing follow-up of PLWS can improve the medical and psychosocial care for each individual patient (with differing medical, physical and psychosocial exposure). In addition, personalizing care may also help reduce the entrenched stigma of psychiatry illness that still persists in many Asian cultures. There is a need to address specific (treatment, physical, psychosocial) exposures and examine combination therapies in line with developing guidelines for categories of PLWS and to evaluate the sustainability of gains beyond the rehabilitation intervention period.

In conclusion, more research work is still needed to evaluate and document the effectiveness of various models of interdisciplinary care and categorizing care for PLWS which have been developed but may not be tested/evaluated. The model tested to be effective but on other long-term non-physical conditions may also be translated and adapted for testing to ensure cost-effective deliveries. Much work is needed along a common battery of measurements (including tools for risk exposure assessments) for better comparisons across interventions and across sub-categories of PLWS. However, in resource-limited countries, strategies that call for the social engagement of communities to support in the management of disability towards recovery and working closely with patients (and their activated families) may be ecologically more feasible. Future research should also examine the interdisciplinary partnership and communication, as well as with the community partners.

## Author details

Siew Yim Loh

Address all correspondence to: syloh@um.edu.my

Faculty of Medicine, University of Malaya, Kuala Lumpur, Malaysia

## References

[1] Schultz SH, North SW, Shields CG. Schizophrenia: A review. American Family Physician. 2007 Jun 15;**75**(12):1821-1829

[2] Fischer BA, Buchanan RW. UpToDate: Schizophrenia in Adults: Epidemiology and Pathogenesis. 2017. Available from: https://www.uptodate.com/contents/schizophrenia-in-adults-epidemiology-and-pathogenesis

[3] Math SB, Chandrashekar CR, Bhugra D. Psychiatric epidemiology in India. The Indian Journal of Medical Research. 2007;**126**:183-192

[4] Avasthi A. Indianizing psychiatry – Is there a case enough? Indian Journal of Psychiatry. 2012;**53**:111-120

[5] Häfner H. The concept of schizophrenia: From unity to diversity. Advances in Psychiatry. 2014, 39 pages. Article ID: 929434. http://dx.doi.org/10.1155/2014/929434

[6] Jacob K, Sharan P, Mirza I, et al. Mental health systems in countries: Where are we now? Lancet. 2007;**370**:1061-1077

[7] WHO. Disease and Injury Regional Estimates for 2004. Geneva, Switzerland: World Health Organization; 2004. http://www.who.int/healthinfo/global_burden_disease/estimates_regional/en/index.html.

[8] WHO. The Global Burden of Disease: 2004 Update. Geneva, Switzerland: World Health Organization; 2008

[9] APA. American Psychiatric Association. Diagnostic and Statistical Manual of Mental Disorders, Fifth Edition (DSM-5). Arlington: American Psychiatric Association; 2015

[10] Koschorke M, Padmavati R, Kumar S, Cohen A, Weiss HA, Chatterjee S, et al. Experiences of stigma and discrimination of people with schizophrenia in India. Social Science & Medicine. 1982;**123**:149-159. http://doi.org/10.1016/j.socscimed.2014.10.035

[11] Chee KY. Determinants of subjective quality of life in first episode schizophrenia: Perspective from Malaysia. Early Intervention in Psychiatry. 2010;**4**(2):111-118

[12] Carmona VR, Gómez-Benito J, Huedo-Medina TB, Rojo JE. Employment outcomes for people with schizophrenia spectrum disorder: A meta-analysis of randomized controlled trials. International Journal of Occupational Medicine and Environmental Health. 2017;**30**(3):345-366

[13] Rathod S, Pinninti N, Irfan M, Gorczynski P, Rathod P, Gega L, Naeem F. Mental health service provision in low- and middle-income countries. Health Services Insights. 2017;**10**:1178632917694350. DOI: http://doi.org/10.1177/1178632917694350

[14] Parkinson S, Morley M, Stewart L, Brockbank H Meeting the occupational needs of mental health service users: Indicative care packages & actual practice. British Journal of Occupational Therapy. 2012;**75**(8);384-389

[15] Corrigan PW, Rao D. On the self-stigma of mental illness: Stages, disclosure, and strategies for change. Canadian Journal of Psychiatry. 2012;**57**(8):464-469

[16] Kelly EL, Fenwick KM, Barr N, Cohen H, Brekke JS. A systematic review of self-management health care models for individuals with serious mental illnesses. Psychiatric Services (Washington, D.C.). 2014;**65**(11):1300-1310. http://doi.org/10.1176/appi.ps.201300502

[17] Lalonde P. Rehabilitation. In: Jones BD, editor. Demystifying Schizophrenia: Navigating Diagnosis, Care and Recovery. Montreal, QC: Grosvenor House Press Inc; 1995. pp. 71-81

[18] Sueiras P, Romano-Betech V, Vergil-Salgado A, de Hoyos A, Quintana-Vargas S, Ruddick W, Altamirano-Bustamante MM. Today's medical self and the other: Challenges and evolving solutions for enhanced humanization and quality of care. PLoS One. 2017;**12**(7):e0181514. http://doi.org/10.1371/journal.pone.0181514

[19] Marzorati C, Pravettoni G. Value as the key concept in the health care system: How it has influenced medical practice and clinical decision-making processes. Journal of Multidisciplinary Healthcare. 2017 Mar 21;**10**:101-106. DOI: 10.2147/JMDH.S122383

[20] Saultz J. The importance of being comprehensive. Family Medicine. 2012;**44**(3):157-158

[21] CFPC. College of Family Physicians of Canada. Standards for Accreditation of Family Medicine Residency Training Programs ("The Red Book"). Mississauga, ON Canada; 2006. Available from: www.cfpc.ca/uploadedFiles/Red%20Book%20English.pdf

[22] Ting JH, Chan BTM, Ahmad HS. Assessment of insight in patients with schizophrenia in Hospital Permai. MJP. 2002;**12**(1):32-37

[23] Sharmilla K, Ahmad HS. A comparison of insight in schizophrenia, bipolar affective disorder with psychosis and major depressive disorder with psychosis. Malaysian Journal of Psychiatry. 2006;**14**(1):35-40

[24] Keltner NL, Schwecke LH, Bostrom CE. Psychiatric Nursing: A Psychotherapeutic Management Approach. St. Louis, MO: Mosby; 1991

[25] Salmi R, Ainsah O, Osman CB, et al. Obesity among patients with schizophrenia, attending outpatient psychiatric clinic, hospital Universiti Kebangsaan Malaysia. ASEAN Journal of Psychiatry. 2007;**8**(2):90-96

[26] Norlelawati AT, Kartini A, Ramli M, et al. Obesity in multiracial schizophrenia patients receiving outpatient treatment in a regionaltertiary hospital in Malaysia. East Asian Arch Psychiatry. 2012;**22**(2):49-56

[27] Fairuz AR, Maniam T, Khalid BA. Prevalence of insulin resistance inschizophrenia in HUKM. The Medical Journal of Malaysia. 2007;**62**(4):290-293

[28] Chee KY. Weight gain and first-generation antipsychotics: experience from a developing country. Journal of Clinical Psychopharmacology. 2008;**28**(5):574-576

[29] Mas Ayu S, Ahmad Hatim S, Mohd Hussain H, et al. Metabolic syndrome and antipsychotic monotherapy treatment among schizophrenia patients in Malaysia. Preventive Medicine. 2013;**57**(Suppl):S50-S53

[30] Mas Ayu S, Ahmad Hatim S, Mohd Hussain H, et al. Metabolic syndrome and cardiovascular risk among patients with schizophrenia receiving antipsychotics in Malaysia. Singapore Medical Journal. 2012;**53**(12):801-807

[31] Loh, Siew Y, Abdullah A, Kadir ABA, Thambu M, Ruzyanei NJN. Structured Walking and Chronic Institutionalized Schizophrenia Inmates www.ccsenet.org. 2016;**8**(1):238-248. DOI: http://dx.doi.org/10.5539/gjhs.v8n1p238

[32] Loh SY, et al Visceral obesity in the normal-weight people-comparing chronic schizophrenia and healthy control subjects. Brain Nerves. 2017;**1**(2):1-6. DOI: 10.15761/JBN.1000111

[33] Kalman N, Waughfield CG. Mental Health Concepts. 2nd ed. Albany, NY: Delmar Publishers Inc.; 1987

[34] Bennett KM. Social engagement as a longitudinal predictor of objective and subjective health. European Journal of Ageing. 2005 Mar;**2**(1):48-55. Published online 2005 Mar 9. DOI: 10.1007/s10433-005-0501-z

[35] Carson VB, Arnold EN. Mental Health Nursing: The Nurse-Patient Journey. Philadelphia: W. B. Saunders Co; 1996

[36] Addington J, Brooks BL, Addington D. Cognitive functioning in first episode psychosis: Initial presentation. Schizophrenia Research. 2003;**62**:59-64

[37] Mohamed S, Paulsen JS, O'Leary D, et al. Generalized cognitive deficits in schizophrenia: A study of first-episode patients. Archives of General Psychiatry. 1999;**56**:749-754

[38] Saykin AJ, Shtasel DL, Gur RE, et al. Neuropsychological deficits in neuroleptic naive patients with first-episode schizophrenia. Archives of General Psychiatry. 1994;**51**:124-131

[39] Guimond S, Chakravarty MM, Bergeron-Gagnon L, Patel R, Lepage M. Verbal memory impairments in schizophrenia associated with cortical thinning. NeuroImage: Clinical, 2016;**11**:20-29. http://doi.org/10.1016/j.nicl.2015.12.010

[40] Meyer EC, Carrión RE, Cornblatt BA, Addington J, Cadenhead KS, Cannon TD, ... the NAPLS Group LJ. The relationship of neurocognition and negative symptoms to social and role functioning over time in individuals at clinical high risk in the first phase of the north american prodrome longitudinal study. Schizophrenia Bulletin. 2014;**40**(6):1452-1461. http://doi.org/10.1093/schbul/sbt235

[41] Rajan KB, Hebert LE, Scherr PA, Mendes de Leon CF, Evans DA. Disability in basic and instrumental activities of daily living is associated with faster rate of decline in cognitive function of older adults. Journal of Gerontology, Series A: Biological Sciences and Medical Sciences. 2013 May;**68**(5):624-30. DOI: 10.1093/gerona/gls208. Epub 2012 Oct 25

[42] Bell MD, Bryson G. Work rehabilitation in schizophrenia: Does cognitive impairment limit improvement? Schizophrenia Bulletin. 2001;**27**:269-279

[43] Twamley EW, Doshi RR, Nayak GV, et al. Generalized cognitive impairments, ability to perform everyday tasks, and level of independence in community living situations of older patients with psychosis. The American Journal of Psychiatry. 2002;**159**:2013-2020

[44] Perlick DA, Rosenheck RA, Kaczynski R, et al. Association of symptomatology and cognitive deficits to functional capacity in schizophrenia. Schizophrenia Bulletin. 2008;**99**:192-199

[45] Green MF. What are the functional consequences of neurocognitive deficits in schizophrenia? The American Journal of Psychiatry. 1996;**153**:321-330

[46] Green MF, Kern RS, Braff DL, Mintz J. Neurocognitive deficits and functional outcome in schizophrenia: are we measuring the "right stuff"? Schizophrenia Bulletin. 2000;**26**:119-136

[47] Fauth EB, Schwartz S, Tschanz JT, Østbye T, Corcoran C, Norton MC. Baseline disability in activities of daily living predicts dementia risk even after controlling for baseline global cognitive ability and depressive symptoms. International Journal of Geriatric Psychiatry. 2013;**28**(6):597-606

[48] Alosco ML, Spitznagel MB, Cohen R, Sweet L, Colbert LH, Josephson R, et al. Cognitive impairment is independently associated with reduced instrumental ADLs in persons with heart failure. The Journal of Cardiovascular Nursing. 2012;**27**(1):44-50. http://doi.org/10.1097/JCN.0b013e318216a6cd

[49] Fong JH, Mitchell OS, Koh BSK. Disaggregating activities of daily living limitations for predicting nursing home admission. Health Services Research. 2015;**50**(2):560-578. http://doi.org/10.1111/1475-6773.12235

[50] Scott WK, Macera CA, Cornman CB, Sharpe PA. Functional health status as a predictor of mortality in men and women over 65. Journal of Clinical Epidemiology. 1997;**50**(3):291-296

[51] Millán-Calenti JC, Tubío J, Pita-Fernández S, González-Abraldes I, Lorenzo T, Fernández-Arruty T, Maseda A. Prevalence of functional disability in activities of daily living (ADL), instrumental activities of daily living (IADL) and associated factors, as predictors of morbidity and mortality. Archives of Gerontology and Geriatrics. 2010;**50**(3):306-310

[52] Gaugler JE, Duval S, Anderson KA, Kane RL. Predicting nursing home admission in the US: A meta-analysis. BMC Geriatrics. 2007;**7**(1):13-26

[53] Wey MC, Loh SY, Doss J, Kadir ABA, Kisely S The oral health of people with chronic schizophrenia: A neglected public health burden. Australia New Zealand Journal of Psychiatry. 2015;**50**(7):1-10. DOI: 10.1177/0004867415615947

[54] Stuart GW, Sundeen SJ. Principles & Practice of Psychiatric Nursing. St. Louis, MO: Mosby; 1995

[55] Mendes de Leon CFM, Rajan KB. Psychosocial influences in onset and progression of late life disability. The Journals of Gerontology Series B: Psychological Sciences and Social Sciences. 2014;**69**:287-302

[56] WHO Methods and data sources for global burden of disease estimates 2000-2011. World Health Organization. 2013. http://www.who.int/healthinfo/statistics/Global DALYmethods_2000_2011.pdf?ua=1. [Accessed: Nov 30, 2017]

[57] Kessler RC, Berglund P, Demler O, Jin R, Merikangas KR. Lifetime prevalence and age of-onset distributions of DSM-IV disorders in the national comorbidity survey replication. Archives of General Psychiatry. 2005;**62**(6):593-602. DOI: 10.1001/archpsyc.62.6.593

[58] Thornton JF, Seeman MV. Schizophrenia Simplified: A Field Guide for Frontline Workers, Families, and Professionals. Toronto: Hogrefe & Huber Publishers; 1993

[59] Mubarak AR, Baba I, Chin LH, Hoe QS. Quality of life of community-based chronic schizophrenia patients in Penang, Malaysia. Australian and New Zealand Journal of Psychiatry. 2003 Oct;**37**(5):577-85

[60] Thornicroft G, Brohan E, Rose D, Sartorius, et al. Global pattern of experienced and anticipated discrimination against people with schizophrenia: A cross-sectional survey. Lancet. 2009;**373**(9661):408-415. DOI: 10.1016/S0140-6736(08)61817-6

[61] Hagelskamp C, Hughes DL. Workplace discrimination predicting racial/ethnic socialization across African American, Latino, and Chinese families. Cultural Diversity & Ethnic Minority Psychology. 2014 Oct;**20**(4):550-60. DOI: 10.1037/a0035321. Epub 2014 Aug 18

[62] Mohd Badli M, Osman CB, Ainsah O. Coping style and clinical factorsin relation to quality of life among patients with schizophrenia. Medicine & Health. 2008;**3**(1):14-21

[63] Bouwmans C, de Sonneville C, Mulder CL, Roijen LH. Employment and the associated impact on quality of life in people diagnosed with schizophrenia. Neuropsychiatric Disease and Treatment. 2015;**11**:2125-2142. Published online 2015 August 18. DOI: 10.2147/NDT.S83546

[64] Hasanah CI, Razali MS. Quality of life: An assessment of the state of psychosocial rehabilitation of patients with schizophrenia in the community. The Journal of the Royal Society for the Promotion of Health. 2002;**122**(4):251-255

[65] Zhang GF, Tsui CM, Lu AJB, Yu LB, Tsang HWH, Li D. Integrated Supported Employment for People With Schizophrenia in Mainland China: A Randomized Controlled Trial. American Journal of Occupational Therapy. 2017 Nov/Dec;**71**(6):7106165020p1-7106165020p8

[66] Modini M, Tan L, Brinchmann B, Wang MJ, Killackey E, Glozier N, Mykletun A. Harvey SB supported employment for people with severe mental illness: Systematic review and meta-analysis of the international evidence. The British Journal of Psychiatry Jul. 2016;**209**(1):14-22. DOI: 10.1192/bjp.bp.115.165092

[67] Occupational Therapists' Use of Occupation-focused Practice in Secure Hospitals Practice Guideline Second Edition Royal College of Occupational Therapists. Available from: https://www.rcot.co.uk/node/397. [Accessed: September 12, 2017]

[68] NIHME. National Institute for Mental Health in England. Guiding Statement on Recovery. Available from: studymore.org.uk/nimherec.pdf;2005

[69] Asher L, Patel V, De Silva MJ. Community-based psychosocial interventions for people with schizophrenia in low and middle-income countries: systematic review and meta-analysis. BMC Psychiatry. 2017;**17**:355. http://doi.org/10.1186/s12888-017-1516-7

[70] Hafizah SWK, Midin M, Kadir AB, Sidi H, Ruzyanei NJ. Das S employment program for patients with severe mental illness in Malaysia: A 3-month outcome. Comprehensive Psychiatry. 2014;**55**:S38-S45

# 4

# Lack of Insight in Bipolar Disorder: The Impact on Treatment Adherence, Adverse Clinical Outcomes and Quality of Life

Cătălina Angela Crișan

**Abstract**

Insight is a multidimensional construct, defined as the awareness of having a mental disorder, of specific symptoms and their attribution to the disorder, the awareness of social consequences, and of need for treatment. Although insight has been studied specifically in schizophrenia and its study in mood disorders has traditionally received limited attention, the evaluation of this concept in mood disorders is also very important because of the impact on treatment compliance and outcome. In bipolar disorder (BD), clinical insight varies substantially over time. Most researchers observed that insight is more impaired during an illness episode than during remission, in mixed than in pure manic episodes, in bipolar II than in bipolar I patients, and in pure mania than in bipolar or unipolar depression. Lack of insight is a consistent factor of non-adherence to medication in bipolar patients, along with severity of BD, side effects of medication, effectiveness, and patient-related factors. Also, impaired insight into treatment and a great number of previous hospitalizations are associated with poorer clinical outcomes (psychiatric hospitalization, emergency room visits, violent or suicidal behavior) among the patients with bipolar I disorder. In the management of bipolar disorder, improving quality of life (QoL) and outcome should be one the most important goals.

**Keywords:** insight, bipolar disorder, adherence, quality of life, outcome

## 1. Introduction

In medicine, the concept of insight into madness seems to have started in early part of the nineteenth century when the clinical descriptions began to include observations about patients' awareness of their pathological state. In 1882, Pick used the term "Krankheitseinsicht" [1], and in 1893, Krafft-Ebing used the term "insightlessness" ("in the later stages of insanity, where delusions have become organized or mental disintegration has ensued, the patient is completely insightless—(einsichtloss) about his disease state") ([2], translated by [3]). In the history of this concept, there were differences in the approach of the most important French, German, and English authors. In the French view, Pinel (1801) referred to the patient's "judgment" and to his capacity to correctly assess his state ("apprécie avec justesse son état") [4]. Baillarger separated the patients into two categories (who were and who were not insane) using insight (the patients with hallucinations, who were convinced of the reality of their hallucinations, were truly mad; on the other hand, the patients with hallucinations who realized that these hallucinations were caused by some derangement in themselves, should not be considered truly mad) [5]. A major debate concerning awareness of mental illness ("la discussion sur les aliénés avec conscience de leur état") and the responsibility of patients for criminal acts was held by the Société Médico-Psychologique in 1869–1870, and then in 1875 Billod observed that the number of patients who were aware about their state of madness was lower than those without the disease awareness [6]. He divided the patients into two categories:

1. Those who were not aware of their pathological state (they were aware of hallucinations and strange experiences but attributed those wrongly).
2. Those who were aware of their pathological state.

a. Patients with incomplete awareness (they were aware of their pathological state but, nevertheless, believed in the reality of their delusions and strange experiences).
b. Patients with complete awareness (they were aware of their pathological state and recognized the falseness of their abnormal experiences).

Billod also observed that insight is a good prognostic factor of the evolution of the disease and for illness recurrence.

Parant classified mentally ill patients, during an episode of illness, into five groups [7]:

1. Those who are aware of their acts and who can discern whether they are good or bad but are not aware of their morbid condition.
2. Those who are aware that they are in an abnormal state but do not understand or admit that this condition is a mental illness.
3. Those who are aware that their mental condition, their acts, and their ideas are the result of a mental illness, but they behave as if they would not do so (patients presenting hallucinations and delusions of persecution, being convinced by the reality of their symptoms, but who also consider themselves to be healthy).
4. Those who are aware of their condition and who understand that this condition is due to a mental illness, but who are incapable of taking an attitude in this regard.
5. Those who are aware of their condition and who understand that this condition is due to a mental illness, but who have committed or been forced to commit dangerous acts.

In the British view, Maudsley believes that the healthy man was incapable of accurately judging the behavior and the experiences of the mental ill; at the same time, the psychic patient could not judge with his healthy psychic functions the phenomenon produced by his psychically impaired functions [8]. Aubrey Lewis, in 1934, distinguished between the change in awareness and the change in judgment, both being mandatory components of the insight [9]. According to his opinion, the patient should be first aware of the change and then form an opinion, a judgment about it. Aubrey Lewis conceptualized the insight as a complex group of judgment types, based on different types of information. Lewis defined the insight as "an attitude adapted to an unhealthy change in itself, and ability to decentralize, and to give a personal judgment on one's own state."

In the German view, Pick argued that for the most part of the mental illnesses (mania, melancholia, obsessive–compulsive disorder, psychosis, dementia, alcohol abuse), the patients were somewhat aware of their affection [1]. He noted that the patients with progressive onset had a better insight time wise, unlike those for whom the disease suddenly started. Pick subdivided the concept of the disease awareness ("Krankheitsbewuβtsein") into the awareness of the phenomenon of being sick ("Krankheitsgefühl") and the disease insight ("Krankheitseinsicht").

Unlike Kraepelin and Bleuler, who did not approached the concept of the insight, Jaspers was the one who studied it for a long time and the one who brought many new elements [10]. He considered that not only the patients become conscious and develop a judgment regarding the symptoms of their illness but also the expression of their illness' symptoms is affected by the patients' awareness and judgment. Jaspers noticed that in the early stages of psychosis, the patients were uncomfortable and embarrassed, having a meaningful reaction to the lived experiences. With the disease progression, the patients tried to make sense of their own experiences, and they elaborated a delusional system. When the disease produced changes in personality, the patient's attitude to the illness was less and less understood.

Even if the concept of insight is widely used, there are important differences between authors regarding his components. In 1989, Greenfeld et al. proposed a model of insight consisting of five distinct and independent dimensions [11]: (1) views about symptoms, (2) views about the existence of an illness, (3) speculations about etiologia, (4) views about the risk of recurrence, and (5) opinions about the opportunity of treatment. This approach is focused more on patients' understanding of what is happening to them and what individual sense they are making of their experiences.

David described three distinct dimensions of insight: (1) the recognition of the presence of a mental illness, (2) the compliance with treatment, and (3) the ability to relabel psychotic symptoms (delusions and hallucinations) as pathological [12].

A more complex multidimensional model of insight is proposed by Amador et al. and consists of the following elements: (1) awareness of the signs, symptoms, and consequences of illness, (2) general attribution about illness and specific attribution about symptoms and their consequences, (3) self-concept formation, and (4) psychological defensiveness [13].

Trying to give a more practical description of the concept, Amador and Strauss proposed two important components: (1) awareness of illness and (2) attribution regarding the illness [14].

Marková [3] summarized in her monography the following components of insight: (1) an attribution of the change to pathology [10, 12, 13], (2) social consequences of illness [13], (3) views concerning etiologia and likely recurrence [11], (4) perception of changes in the self and one's interaction with the world [15], (5) need for medical treatment [12, 13, 16], (6) attitudes toward experiences [17], (7) comparison with the previous function [18], (8) predictions of performance on specific tests [19, 20], and (9) resemblance of own experiences to hypothetical cases [21].

Most studies about insight were conducted with patients suffering from schizophrenia and other psychotic disorders, neglecting patients with mood disorders. However, in the last few years, there has been an increase in interest about insight in patients with bipolar disorder [22]. The awareness of illness can be quite impaired in mania, second only to schizophrenia, even in the absence of psychosis [23].

Given the importance of insight to diagnosis, treatment adherence, and psychosocial outcome, we considered that it is appropriate to pay attention to this phenomenon. This chapter presents few remarks about the history of the concept, different models of insight, the most important psychometric tools in assessing insight and clinical implications of poor insight in patients diagnosed with bipolar disorder. Taking into account that clinical insight varies substantially over time in bipolar patients, the relationship of insight to episode subtypes and symptom dimensions is analyzed in detail. Than other important themes are addressed: the impact of unawareness of illness on non-adherence to medication, on outcome, and quality of life (QoL).

## 2. Measurement of insight

Over the past 15 years, semi-structured interviews with systematized scoring systems and proven psychometric strengths have been devised to measure insight. The first such measure to be used widely was The Insight and Treatment Attitudes Questionnaire (ITAQ) developed by McEvoy et al. [24]. The ITAQ has been used in large samples of patients with schizophrenia and has been shown to be reliable and valid. The questionnaire comprises 11 items designed to assess patients' recognition of illness and the need for treatment. The response of the patient is scored as 2 = good insight, 1 = partial insight, and 0 = no insight. The ITAQ employs a narrow definition of insight and does not assess many of the psychological domains that are believed to comprise insight into illness more generally.

David's Schedule for the Assessment of Insight (SAI) assesses insight based on a patient's recognition of having a mental illness, compliance with treatment, and ability to label unusual events, such as delusions and hallucinations, as pathological [12]. The Schedule for the Assessment of Insight explores insight beyond the acknowledgment of illness and the need for treatment. This measure does not, however, consider how insight may vary from symptom to symptom, nor does it consider differences between current and retrospective insight into illness.

Similarly, the Insight Scale (IS) devised by Birchwood et al. is an alternative direct translation from David's three-dimensional model of **insight, but in this case,** the empirical form is presented as a self-report measure (scoring 0–4 on each dimension, maximum: 12) [25].

Kemp and David, back in 1995, developed The Schedule for Assessment of Insight—Expanded version (SAI-E) [26], a three-dimensional scale designed to measure insight into mental illness. The questionnaire contains 10 items on three apparently separated but actually overlapped extents, as follows: the first three questions evaluate the awareness of the illness, questions 4–7 measure the capacity to relabel psychotic experiences as abnormal and the awareness of symptoms, while the latter questions rank the treatment compliance of the evaluated patient. The clinician conducts the survey by asking the patient a set of questions and then calculates the result: a higher-attained score indicates an increased level of insight.

Amador and Strauss developed the Scale to assess Unawareness of Mental Disorder (SUMD) [27], which distinguishes current and retrospective awareness of (1) having a mental disorder, (2) the effects of medication, (3) the consequences of mental disorder, and (4) the specific signs and symptoms. Since its development, this scale has gained widespread acceptance as a multidimensional measure of insight and has been validated and studied on a range of clinical samples. SUMD consists of 20 items: the first three evaluate general aspects, such as awareness of the mental disorder, of the attained effects of medication, and of the social consequences of having a mental disorder, while the latter inquire more specific topics: hallucinations, delusions, thought disorder, inappropriate affect, unusual appearance and eye contact, stereotypic or ritualistic behavior, poor social judgment and relationships, poor control of aggressive and sexual impulses, poverty of speech, flat or blunt affect, avolition, apathy, presence of anhedonia, diminished attention, and confusion-disorientation. The survey is administered by the clinician or by a trained reviewer and it can take up to 40 min. Evaluation is performed through a five-level Likert scale, a value of 0 showing intact insight.

In 1992, Carsky et al. developed Patient's Experience of Hospitalization (PEH), an 18-item self-report scale, which reflects predominantly views about being in hospital [28]. The instrument is focused on a narrow definition of denial, specifically limiting this to a failure to acknowledge: (1) having an illness or that the illness has a name or a cause, (2) any need for hospitalization, and (3) that the illness has personal impact. Each item is rated on a four-point scale of severity or level of agreement with a higher total score indicating greater denial.

Using the same concept, Marks et al. developed the Self-Appraisal of Illness Questionnaire (SAIQ) based closely on the PEH but designed for use in community settings. SAIQ is a 17-item self-report scale following the format of the PEH but substituting items about hospitalization with similar items about the need for treatment [29]. Olaya et al. developed a multidimensional scale, the Insight Scale for Affective Disorders (ISAD), a hetero-evaluation instrument for patients with mood disorders [30]. The scale evaluates dimensions like insight into illness, treatment needs, and social consequences [31]. The instrument, based on the Scale to Assess Unawareness in Mental Disorders (SUMD) [27], consists of 17 items. Scores may range from 1 (absence of symptom or full insight) to 5 (no insight) for each item, meaning that any score above 1 indicates insight alteration for that item. This scale allows for a more complex assessment of insight, addressing BD in a comprehensive manner.

## 3. Clinical implications of poor insight in bipolar disorder

### 3.1. The relationship of insight to episode subtypes and symptom dimensions

Even if the researcher's attention was focused mainly on patients diagnosed with schizophrenia, and there is far less research on insight in bipolar disorder, a number of studies have shown that individuals with bipolar disorder frequently experience impairments in insight [32–36]. While in schizophrenia insight is viewed as more of a stable trait [37], in bipolar disorder it has been conceptualized as more of a state-dependent construct, with alterations dependent on illness phases [38–40].

Results are mixed when comparing insight of patients with schizophrenia and of bipolar patients. Some studies show that schizophrenic patients have less insight than those suffering of psychotic or mixed mania [41], while other researches show that schizophrenic patients have a similar insight deficit with patients who have been diagnosed with acute-phased bipolar disorder [32, 42–44] and to bipolar disorder with psychotic features [23, 45, 46]. The reason for the mixed results is not very clear, but one of the possible explanations could be that these studies have not taken comorbid alcohol use disorder into consideration.

Peralta and Cuesta reported in their study that the presence of psychotic features did not significantly affect insight level in manic patients at discharge from the acute ward [47]. However, Yen et al., comparing insight in-patients with schizophrenia and bipolar disorder in remission, reported that bipolar patients with psychotic features had lower levels of insight than those without psychotic features [48].

In another study, Yen et al. analyzed a cohort of 65 patients with type-I bipolar disorder and observed them over a 2-year period [49]. During this period, patients received six follow-up assessments. SAI-E was used for establishing their insight levels, along with the Young Mania Rating Scale (YMRS) and the Hamilton Rating Scale for Depression (HAM-D), for determining affective tendencies. It was observed that insight was constant during the 2-years period in continuously-stable patients. A decreased insight could be associated with the presence of the manic phase, in both single manic and repeated manic episodes. The insight returned to the pre-episodic level for patients with a single manic episode, but it remained altered in most of patients with multiple manic episodes. Depressive episodes have shown no change of insight, regardless of the number of episodes.

In 2010, Cassidy examined lack of insight in 156 bipolar patients in all phases of the illness. A total of 86 patients were evaluated during pure manic episodes, 29 during mixed manic episodes, 14 during bipolar depressed episodes, and 27 in remission [38]. The purely manic group scored a mean (SD) lack of insight of 2.39 (1.62), the bipolar depressed group had a score of 0.57 (0.85) ($p < 0.001$), while the euthymic group has shown a mean of 0.444 (0.934) ($p < 0.001$).

Differences between the mixed-manic, bipolar-depressed, and euthymic groups were null. The author findings (84.9% subjects during pure mania had scores of 1 or greater) indicated at least a moderate denial of illness in manic patients. Psychomotor agitation and irritability, both core features of mania, were predictive of lack of insight during acute episodes.

De Assis da Silva et al. included in their study from 2015 95 patients with bipolar disorder and divided them into two different groups according to the mood state presented during assessment (i.e., euthymia, mania, and depression) [36]. Insight was evaluated using the hetero-evaluation questionnaire ISAD developed by Olaya et al. [30]. Patients with bipolar disorder in mania show less insight about their condition than patients in depression or euthymia, and less insight about their symptoms than patients with depression, with the exception of awareness of weight change. The advantage of this study is that the scale used to assess insight (ISAD) is a specific scale tailored to mood disorders, which allowed the authors to conduct a detailed evaluation of insight into specific symptoms of mood disorders.

There are some longitudinal studies of insight in the acute depressive episode [23, 44, 47, 50]. These studies suggest that insight is not very impaired in the acute non-psychotic depressive episode, and that insight may increase as depression worsens. However, insight is moderately impaired in psychotic depression [23]. Insight appears to improve markedly upon acute recovery from psychotic depression.

The relationship between insight and suicidality is complex. Amador et al. [51] and Schwartz and Petersen [52] found in their studies an association between intact insight and increased risk of suicide in patients diagnosed with schizophrenia. The results are not similar when analyzing patients with mood disorders.

In 2017, throughout the year, de Assiss da Silva et al. [53] followed a group of 165 bipolar patients, 53 of whom had depressive episodes according to DSM-5 criteria. Insight was evaluated through the Insight Scale for Affective Disorder (ISAD). ISAD total scores and sub-scores based on the four factors of the scale (insight into symptoms, the condition itself, self-esteem, and social relationship were generated for the analysis. Worse total insight correlated with suicide attempt/ideation. An altered self-esteem insight was associated not only with suicidal ideation or suicide attempt but also with activity reduction and psychomotor retardation. Altered symptom-related insight correlated also with psychomotor retardation. It was shown that a better insight into having an affective disorder determines more intense hypochondriac symptoms. Worse insight into having an illness was associated with psychotic episodes. The study concluded by exposing that symptoms other than psychosis, that is, suicidal ideation, psychomotor retardation, and reduction of activity, correlate with insight impairment in bipolar depression.

Focusing on the correlation between insight level and suicidal behavior/ideation in bipolar depression, de Assiss da Silva et al. [54] observed in the same group of 165 patients who were followed during one year that a history of suicidal attempts was associated with worse insight in 60 patients with one episode of bipolar depression. No correlation between current suicidal ideation and insight level was found. The results of this study suggest that a history of suicide attempts may correlate with higher impairment of insight in bipolar depression.

### 3.2. The impact of insight on non-adherence

One of the greatest problems clinicians face when dealing with chronic illnesses is the effectiveness of treatment. This is influenced by different factors such as patient tolerance of the drug, the appropriateness of the regimen [55], and adherence to treatment. Studies demonstrated that antipsychotic medication reduces the severity of serious mental illness and improves patient outcomes if medicines are taken as prescribed. Medication adherence previously known as compliance [56], is a process of collaboration between the physician and the patient (if during the compliance, the physician is omniscient, the patient must strictly follow the medical prescription; in case of adherence, the patient has an active role in decision-making regarding the type of agreed medication, the way of administration, and the therapy duration). In this case, the patient may refuse to check-in for appointments or may begin to discontinue his medication. Such behavior has a negative impact on the outcome and leads to higher rates of recurrence and hospitalization [57]. The non-adherence may be deliberate (the patient reduces or stops deliberately the medication, being convinced that he does not need medication for feel good and the medication is harmful for him due to possible side effects) or unintentionally (the patient skips some medication doses, either by forgetting them or because they do not check-in in time for a new recipe).

Medication adherence is a dynamic behavior, influenced by multiple factors [58]: factors related to patients (adverse effects of medication, lack of insight), their social relationships (family support and therapeutic alliance), cognitive problems (impaired memory or attention) [59], and the system for providing health services [60]. Rates of low adherence have been reported to be as high as two-thirds in patients with schizophrenia [61]. Bipolar patients have also low rates of adherence [62–64].

In their review about adherence to antipsychotic medication in two serious psychiatric disorders, bipolar disorder and schizophrenia, Garcia et al. systematized (**Table 1**) factors common for both pathologies and specific factors by diagnosis [65].

Lack of insight seems to be the most crucial factor impacting adherence [66]. Lack of awareness may fluctuate from complete denial of illness and full rejection of the diagnosis to minimization and rationalization of symptoms along with disapproval of medication's beneficial effects, such as treating specific symptoms and minimizing the relapse risk. A considerable number of patients with schizophrenia exhibit a diminished or completely absent insight into their ailment, being more likely to completely reject their need for treatment, therefore being sustainably noncompliant. Hence, it is essential to assess patients' insight on a continuum and not just to rate it as "good" or "poor." Is the patient aware of the disease, its nature, its symptoms, and the need of undergoing antipsychotic treatment for both acute and maintenance treatment? Lacks in the capability of recognizing the presence of a mental illness and the beneficial effect of antipsychotic medication would definitely increase the likelihood of altered compliance. Also, insight has a beneficial impact over the therapeutic relationship [67].

There are several studies which proved the importance of insight (as patient-related factor) on adherence in patients diagnosed with bipolar disorder. González-Pinto et al. [68], analyzing 1831 patients with bipolar disorder (in the EMBLEM Project), found that the following

| SCHIZOPHRENIA | COMMON FACTORS | BIPOLAR DISORDER |
|---|---|---|
| • positive symptoms<br>• highly-severe depression at baseline<br>• early dysphoric response<br>• brief illness duration<br>• presence of adverse effects (extrapyramidal syndrome, neuroleptic-induced dysphoria, akathisia, sexual impairment, weight gain)<br>• poor therapeutic response or tolerance development<br>• early treatment cessation rate<br>• hostility to treatment | • low levels of education<br>• young age<br>• cognitive impairment<br>• high intensity of delusional symptoms and suspiciousness<br>• substance abuse/dependence<br>• minority ethnicity<br>• poor insight<br>• poor therapeutic alliance<br>• low socioeconomic status<br>• barriers to treatment, bad patient experience of admission | • psychotic symptoms<br>• highly-severe depressive episodes<br>• presence of rapid-cycling<br>• increased affective morbidity<br>• comorbidities (anxiety, obsessive-compulsive disorder)<br>• adverse effects: weight gain, cognitive impairment<br>• longer duration of suicide attempts episodes |

**Table 1.** Factors influencing adherence to antipsychotic medication in bipolar disorder and schizophrenia [65].

factors were significantly positively associated with good adherence: good illness awareness (good adherence from the start of treatment) and a short duration of episodes. In contrast, high scores in the Clinical Global Impressions hallucinations/delusions scale at baseline and depressive symptoms during mania were related to poor adherence.

An observational study, conducted in Europe by Novick et al. [69], included 903 patients, out of which 612 were diagnosed with schizophrenia and 291 with bipolar disorder. Its design was meant to evaluate the outcome of patients treated with two oral formulations of olanzapine over a 1-year period through several evaluation tools, as follows: Clinical Global Impression (CGI), Global assessment of Functioning (GAF), Scale to Assess Unawareness of Mental Disorder (SUMD), Medication Adherence Rating Scale (MARS), and Working Alliance Inventory (WAI). The results have shown that medication adherence had higher levels in bipolar patients (mean MARS score (SD) 6.5 (2.8)) versus schizophrenic patients (mean MARS score (SD) 5.8 (2.7)) ($p < 0.0001$). An increased insight was associated with a better treatment adherence. Higher levels of insight were related to a powerful therapeutic alliance (SCC ranging from 0.38 to 0.48, $p < 0.0001$). The research has also shown that, 1 year after the follow-up, the improvement of patients' awareness of their mental disorder (gain of insight) or an improvement in the patient-physician relationship was directly associated with a better medication adherence, an improvement of the overall functioning, and a better outcome.

Copeland et al. [70] conducted a cross-sectional survey of patients recruited into the Continuous Improvement for Veterans in Care-Mood Disorders, assessing therapeutic insight and two measures of medication adherence: the Morisky scale of interpersonal barriers and missing any doses the previous four days. A total of 435 patients were included. Greater insight into medication was negatively associated with both measures of poor adherence. Poor adherence was increased for women, African Americans, mania, and hazardous drinking. Moon et al. investigated dropout patterns and their associated factors in 275 patients with bipolar disorders who were prospectively examined for 3 years [71]. The authors observed that the dropout rates increased rapidly during the first three months and slowed after 12 months. Past psychotic symptoms, longer illness duration, past psychiatric diagnoses, and a past history of dropouts significantly influenced the time to dropout in bipolar patients. The main reasons for dropout were denial of therapeutic need and lack of treatment efficacy.

A cross-sectional study, conducted by Medina et al. [72] in five Spanish mental health community centers, was aimed to establish the various attitudes toward antipsychotics at the moment of discharge in both patients with schizophrenia and bipolar disorder and, as a secondary aim, to analyze the connection between patients' attitude and sociodemographic and clinical data. A total of 86 patients (45 with a diagnosis of schizophrenia and 41 with bipolar disorder) were initially included in the study. Patients' attitude toward treatment was assessed with the 10-item Drug Attitude Inventory (DAI-10) [73], aspects of treatment adherence with Rating of Medication Influences (ROMI) scale [74], insight with SUMD scale [27]. A total of 26% of the patients presented a negative attitude toward antipsychotic treatment (mean DAI-10 score of −4.7, SD 2.7). Most of them were diagnosed with schizophrenia. Patients with a negative attitude obtained insight scores at discharge indicative of poorer disease awareness ($r = -0.31$, $P = 0.0039$) and had a greater number of previous acute episodes.

The determinant reasons of non-adherence to medication in patients with serious mental illness were evaluated by Velligan et al. through a systematic literature review [75]. Intentional and unintentional adherence was evaluated through several indicators for each category, as follows: poor insight, disavowal toward medication, distressful effects of medication, family or social support, access to mental health-care providers, poor therapeutic alliance, and stigma for the first category and substance abuse, cognitive impairment, depression, family and social support, access to mental health care, and social functioning for the second category. A total of 20 insight-related studies (11 prospective and 9 cross-sectional) analyzed the relationship between insight and adherence. Several prospective studies have shown that a better insight, evaluated through three insight scores, was associated with an improved adherence in both schizophrenic and bipolar patients [69]. Patients with bipolar disorder presented poor awareness of their disease after acute mania treatment, associating a higher probability of non-adherence during the maintenance therapy [68]. Cross-sectional studies have shown that, in patients over 50 years old diagnosed with bipolar disorder, a poor insight is associated with non-adherence [76]. Poor insight was identified as a cause for non-adherence in more than half of the studies, followed by substance abuse, a negative attitude toward medication, side effects, and cognitive impairments. Having a negative attitude toward medication is a determinant factor of intentional non-adherence, being considered to mediate effects of insight and of the therapeutic alliance.

Taking into account the major impact that adherence to medication has on the outcome of bipolar patients and the strong correlation between three factors—awareness of illness, adherence to medication and therapeutic alliance—García et al. [65] summarize in their systematic review the potential areas for intervention to improve adherence:

- *factors associated with patients*
  - early intervention programs for young patients.
  - treatment for different dependencies (on alcohol or other drugs), encouraging cessation.
  - increase awareness of the illness and of the benefits of antipsychotic treatment through psycho-education and psychotherapy interventions.
  - prevent or minimize adverse effects of antipsychotics, personalized treatment.
  - programs and/or technical devices to support treatment adherence for patients with cognitive dysfunctions.
  - assess patient education and quality of life.
  - analyze the symptoms at onset and during the course of illness.
  - consider patient ethnicity as a potential risk factor for non-adherence
- *factors associated with pharmacological treatment*
  - explanation about treatment plan.
  - simple posology
- *factors associated with social relationships*
  - improve the patient-physician relationship.
  - involve the family in the illness of the patient
- *factors associated with the service provision system*
  - avoid patients' first contact with the health system being a traumatic experience.
  - facilitate the access to treatment and health centers.

### 3.3. Quality of life and its association with insight in bipolar patients.

It is important to note that the impact of insight on quality of life may be subtle during remission and may be more substantially affected in full-blown manic symptoms. Impaired insight into treatment and a greater number of previous admissions significantly increased the risk of adverse clinical outcomes with bipolar disorder.

Dias et al. evaluated in their study the relationship between insight, quality of life, and cognition in bipolar disorder [77]. A neuropsychological battery assessing attention, mental control, perceptual-motor skills, executive functions, verbal fluency, abstraction and visuospatial attention was administered to 70 remitted bipolar patients and 50 healthy controls. No differences in quality of life and cognitive performance were observed between bipolar patients with impaired and preserved insight. Insight was found to be correlated with poorer psychological and environmental quality of life.

Gazalle et al. [78] studied 120 type-I bipolar patients (40 manic, 40 depressed, 40 euthymic), and 40 matched controls. Manic patients presented the lowest GAF measures but reported same overall QoL as euthymic patients and controls, and better QoL than depressed patients. Authors suggested that this mismatch between objective and subjective measures during acute mania may be associated with a lack of insight or awareness of their own illness.

Quality-of-life levels were compared by Yen et al. among two groups: remissive schizophrenic and bipolar patients and healthy control subjects. The impact of insight, adverse effects of medication, and use of atypical antipsychotics over the quality of life was analyzed [79]. A total of 96 subjects with bipolar disorder in remission, 96 subjects with schizophrenia in remission, and 106 healthy control subjects were included in the study. The results demonstrated that the subjects with bipolar disorder in remission had similarly poor levels of quality of life in all four domains as those with schizophrenia in remission, and both groups had poorer quality of life than subjects in control group. Insight was negatively associated with quality of life on the physical domain in schizophrenia and bipolar patients in remission. The results indicate that subjects with bipolar disorder are dissatisfied with their quality of life, even when they are in remitted state.

### 3.4. Insight and outcome in bipolar disorder

Research has revealed that a lack of insight is associated with poorer clinical outcomes in both schizophrenia and bipolar disorder.

Ghaemi et al. performed a study to assess the relationship between impairment in insight and long-term outcomes in affective and anxiety disorders [80]. They included 101 patients and the mean follow-up period was 3.9 months. Initial impairment in insight did not correlate with poor outcome. However, improvement in insight correlated with good outcome, particularly in bipolar disorder type I ($r = 0.56–0.67$, $P = 0.0005$).

Yen et al. followed 65 remitted bipolar I disorder patients over a 2-year period. Assessments were performed at 3, 6, 9, 12, 18, and 24 months to detect the adverse clinical outcomes defined by the incidence of bipolar-related psychiatric hospitalization, emergency room visits, and violent or suicidal behavior. Impaired insight into treatment and a greater number of previous hospitalizations significantly increased the risk for adverse clinical outcomes. However, insight into recognition of the illness and relabeling of psychotic phenomena did not have any significant effect on adverse clinical outcomes. Bipolar patients' insight into treatment is an independent predictor of adverse clinical outcomes [81].

It was shown that, in order to target a better patient outcome, treatment-related insight should be improved. The Health Belief Model, a proposed psychological model, aims to explain and predict health behaviors by focusing on individuals' attitudes and beliefs that may influence adherence [82]. The aforementioned model stipulates that two behaviors are playing an essential role in medication acceptance, that is, patients' awareness of their condition and patients' acknowledgement of the benefits provided by their treatment adherence.

Psycho-education became a common practice in mental health settings, especially for patients diagnosed with bipolar disorder. Its aim is to increase patients' ability of managing their life during a long-term illness. Specifically designed psychological interventions for relapse prevention, associated with mood stabilizers, are useful in patients with bipolar disorder.

Most recently published psychotherapy studies describe positive maintenance results as an add-on treatment, with efficiency in the treatment of depressive episodes. Interestingly, several groups from all over the world described similar results and reached similar conclusions; almost all tested interventions contain psycho-educative tools for compliance enhancement and early identification of prodromal signs, stating the importance of a regular lifestyle, and exploring patients' health beliefs and the awareness of illness [83].

## 4. Conclusions

In bipolar disorder, awareness of illness is not the same in manic, mixed, or depressive episodes. In acute mania, patients lack insight, while depression, viewed either syndrome wise or dimensionally, appears to preserve insight during acute episodes. Thus, insight impairment is less severe in bipolar depression than in mania. However, psychotic depression, compared to nonpsychotic depression, is associated with a worsened insight. Evidence shows that depression-related insight might be augmented by the severity of the depressive symptoms, possibly approving the depressive realism hypothesis. Insight of remissive bipolar patients seems to be recovered. Therefore, lack of insight in bipolar disorder appears to be a mood range-related phenomenon, unlike schizophrenia.

Poor insight is associated with non-adherence. Insight impacts on the therapeutic alliance with mental health professionals (this association may be bidirectional: while insight may influence therapeutic relationship, therapeutic relationship may also influence insight). Insight, therapeutic alliance with the treating psychiatrist, and medication adherence are highly correlated in bipolar patients as in patients diagnosed with schizophrenia. The three factors covary during the course of illness and an improvement in one leads to improvements in the others. Patient's insight into treatment is a significant predictor of adverse clinical outcomes. It may be essential to include that improving insight into treatment might be a promising objective for final outcome.

At present, the usefulness of psychotherapy (family-focused therapy, interpersonal and social rhythm therapy, cognitive-behavioral therapy) for improving treatment adherence and clinical outcome of bipolar patients is unquestionable, and future treatment guidelines should promote its regular use among clinicians. As clinicians, we are responsible to offer the best treatment available to our patients, and this includes both evidence-based psycho-education programs and newer pharmacological agents.

## Author details

Cătălina Angela Crişan[1,2*]

*Address all correspondence to: ccrisan2004@yahoo.com

1 Department of Neurosciences, Discipline of Psychiatry and Pediatric Psychiatry, Iuliu Haţieganu University of Medicine and Pharmacy, Cluj-Napoca, Romania

2 Psychiatric Clinic I, Emergency County Hospital, Cluj-Napoca, Romania

## References

[1] Pick A. Über Krankheitsbewusstsein in psychischen Krankheiten. Archiv für Psychiatrie und Nervenkrankheiten. 1882;**13**:518-558

[2] Krafft-Ebing. Lehrbuch der Psychiatrie. 5th ed. Stuttgart: F Enke; 1893

[3] Marková IS. Insight in Psychiatry. Cambridge, UK: Cambridge University Press; 2005

[4] Pinel P. Traité Medico-Philosophique Sur l'aliénation Mentale, Ou la Manie. Paris: Richard, Caille et Ravier; 1801

[5] Baillarger JGF. Essai Sur Une classification des différents genres de folie. Annales Médico-Psychologiques. 1853;**5**:545-566

[6] Billod E. Discussion Sur les aliénés avec conscience. Annales Médico-Psychologiques. 1870;**3**:264-281

[7] Parant V. La Raison Dans la Folie. Paris: Doin; 1888

[8] Maudsley H. Responsibility in Mental Disease. London: Kegan Paul & Trench; 1885

[9] Lewis A. The psychopathology of insight. Journal of Medical Psychology. 1934;**14**:332-348

[10] Jaspers K. Allgemeine Psychopathologie. 5th ed. Berlin: Springer; 1948

[11] Greenfeld D, Strauss JS, Bowers MB, Mandelkern M. Insight and interpretation of illness in recovery from psychosis. Schizophrenia Bulletin. 1989;**15**:245-252

[12] David AS. Insight and psychosis. British Journal of Psychiatry. 1990;**156**:798-808

[13] Amador XF, Strauss DH, Yale SA, Gorman JM. Awareness of illness in schizophrenia. Schizophrenia Bulletin. 1991;**17**:113-132

[14] Amador XF, Strauss DH. Poor insight in schizophrenia. Psychiatric Quarterly. 1993; **64**:305-318

[15] Marková IS, Berrios GE. The assessment of insight in clinical psychiatry revisited. Comprehensive Psychiatry. 1992;**86**:159-164

[16] McEvoy JP, Freter S, Everett G, Geller JL, Appelbaum P, Apperson LJ, Roth L. Insight and the clinical outcome of schizophrenic patients. The Journal of Nervous and Mental Disease. 1989;**177**:48-51

[17] Marks KA, Fastenau PS, Lysaker PH, Bond GR. Self-appraisal of illness questionnaire (SAIQ): Relationship to researcher-rated insight and neuropsychological function in schizophrenia. Schizophrenia Research. 2000;**45**:203-211

[18] Sherer M, Bergloff P, Boake C, High W, Levin E. The awareness questionnaire: Factor analysis structure and internal consistency. Brain Injury. 1998;**12**:63-68

[19] Schacter DL. Unawareness of deficit and unawareness of knowledge in patients with memory disorders. In: Prigatano GP, Schacter DL, editors. Awareness of Deficit after Brain Injury. Oxford: Oxford University Press; 1991. pp. 127-151

[20] Correa DD, Graves RE, Costa L. Awareness of memory deficit in Alzheimer's disease patients and memory-impaired older adults. Aging, Neuropsychology and Cognition. 1996;**3**:215-228

[21] McEvoy JP, Schooler NR, Friedman E, Steingard S, Allen M. Use of psychopathology vignettes by patients with schizophrenia or schizoaffective disorder and by mental health professionals to judge patients' insight. American Journal of Psychiatry. 1993;**150**:1649-1653

[22] de Assiss da Silva RA, Mograbi DC, Landeira-Fernades J, Cheniaux E. O insight no transtorno bipolar: Uma revisão sistemática. Jornal Brasileiro de Psiquiatria. 2014;**63**:242-254

[23] Amador XA, Flaum M, Andreasen NC, Strauss DH, Yale SA, Clark SC, Gorman JM. Awareness of illness in schizophrenia and schizoaffective disorders and mood disorders. Archives of General Psychiatry. 1994;**51**:826-836

[24] McEvoy JP, Aland J Jr, Wilson WH, Guy W and Hawkins L. Measuring chronic schizophrenic patients's attitudes toward their illness and treatment. Hospital and Community Psychiatry. 1981;**32**:856-858

[25] Birchwood M, Smith J, Drury V, Healy J, Macmillan F, Slade MA. A self-report insight-scale for psychosis: Reliability, validity and sensitivity to change. Acta Psychiatrica Scandinavica. 1994;**89**:62-67

[26] Kemp RA, David A. Psychological predictors of insight and compliance in psychotic patients. British Journal of Psychiatry. 1996;**169**:444-450

[27] Amador XF, Strauss DH. The Scale to Assess Unawareness of Mental Disorder (SUMD). New York, USA: Columbia University and New York State Psychiatric Institute; 1990

[28] Carsky M, Selzer MA, Terkelsen K, Hurt SW. The PEH: A questionnaire to assess acknowledgment of psychiatric illness. Journal of Nervous and Mental Disease. 1992;**180**:458-464

[29] Marks KA, Fastenau PS, Lysaker PH, Bond GR. Self-appraisal of illness questionnaire (SAIQ): Relationship to researcher-rated insight and neuropsychological function in schizophrenia. Schizophrenia Research. 2000;**45**:203-211

[30] Olaya B, Marsà F, Ochoa S, Balanzá-Martínez V, Barbeito S, García-Portilla MP, González-Pinto A, Lobo A, López-Antón R, Usall J, Arranz B, Haro JM. Development of the insight scale for affective disorders (ISAD): Modification from the scale to assess unawareness. Journal of Affective Disorders. 2012;**142**:65-71

[31] Amador XF, Strauss DH, Yale S, Flaum MM, Endicott J, Gorman JM. Assessment of insight in psychosis. The American Journal of Psychiatry. 1993;**150**:873-879

[32] Pini S, Cassano GB, Dell'Osso L, Amador XF. Insight into illness in schizophrenia, schizoaffective disorder, and mood disorders with psychotic features. The American Journal of Psychiatry. 2001;**158**:122-125

[33] Latalova K. Insight in bipolar disorder. The Psychiatric Quarterly. 2012;**83**(3):293-310

[34] Van der Werf-Eldering MJ, Van der Meer L, Burger H, Holthausen EA, Nolen WA, Aleman A. Insight in bipolar disorder: Associations with cognitive and emotional processing and illness characteristics. Bipolar Disorders. 2011;**13**:343-354

[35] Trevisi M, Talamo A, Bandinelli PL, Ducci G, Kotzalidis GD, Santucci C, Manfredi G, Girardi N, Tatarelli R. Insight and awareness as related to psychopathology and cognition. Psychopathology. 2012;**45**:235-243

[36] de Assis da Silva R, Mograbi DC, EVM C, Bifano J, Wainstok, Silva Silveira LA, Cheniaux E. Insight in bipolar disorder: A comparison between mania, depression and euthymia using insight scale for affective disorders. Trends in Psychiatry and Psychotherapy. 2015;**37**(3):152-156

[37] Wiffen BD, Rabinowitz J, Lex A, David AS. Correlates, change and 'state or trait' properties of insight in schizophrenia. Schizophrenia Research. 2010;**122**:94-103

[38] Cassidy F. Insight in bipolar disorder: Relationship to episode subtypes and symptom dimensions. Neuropsychiatric Disease and Treatment. 2010;**6**:627-631

[39] Depp AC, Harmell AL, Savla GN, Mausbach BT, Jeste DV, Palmer BW. A prospective study of the tracjectories of clinical insight, affective symptoms, and cognitive ability in bipolar disorder. Journal of Affective Disorder. 2014;**0**:250-255

[40] Ghaemi SN, Rosenquist KJ. Is insight in mania state-dependent?: A meta-analysis. The Journal of Mental and Nervous Disease. 2004;**192**(11):771-775

[41] Pini S, DeQueiroz V, Dell'Osso L, et al. Cross-sectional similarities and differences between schizophrenia, schizoaffective disorder and mania or mixed mania with mood-incongruent psychotic features. European Journal of Psychiatry. 2004;**19**:8-14

[42] Fennig S, Everett E, Bromet EJ, et al. Insight in first admission psychotic patients. Schizophrenia Research. 1996;**22**:257-263

[43] Weiler SN, Boiman E, Goodwin FK. Insight and outcome in bipolar, unipolar, and anxiety disorders. Comprehensive Psychiatry. 2000;**41**:167-171

[44] Michalakeas A, Skoutas C, Charalambous A, Peristeris A, Marinos V, Keramari E. Insight in schizophrenia and mood disorders and its relation to psychopathology. Acta Psychiatrica Scandinavica. 1994;**90**:46-49

[45] Arduini L, Kalyvoka A, Stratta P, Rinaldi O, Daneluzzo E, Rossi A. Insight and neuropsychological function in patients with schizophrenia and bipolar disorder with psychotic features. Canadian Journal of Psychiatry. 2003;**48**:338-341

[46] Dell'Osso L, Pini S, Tundo A, Sarno N, Musetti L, Cassano GB. Clinical characteristics of mania, mixed mania, and bipolar depression with psychotic features. Comprehensive Psychiatry. 2000;**41**:242-247

[47] Peralta V, Cuesta M. Lack of insight in mood disorders. Journal of Affective Disorders. 1998;**49**:55-58

[48] Yen C-F, Chen C-C, Cheng C-P, Yen C-N, Lin H-C, Ko C-H, Yen J-Y, Chen C-S. Comparison of insight in schizophrenia, bipolar I disorder, and depressive disorders with or without comorbid alcohol use disorder. Psychiatry and Clinical Neurosciences. 2008;**62**:685-690

[49] Yen C-F, Chen C-S, Ko C-H, Huang C-F. Changes in insight among patients with bipolar I disorder: A 2-year prospective study. Bipolar Disorders. 2007;**9**(3):238-242

[50] Ghaemi SN, Sachs GS, Baldassano CF, Truman CJ. Insight in seasonal affective disorder. Comprehensive Psychiatry. 1997;**38**:345-348

[51] Amador XF, Friedman JH, Kasapis C, Yale SA, Flaum M, Gorman GM. Suicidal behavior in schizophrenia and its relationship to awareness of illness. American Journal of Psychiatry. 1996;**153**:1185-1188

[52] Schwartz R, Petersen S. The relationship between insight and suicidality among patients with schizophrenia. The Journal of Nervous and Mental Disease. 1999;**187**:376-378

[53] de Assiss da Silva R, Mograbi DC, Camelo EVM, Santana CMT, Landeira-Fernandez J, Cheniaux E. Clinical correlates of loss of insight in bipolar depression. Trends in Psychiatry and Psychotherapy. 2017;**39**(4):264-269

[54] de Assiss da Silva R, Mograbi DC, Bifano J, Santana CM, Cheniaux E. Correlation between insight level and suicidal behavior/ideation in bipolar depression. Psychiatric Quarterly. 2017;**88**(1):47-53

[55] Lindenmayer JP, Liu-Seifert H, Kulkarni PM. Medication non-adherence and treatment outcome in patients with schizophrenia or schizoaffective disorder with suboptimal prior response. Journal of Clinical Psychiatry. 2009;**70**:990-996

[56] Nosé M, Barbui C, Tansella M. How often do patients with psychosis fail to adhere to treatment programmes? A systematic review. Psychological Medicine. 2003;**33**:1149-1160

[57] Jeste SD, Patterson TL, Palmer BW, Dolder CR, Goldman S, Jeste DV. Cognitive predictors of medication adherence among middle-aged and older outpatients with schizophrenia. Schizophrenia Reasearch. 2003;**63**:49-58

[58] Day JC, Bentall RP, Roberts C, Randall F, Rogers A, Cattell D, Healy D, Rae P, Power C. Attitudes toward antipsychotic medication: The impact of clinical variables and relationships with health professionals. Achives General Psychiatry. 2005;**62**:717-724

[59] Martinez-Aran SJ, Colom F, Torrent C, Tabares-Seisdedos R, Daban C, Leboyer M, Henry C, Goodwin GM, Gonzalez-Pinto A, Cruz N, Sanchez-Moreno J, Vieta E. Treatment non-adherence and neurocognitive impairment in bipolar disorder. Journal of Clinical Psychiatry. 2009;**70**:1017-1023

[60] Velligan DI, Weiden PJ, Sajatovic M, Scott J, Carpenter D, Ross R, Docherty JP, Expert Consensus Panel on Adherence Problems in Serious and Persistent Mental Illness. The expert consensus guideline series: Adherence problems in patients with serious and persistent mental illness. Journal of Clinical Psychiatry. 2009;**70**(Suppl 4):1-46

[61] Oehl M, Hummer M, Fleischhacker WW. Compliance with antipsychotic treatment. Acta Psychiatrica Scandinavica Suppl. 2000;**407**:83-86

[62] Lingam R, Scott J. Treatment non-adherence in affective disorders. Acta Psychiatrica Scandinavica. 2002;**105**:164-172

[63] Montes JM, Maurino J, de Dios C, Medina E. Suboptimal treatment adherence in bipolar disorder: Impact on clinical outcome and functioning. Patient Preference and Adherence. 2013;**7**:89-94

[64] Leclerc E, Mansur RB, Brietzke E. Determinants of adherence to treatment in bipolar disorder: A comprehensive review. Journal of Affective Disorders. 2013;**149**:247-252

[65] García S, Martínez-Cengotitabengoa M, López-Zurbano S, Zorrilla I, López P, Vieta E, González-Pinto A. Adherence to antipsychotic medication in bipolar disorder and schizophrenic patients. A systematic review. Journal of Clinical Psychopharmacolgy. 2016;**36**(4):355-371

[66] Buckley PF, Wirshing DA, Bhushan P, Pierre JM, Resnick SA, Wirshing WC. Lack of insight in schizophrenia: Impact on treatment adherence. CNS Drugs. 2007;**21**:129-141

[67] Higashi K, Medic G, Littlewood KJ, Diez T, Ganström O, Hert D. Medication adherence in schizophrenia: Factors influencing adherence to antipsychotic medication in schizophrenia-spectrum disorders. Psychiatry Research. 2014;**854-863**:S0165-S1781

[68] González-Pinto A, Reed C, Novick D. Assessment of medication adherence in a cohort of patients with bipolar disorder. Pharmacopsychiatry. 2010;**43**:263-270

[69] Novick D, Montgomery W, Treuer W, Aguado J, Kraemer S, Haro JM. Relationship of insight with medication adherence and the impact on outcomes in patients with schizophrenia and bipolar disorder: Results from 1-year European outpatient observational study. BMC Psychiatry. 2015;**15**(189):1-8

[70] Copeland LA, Zeber JE, Salloum IM, Pincus HA, Fine MJ, Kilbourne AM. Treatment adherence and illness insight in veterans with bipolar disorder. Journal of Nervous Mental Disease. 2008;**196**(1):16-21

[71] Moon E, Chang JS, Kim MY, Seo MH, Cha B, Ha TH, Choi S, Cho HS, Park T, Ha K. Dropout rate and associated factors in patients with bipolar disorders. Journal of Affective Disorders. 2012;**141**(1):47-54

[72] Medina E, Salvà J, Ampudia R, Maurino J, Larumbe J. Short-term clinical stability and lack of insight are associated with a negative attitude towards antipsychotic treatment at discharge in patients with schizophrenia and bipolar disorder. Patient Preference and Adherence. 2012;**6**:623-629

[73] Hogan TP, Awad AG, Eastwood R. A self-report scale predictive of drug compliance in schizophrenics: Reliability and discriminative validity. Psychological Medicine. 1983;**13**:177-183

[74] Weiden P, Rapkin B, Mott T, Zygmunt A, Goldman D, Horvitz-Lennon M, Frances A. Rating of medication influences (ROMI) scale in schizophrenia. Schizophrenia Bulletin. 1994;**20**:297-310

[75] Velligan DI, Sajatovic M, Hatch A, Kramata P, Docherty JP. Why do psychiatric patients stop antipsychotic medication? A systematic review of reasons for non-adherence to medication in patients with serious mentall illness. Patient Preference and Adherence. 2017;**11**:449-468

[76] Pratt SI, Mueser KT, Driscoll M, Wolfe R, Bartels SJ. Medication non-adherence in older people with serious mental illness: Prevalence and correlates. Psychiatric Rehabilitation Journal. 2006;**29**(4):299-310

[77] Dias VV, Brissos S, Frey BN, Kapczinski F. Insight, quality of life and cognitive functioning in euthymic patients with bipolar disorder. Journal of Affective Disorders. 2008;**110**(1-2):75-83

[78] Gazalle FK, Frey BN, Hallal PC, Andreazza AC, Cunha AB, Santin A, Kapczinski F. Mismatch between self-reported quality of life and functional assessment in acute mania: A matter of unawareness of illness? Journal of Affective Disorders. 2007;**103**(1-3):247-252

[79] Yen C-F, Cheng C-P, Huang C-F, Yen J-Y, Ko C-H, Chen C-S. Quality of life and its association with insight, adverse effects of medication and use of atypical antipsychotics in patients with bipolar disorder and schizophrenia in remission. Bipolar Disorders. 2008;**10**(5):617-624

[80] Ghaemi SN, Boiman E, Goodwin FK. Insight and outcome in bipolar, unipolar, and anxiety disorders. Comprehensive Psychiatry. 2000;**41**(3):167-171

[81] Yen CF, Chen CS, Yen JY, Ko CH. The predictive effect of insight on adverse clinical outcomes in bipolar I disorder: A two-year prospective study. Journal of Affective Disorders. 2008;**108**(1-2):121-127

[82] Lacro JP, Dunn LB, Dolder C, Leckband S, Jeste DV. Prevalence of and risk factors for medication non-adherence in patients with schizophrenia: A comprehensive review of recent literature. Journal of Clinical Psychiatry. 2002;**63**:892-909

[83] Colom F, Lam D. Psychoeducation: Improving outcomes in bipolar disorder. European Psychiatry. 2005;**20**(5-6):359-364

# 5

# Descent into Darkness

Susan Weiner

**Abstract**

This personal narrative of a time with schizophrenia will cover one patient's descent into madness and ultimate recovery from a period that felt like a sentence in a prison of hell and irrationality. Following a breakdown that led to the patient's withdrawal from graduate school, this narrative covers the experience of madness that led to delusions and hallucinations which tyrannized the patient's world. The narrative not only follows the breakdown of humanity that cursed the patient's understanding but also provides for the highlights of recovery that brought about a return to intellectual activities and a full comprehension of experience in the world. Though this patient's life was destroyed by schizophrenia, including the loss of all worldly goods and a career in academia, her experience of caring psychiatrists and a loving family redeemed her life and brought about solace and renewal at last.

**Keywords:** schizophrenia, madness, delusions, hallucinations, recovery, sanity

## 1. Introduction

The scientific basis of benefits in autobiographical recall in psychosis is suggested in some recent research and review papers [1–3]. It may also be noted that some books on autobiographical issues in psychosis indicate how important personal memories are in self-help and in explaining the subjective sense of the illness [4–6]. To this end, I offer a narrative of my time in insanity. I hope that it may be illustrative of one person's experience with schizophrenia and thus useful to psychiatrists and others who study not only the neurological changes in the brain but also the subjective experience of an altered reality and its consequences on outlook and behavior.

## 2. Heading

In the spring of 1993, I came down with schizoaffective disorder. At the time, I was a graduate student in history at a West Coast University in the United States. This disorder took me by the neck, shook out my life and utterly destroyed my career along with my hopes and dreams. To be honest, it shook up my humanity most of all and reduced me to what I now feel was a state of less than an animal. I would say I felt like a cornered beast, alienated from my friends and family and wholly cut off from the human race.

I interacted solely with dreams and created a whole world of delusions that determined how I spent my time and what I understood of reality, such as it presented itself to me. Because I had money to pay for my next year of graduate study, I was able to live off the proceeds and disappear into a large city leaving the real world and my relationships behind as I struggled to understand what I felt was the real truth of the world revealed to me at last.

What I remember most of my time alone with psychosis was how harrowing it was. I lived my days in what I considered a war zone, terrorized by an enemy I believed to be an Adolf Hitler or Saddam Hussein of dictators bent on world domination. In my opinion, I was a spy, modeled on the French Resistance. I thought I was working with a shadowy organization to undermine the growing influence and power of a madman who would surely destroy the world.

In this capacity, fear was my constant companion, my warm blanket in a dark forest of the unknown, helping to manage my response against the biting cold of evil. I regarded it as a necessary implement, useful as wool against a blizzard of pure, unadulterated madness that consumed my days. Though I was insane, I believed I was only now in possession of the real truth of the world. You could not have argued me out of my beliefs. I would have considered you pernicious and in league with the devil. In some ways, it was like being brain-washed.

In reality, I already considered most people in league with the Evil Dictator as I thought of him. Therefore, I avoided people as if they were indeed devils and only interacted with them when absolutely necessary. I lived in a world accentuated with horror as if some SS Storm Troopers followed close behind me threatening torture and medical experiments if I were caught. Because that is how I interpreted the new data of the world, represented to me in terms of code placed in newspapers and the radio that spoke to me alone of all the millions of people in the world. It never occurred to me to question this data that suddenly presented itself to me. It seemed only reasonable that truth should be given to me alone. It seemed as clear to me that the world might be flat when all along I had information that it is round. I was as certain of this new information as if I were Ptolemy mistakenly describing the circuits of the planets and stars.

In my opinion, madness came on me suddenly. Although I had early symptoms that friends began to observe, to me the break between sanity and insanity came as a matter of a moment. I can pinpoint that minute to the very instant. I was crying. Something had upset me. Something I would have coped with in my right mind. But now my emotions had become so labile. I cried and cried and cried some more. Even I wondered why I was crying so hard. It was as though I was engaged in an inebriated crying binge. And then I had a thought, a brief weird and poignant thought "This person has hurt me so much that I will go insane over it." I would strike at this individual for upsetting me, though in reality, it was at myself I unknowingly struck. And so it began: in that moment of unwarranted grief, I went completely and clinically insane. In effect, I announced the beginning of a psychotic episode to myself.

Without warning I began to believe the disc jockey on the radio was speaking to me. It shocked me. Could this be true? Something like this had never happened before. But now it seemed quite reasonable that it might. I never thought to question how in the world it was happening or even that it occurred. It never struck me that anything was wrong with my perspective beyond the fact that I had been wronged and now here was information confirming it.

The disc jockey seemed to relate my opinion right back at me. He played a song, "Breaking the Girl," from the rock group the Red Hot Chili Peppers. I felt vindicated. Someone else agreed that I was wronged and showed it by playing a song that spoke to that effect. So it was that the radio corroborated my feelings. A sort of coincidence became substantiated fact in the whirling insanity in my head. Of course representatives spoke to you from the radio. Can you see how tentative this relation was? But this supposed point held for me the very height of plausibility. I wondered to myself why had I never listened carefully to the radio before. In that moment of consideration, I was lost. I, as I knew myself, was gone. Long gone.

And yet many of my memories of this time remain vivid. I try to forget them as they are embarrassing and the terror of insanity is as frightening now as when it began. The memories worry me. Like epileptic fits, I worry the insanity will reoccur as if no time had passed, as if 20 years had not intervened to distance me from the consequences of irrationality. I know some people romanticize mental illness [7]. A removal of the veil of rational thought they think imprisons us in the world. This is frankly absurd. Only someone who is not a responsible psychiatrist could make such a damaging assessment.

In reality, irrationality is an invitation to hell where nothing is as it seems. There is no freedom in irrational thinking. When you cannot care for yourself or even brush your teeth regularly, when you are incredibly vulnerable to all sorts of real evil such as theft, rape or murder, the free workings of the imagination unencumbered by rational structures threaten your daily existence. Without rationality, we are unable to examine and make sense of world, of the myriad bits of data that we experience and act upon without conscious thought. Irrationality alone is as dangerous and destructive to the mind as a tornado that tears across an urban landscape. You are forced to ask, like the poet, Sylvia Plath in *Poppies in October*, "Oh my God, what am I/That these late mouths should cry open/In a forest of frosts, in a dawn of cornflowers"? [8].

Once ruptured by such an earthquake in your mind, you are forever imprisoned by the knowledge that it continues to exist underground ready to tear open a gaping hole in your existence again. I am unable to forget the cracked hermeneutical system that governed my days. Secret codes became my life. Found in all kinds of media from television, radio, to newspapers, I felt that only I (and a special Illuminati-like few) could decode their meaning. I lived for seven long months alone with only my delusions to guide me. How I paid rent on a small, dingy room and managed to appear at least semi-normal amazes me to this day. I spent my time engaged in what I thought was deep cover as a master spy decoding messages from the shadowy organization that would alert me to secret operations and strategy against the Evil Dictator. Naturally I was a highly valued employee and most in demand. Insanity is nothing if not grandiose and vainglorious. I even went on a countrywide road trip to break down defenses that the Evil Dictator and his minions had placed in otherwise unsuspecting communities. In some respects, I felt I was successful.

See how I slip into first-person narration of the events as if they really happened? It was all so real to me that in my memory, it is not what supposedly happened but what really did. The psychotic episode lasted so long (and in a later episode continued unabated for almost a year) and was of such heightened experience, like a visit to a circus, that it feels as real to me as if it was true. I did fight against an unimaginable horror and evil that threatened my country. I was engaged in clandestine activities that led me to withdraw from my PhD program and break from all my family and friends. I feel as if the line between reality and insanity is blurred in my head. It felt so true. And that feeling remains if not the thoughts that promoted it.

For that reason, I am leery of these memories. When I approach them in depth again, the delusions make an entrance. They wander into my mind as if they had been gone only a little while and not for whole decades. Perhaps as I watch the evening news tonight, it will come to me that there is a hidden message within the supposedly objective presentation of the day's events? Perhaps I will wonder if there is a code written as if in invisible ink that I need to decipher and respond to? Maybe I will take notes again on words that strike me as important in the anchor's speech? Maybe I will search out the hidden meaning in the segments they choose to present on the news? Because I became so habituated and accustomed to this line of thought it comes back as naturally as riding a bike. What took 7 months to develop into a full-fledged world view seems to threaten me again like a destabilizing virus.

Thoughts like these remain under the surface of my conscious life like tiny ants nesting in the timber of a house. It is incumbent on me now to live with this now as there is no amount of talk or medicine that will rid me of a decay that threatens the very pillars of my mind. Yet, despite the remaining embers of irrationality, I have made so much progress. For this reason, I worry insanity will return and devastate the otherwise full plains of my mind. Memories will start the tapes running all over again. I live with this uneasiness, with the apprehension that I will lose years of back-breaking work to regain my life. I worry I will begin to attend to conversations again looking to find that nugget of information to organize my thoughts and actions on any given day. In my mind, I cringe from the idea that there is a full world of meaning hidden beneath the daily patterns of our everyday speech and concerns that occupy so much of our time. I remember too well where that deceptively interesting consideration leads.

That is why I am fully compliant with medication. Though my antipsychotic makes me feel as if my head has a bucket of concrete in its cavity rather than a brain, I endure it. Though I am cognitively impaired by more medication than a cancer patient takes, I put up with it being almost impossible to read nonfiction and with it being difficult to engage in social activities. Because in my first years of illness I often refused to take enough medication to mediate the insanity, I had to learn through bitter experience that the crippling sedation of antipsychotics is the most logical choice to be made in this predicament. Agonizing boredom is preferred over insanity. Loneliness is better than a whole host of delusions. I would rather be severely disabled than to be insane where the truth is never to be found and peace is not offered for any price. In fact, in my experience, the difficulties of psychotropic medications are well worth the trade-off in sanity. If you can accept the diminishment in your life of all you once held dear you can begin to build another world that may present its own joys, its own wonder in the end. It took me a while to learn this. But, fortunately, in time I learned it well.

It seems to me that one of the most difficult aspects of insanity was how upside down my world appeared to me at first. It was like being thrown into a lake and learning to swim or sink beneath fiery waters. I had never heard of nor had any experience with the symptoms of psychosis so when they presented I was unable to recognize them. Out of nowhere, I began to believe my phone was tapped. Soon, I thought someone or some persons were watching me. Can you imagine how disconcerting and alarming such concerns might be? These ideas seemed as legitimate to me as knowing who the president of my United States was, facts that sustained the essential background of my reality.

I even believed I fact checked them to determine their legitimacy. Did graffiti on a wall seem to have a message that spoke directly to me? Did flyers on a bulletin board acknowledge some truth about my reality? I related all this to my burgeoning belief system, and it seemed to synchronize with my concern that unknown persons were trying to communicate with me. Despite the obviously loose correlation of reference, why these people never spoke to me outright was a question I never thought to pursue. It was just a given of the situation, like rain comes from clouds—a fact you learn and expect to occur with some regularity.

Although flyers and graffiti might be twisted into any kind of significance, it seemed obvious to me that the meaning related directly to myself alone. The abbreviation for the World Wide Web (the "www" introducing any email address on a flyer) held a special significance for me. It seemed to have a connotation that lay in what seemed to be a simple play on letters and words: "www" spoke to me obscurely of World War III. I thought it contained a reference to the oncoming of a new and terrible worldwide war. To say that I was stunned and horrified, is to understate the obvious. I was in a panic. It began to dawn on me that war was on the brink of happening in what I had otherwise believed was a promising horizon and future as a history professor. All I knew about the world was wrong, and I thought if I only looked carefully enough, there was proof of what was true right beneath my nose.

The repetition of email addresses that appeared with the public unveiling of the Internet in the early 1990s alarmed me and caused me to rethink my position on what was really and even factually accurate. As it dawned on me that evil was about to enter my existence, and that of my fellow citizens, I was distraught. What was going on and how did it relate to my life, I thought? Although my understanding of the connotation of "www" was hardly reasonable or comprehensible, I was certain of its legitimacy. What do you do when you think world war is coming? Do you continue to pursue the studies you love or do you join in the offensive? Obviously, you do your duty by humanity like any other soldier in any other conflict. You pursue the defense of those you love and those in your country whom you value.

At first, I was furious with my friends and family who I sometimes thought understood everything that was happening long before I did. Why had no one informed me of the real state of being in the world? Instead I had been allowed to live in ignorance of a terrifying massacre that loomed in the near future. It was like some dystopian nightmare. Because no one spoke to me in what I felt was an honest and direct way about the real truth of the world, it occurred to me I was being asked to be a special operative who could work *in cognito* to help save my country from the jaws of sheer evil. Again, paranoid delusions lead to big dreams. You are never just a cog in the wheel. You are the main spoke around which the rest of the world looms. A Hitler of a dictator pursued me of all the people in the world (who might or might not know they were threatened with imminent destruction).

My undergraduate degree was in English Literature. I think the critical analysis of works you learn most was my undoing in psychosis. I began to believe that structures of meaning were layered into reality as they were in a book. Deep meanings took on the most important aspect of my time trying to understand the world. In this case, I had to learn to read beneath the obvious denotation of any statement or sentence. This was exhausting. Everything I heard, everything I read, everything I saw had to be decoded for its ultimate implication. What was it trying to say to me? What was the message hidden in the puzzle for me to learn and act on in my day?

I took notes. I studied advertisements, even cosmetic banners in department stores. I actually drove around and regarded numbers and letters on license plates. And even though it seems ridiculous now, everything held meaning that I had to decode. At night, I sat home and put together the layers that had been offered to me on any particular day. From this I learned (or believed I learned) about the malevolent force bent on world conquest and that I faced horrifying dangers that included the very real threat of torture and execution. I was shocked and even horror-struck. Why had I had remained innocent to the very present dangers of this world before? I came up with a complicated answer to that question, but it only frightened me more and convinced me that my series of delusions were deeply and absolutely authentic. I never shared my belief system with others though. What kind of spy would give away their intelligence I reasoned?

I even determined that my father and sister were trying to sell me to the Saudis for medical experiments. I was pretty upset with them. In general, I was pretty upset most of the time. I felt I was pursued by evil and if it won the world would come to pieces. Really, it was like one of those video games your children play. Ironically, it would have been exciting if it were not so real, I thought. None of it seemed crazy to me. It appeared all too rational and real. Despite my education, I had absolutely no insight into my disease at all.

How else did I construct these seemingly random theories about reality as I knew it? Here is an example. In 1993, a movie came out in the United States called *The Net*, starring Sandra Bullock. She and I had shared some similar traits. We both had moderately long brown hair. We both had brown eyes and were of similar height. Can you see where this is going? Based on a few corresponding features I began to identify with her. I felt she represented me in this movie. Movie advertisements on bus stop billboards called out to me and tugged at the recesses of my mind. I decided to go see the film. Perhaps I should have been working on a paper that was dwindling in importance to me? Instead, I paid my movie money, drank the poison, and fully submitted to the full force of insanity that was to follow.

In *The Net*, Sandra Bullock's character was stripped of civilization and the accoutrements of middle-class life. Her identity was stolen from her as well as her career, home and friends. In this thriller movie, she was made to live and act underground to save her life and that of the freedom of her country which was threatened by an evil CEO of a large corporation. Can you see the parallels between some of my own hard-won beliefs and that of the fate of Sandra Bullock in the movie?

After sitting through the film, I realized I was being asked to give up my comfortable life to battle evil where it showed itself in my country. Because I resembled Sandra Bullock (in my mind), it was clear I was supposed to divest myself of attachments, including family, friends and even furniture and clothing. This would allow me to be mobile like the character in the film. It was necessary to conduct guerilla warfare with no goods to tie me to a place or family relations to threaten my commitment to being a spy. I resisted for a while but finally I gave in. I made a tearful break with my relations and the university where I was so happy. Then, I gave away most of my household items and jewelry to a charity organization. It was an awful time for me. I disappeared from my life as a graduate student into the big city where I lived. No one knew where I had gone or how I was. Imagine the distress my parents experienced. I was gone for 7 months. Who knew if I was ever coming back?

However, I thought a break was necessary to prosecute war against the worst viciousness America had seen since Hitler. Following my introduction to texts within texts, I went to a lot of movies and drew similar conclusions about how to fight an under-the-table war that might damage the standing of a rising dictator. Such conclusions reminded me of Elie Wiesel in Auschwitz who said, "Could this just be a nightmare? An unimaginable nightmare … We must do something. We can't let them kill us like that, like cattle in the slaughterhouse. We must revolt." [9]. Although Jews in concentration camps were unable to revolt, I felt it was incumbent on me to fight back, to fight against the madness in the deepest of nights in my head that I only assumed was real.

To be honest, I engaged in a lot of magical thinking and ritual actions. I would say I was essentially engaged in casting spells that I thought would safeguard my well-being and threaten wickedness as it loomed. If I said a ritual incantation correctly, it would bar the Evil Dictator from acting. I spent a lot of time interpreting the code I found in newspapers and daily life, such as advertisements on display cases in stores. From this code, I extracted pieces of information that told me what words and in what order to recite them to counter the evil perpetuated by those who would oppress my nation and its vulnerable and innocent civilians. As far as I knew, I was engaged in my duty to my country for those 7 months until in the real world I was finally caught and hospitalized by the police. The only threat I presented to anyone was to myself. Violence against others was against my code of conduct.

In my altered state, I believed danger threatened me from all sides. Perhaps it is easy to see how frightened and disoriented I felt and became. Sheer panic and anxiety became my closest friends. What was left of my world was shattered with the development of the disease. As time went on, madness became more of a tyrant and ruled my hours and days like an emperor controlling his court. It was not only perceived physical danger that threatened me. There was also the severe mortification of my humanity as the disease preyed upon and destroyed my mind.

At a certain point, I decided that anyone and everyone could read my mind. Though I could not see into anyone else's head, I believed my thoughts were as visible as if seen through clear glass. Truly, this belief was daunting and disturbing. Many of our thoughts are not fit for public consumption. It is the nature of consciousness. We are torn by drives, aggressions and feelings we barely understand. Should they become public knowledge we might well be considered anathema. So the disease also ripped away at my humanity. It felt as if I was beset by devils: one day, racial epithets became engaged in my brain and from that day forward they never stopped. I was appalled. I had not heard words like this unless delivered by ignorant, bellicose morons. And I believed that everyone could hear them as I passed by. It was as true for Italians or Middle Eastern peoples. No gender was safe from the viciousness I hurled at people as I passed by. On streets I called women whores and worse. I tore into Eastern Europeans as Pollacks. I was completely unable to repress these thoughts in my head. And I thought that everyone heard them. I was mortified and distraught. I used the utmost of my energy to repress these ideas and to kill them off but it was of no avail. They occurred and recurred like hiccups, rising to the surface and bubbling forth with no help for them but to apologize profusely in their wake.

One day I took a cab ride. I decided the cab driver looked like a child molester. In my head I told him so. Naturally, I believed he heard this judgment as loud and clear as if I spoke through a megaphone. Fortunately, I was unable to register how he replied in his own brain. Notwithstanding I apologized in my head. Over and over again, I begged him to forgive me for thinking such an awful thing about a stranger who had done me no harm. Once the thought had come, it repeated itself as if on a loop. I had no control over it. I believed the thought was offered as loudly as if in spoken word. In essence, I insulted this poor man repeatedly and violently. He continued to be polite despite my repeated denigration of his looks. I was not fooled. I knew he heard me and that he was as strictly offended as I was desirous of not causing offense. This happened to me every day, and it came without warning. I found it terribly hard to bear. Essentially, I believed I was hurling damaging racial vulgarities and insults to anyone at any time on the street. I have left out the worst of these experiences as they remain unprintable. This was another reason I began to avoid people like the plague.

At once I was being asked to exist on two planes. On one level I spoke out loud to people. "Will you show me that camera in the case," I might ask? And then, since the clerk could read my mind, another thought came to me which I only believed was heard out loud. "Are you being sold as a slave to an overlord," I might conclude in my head? Whatever reply the clerk gave in spoken language would be my clue as to what I was supposed to learn from the shadowy resistance organization I worked for. This kept up month after month. After some time, the dual nature of the labor left me completely exhausted and broken down. However, although I believe I asked for it, I found no recourse, no relief; I had to run to keep up and never stop running. Also, I was no longer sleeping much. I felt on the verge of a breakdown. As I recount these memories, I remember just how painful they were and yet how absurd and outlandish they may appear today. Yet, imagine this is your very reality. You sincerely believe you have just called someone an unforgivable name. Right to their face. How do you cope with that and still feel human? I sincerely believed my humanity was being undermined and deposed. I fought vainly to retain my decency in the face of the inner violence that surrounded me at all times.

I felt keenly the breakdown in my humanity that is involved in psychosis. Not only was I besieged by a fear of physical danger in my external world, but I was overwhelmed by the changes in my mind that invaded my inner world and left me no place of safety or peace. Coming near on 7 months of uninterrupted insanity, I began to understand I was being pursued by the Evil Dictator so I could be transformed into a monster-like, zombie serial killer. This sounds like an advertisement for the year's most frightening horror flick. Instead, it was a belief that terrorized me and caused me to become frantic and desperate. I was in great danger of harming myself as I tried to avoid a fate that I thought ran me down like a shadow.

After about 5 or 6 months of psychosis, I developed anhedonia. I remember when it came on quite vividly. I was engaged on my road trip to try to save the United States from booby traps set like land mines by the Evil Dictator and his ruthless, unorthodox government. I drove from state to state across the country intent on and invested in my magical thinking where I had only to speak to dismantle snares set for an innocent population. I never knew exactly what sort of traps these might be. It never occurred to me to wonder. It was only my duty to proceed according to the information I thought accrued from codes left in the media or in spoken word by various informants (from hotel clerks to cashiers in gas stations and grocery stores). The whole world was involved in my madness and that seemed quite logical to me. I can only imagine how I presented myself to various people with whom I interacted. In essence, I was on a giant treasure hunt with a return to the status quo of the country as my golden statue.

I was driving through Utah when I first noticed the anhedonia. As I wound my way through canyons, there were picturesque or scenic pullovers on the shoulder of the freeway. I drove into one and walked out onto a cliff to view the beautiful striations of color that curved their way in rippling stripes along the canyon beyond me. I had seen pictures of Utah ravines and chasms. Now, I found myself with an opportunity to really observe them in their glory. I anticipated the joy I would find in taking a moment for myself in a day I regarded as full of hard and intense work (remember, license plates absorbed my attention at all times, I took notes on them as I drove).

Only nothing happened. I could see the mineral deposits in the side of the cliff were gorgeous. I could see the various colors that stippled the rock before me. Yet I encountered no emotional reaction in response to this view. I felt no pleasure or joy in seeing the beauty I knew was there but to which I could no longer respond to or even feel. I was astonished and sick at heart. I really began to feel my humanity was being stolen from me piece by piece. As in truth it was, but by the breakdown in my own brain not through the machinations of another. I attributed the anhedonia (a condition I had never heard of before) to plans for my utter destruction. What could I do but continue the morning along with my significant work? Although I felt like others before and after who might say, "It was like I was no longer a person," [10]. I was attuned to duty and felt its claim on me.

There were other times I experienced hallucinations that terrified me. I understood they were not real but the experience was painful nonetheless. In fact, I believed I was being tortured but I did not know how to stop it. For a while when I closed my eyes, cartoon characters appeared in the black darkness before my eyes. These characters were bright as neon strobe lights and in all colors of a crayon box. They streamed before me back and forth like ghosts on a Halloween string. They were so bright it actually hurt my eyes. The only way I could modify or impede them was by keeping my eyes wide open no matter how fatigued I felt. Of course, this made sleep particularly difficult. And I was so afraid. I was afraid I would go blind from the intensity of the figures before me. For some time at night, I kept my eyes open until I could fall asleep from sheer and utter exhaustion.

There were also periods where I experienced strange auditory hallucinations. I knew these sounds were just as unreal as the cartoon images that plagued me. And yet in their own way, they too were frightening. I heard murmurings in back rooms that sounded like low voices on the radio. Murmur, murmur, murmur they went like a broken record, like a recording or stimulus designed to drive you insane. Many rumbling voices muttering words just below my range of hearing. I also attributed this hallucination to a form of torture. I believed the Evil Dictator was threatening me with what I might encounter next if I continued to oppose his reign and to work actively to resist him. Ironically, I believed he was threatening me with insanity. At that time, though I was sure I was sane, I was concerned that evil might undermine my grasp of reality. I continued to feel that my grip on sanity was good though in reality I was disintegrating beneath the unimpeded development of madness.

It was late into the development of schizoaffective disorder that my experience of anhedonia and these series of hallucinations led me to reason that my soul, my very humanity was under attack by the evil enemy. Over time I concluded that I was being transformed into the zombie serial killer who would roam the streets and assassinate individuals according to the will of the Evil Dictator. It seems a little bit like a Star Wars plot to me. In this case, good was being ravaged by a terrible, spreading evil. Already I could not experience beauty anymore. An afternoon breeze on my cheek left me feeling nothing. I no longer took pleasure in its soft touch through my hair. I could feel the light wind, but I did not have a reaction to it in my own heart anymore.

To be transformed into a zombie serial killer is a conclusion that sounds almost laughable when put into print. Yet, I believe it shows the propensity toward magical thinking that pervades our unconscious when no one is looking. From these experiences, I drew conclusions that led me to believe the loss of humanity I experienced was due to an external force bent on my destruction. One experience led to another until I felt that I was being threatened with becoming an inhuman creature. So that one night when I looked out a window on the ground floor of a hotel and saw a ragged drug addict or alcoholic stumbling through the street I believed he was one of those killers searching for me through darkened streets. To me he was the walking dead. It seemed a horrible confirmation of accumulated fears in which I believed I was marked for death. Some zombie assassin would savagely murder me, and then, like a vampire, my transformation into one among a vast serial killer army would be complete. I would be as devoted to the Evil Dictator as any SS officer in Hitler's army. You can see the fairy tale-like thinking that pervaded my conclusions. The good versus evil duality that defined my days. And especially the externalization of cause and effect of symptoms that were really creating havoc in my own brain.

And then one day, to my great surprise, I was what you can call sane. It happened that I was finally cornered and apprehended by the police and sometime later, fell under the care of a wonderful, caring psychiatrist who attended to my diagnosis with what was the newest and most radical psychotropic medication of the time, Risperidone. Suddenly, I could understand, I felt, I could reason again. I might end my story here but it would be the wrong position from which to close my account. It took many years and several extended periods of delusions for me to recover from mental illness. As much as one might say they are able to recover. I want to point out, however, the crucial role psychiatrists play in the recovery of sanity and humanity again after long stretches of madness. I have had two devoted psychiatrists for over 20 long years now. In this, I know I am blessed. Their long experience and strength of character have been instrumental in my recovery from delusions and return to a life beyond that of solipsistic ideas dreamt up in nightmares. I believe both of them helped me to become a better person than I was going in to psychosis.

I think my psychiatrists focused their efforts on the recovery of humanity whose loss was so traumatic for me when I was ill. Both have consistently treated me with dignity, charity and compassion. They behaved toward me as if my delusions were never an irritant or imposition. They worked as the people do who love me, with a concern for my state of mind, my happiness and my overall well-being. When I could not reason, they were the voice of reality. When I considered myself an aberration and a monster on the very edge of society, they reminded me of what I had accomplished and perhaps could achieve again in small measure. They stood by me just as a parent will and supported my dreams. They never discouraged me from being able to function at any level. They saw me through every struggle, every failure, and every time I felt lost and adrift in my world. In conclusion, they behaved toward me as if I were as important to them as a loved one is to a family member. They insisted on my humanity and sought to save my soul even when I was as torn and shredded as a sick animal.

An example may suffice. Today, my current psychiatrist is sensitive to the fact that I still feel overwhelmed by irrational fears. I believe at least some of these fears are a side effect of the dose of Risperidone. They increase or decrease with the level of the antipsychotic medication. But because of these irrational fears, cold winter snow days and icy stretches of road terrify me. I am consumed with fear of some conflagration of an accident on slick, ice-covered pavement. Although such fears have little basis in reality, my psychiatrist remains flexible if I ask to change an appointment away from a date that calls for snow. She has always reacted with kindness and sympathy if I would like to change an appointment according to the images of death and violence that crowd in on my imagination. These fears are not amenable to reason and continue to haunt me year after year.

Honestly, her response has been a great relief to me and has helped me to function better than if she ignored my plea or were uncompromising in her reaction to my very pressing fears. My psychiatrist cares for me. It shows and is significant in how I approach other people as I aspire to pick up the pieces of my life. I know she does not think of me as a freak she studies or is saddled with. This has a great impact on my confidence in reaching out to other people. It is also a balm for my heart that has been ravaged by illness. I am fragile now. Both of my psychiatrists have never questioned this fact or challenged me to rise before I could stand. Instead they have held out a hand. It is the very dignity they offer that has reached into my heart and touched my soul. In conjunction with pharmaceuticals, I believe this has laid the foundation for my return to health.

In addition, I will never forget, nor cease to be grateful for, my first psychiatrist [11]. When I first met him, I believed he was a covert member of the CIA who intended to inflict painful, Dr. Mengele-like, medical experiments on me. Of course, I was alarmed, and I hated and distrusted him on the spot. I held every grudge against him that could be imposed by a paranoid mind. In the interests of self-preservation, I meant to deceive him at every turn and to mislead him both of my intentions (at that time to harm myself) and as to how I hoped to escape what I thought were his dangerous clutches. Yet, his attitude of decency and kindness seeped into my conscious mind. He treated me with patience and kindness. He asked me questions about what I believed. He spoke quietly and reassuringly about what was going to happen to me now and how he wanted to treat me for illness. Although I was sure I was sane and that my psychiatrist was a genuine, threatening representation of evil, I made note of his apparent unconditional support. Despite myself he was soothing to me, and when medical experiments did not materialize I began to trust him.

My first psychiatrist switched my antipsychotic from Haldol (prescribed for me in a hospital) to Risperidone. The only effect Haldol had on me was to make me feel sick. But use of the Risperidone immediately had an effect and right away I began to understand something was desperately wrong with my world view. You cannot imagine how grateful I was at this turn of events. At the time, I was petrified that the end of the world was at hand. The calm manner of my psychiatrist emboldened me, and I was able to take what seemed a tremendous chance to talk to him about what I really believed was happening in the world. My psychiatrist was so quiet and unassuming. He never made a fuss or tried to force me into understanding that my belief system was illegitimate. Instead, he simply told me that what I believed to be true was a fantasy. Within a week of being on this new medication, I could see what he said was true. So I began my back breaking climb away from the valley of hell.

The point I want to make is that I haven't made that climb alone. In conjunction with my parents and psychiatrists I have forced myself to take one step after another. They were the hands that steadied me. So one leaves perdition behind, on the faith of others that you can rise. With the faith that the devil's playground is not your ultimate resting place. Without them I believe I would be less myself, less the human being I was before and who I became. It is with gratitude for kindnesses and love that I have stood up once again and planned for the refoundation of a home on fertile plains.

## 3. Conclusion

I write this account not to gain sympathy but in solidarity with those who remain ill, with those who find themselves on the street, who do not know the helping hand of compassion. Without a cure for the delusions I too might have become homeless and in and out of penal institutions. In my case, the police rescued me. My doctors brought about salvation and protection. Medication worked effectively for me and revived me. My parents made possible this life we have constructed together in the wake of destruction. So, I am always mindful of those who refuse treatment and remain hopelessly insane. May we remember them when we vote for politicians or city councils who support mental health treatment and outreach to those who remain in their own private corner of hell.

## Author details

Susan Weiner

Address all correspondence to: suskweiner@aol.com

Private Residence, North Potomac, MD, USA

## References

[1] Watson A, Barker V, Hall J, Lawrie SM. British Journal of Psychiatry. 2012;**211**:423-424

[2] Berna F, Potheegadoo J, Aouadi I, Ricarte JJ, Allé MC, Coutelle R, Boyer L, Cuervo-Lombard CV, Danion JM. A meta-analysis of autobiographical memory studies in schizophrenia spectrum disorder. Schizophrenia Bulletin. 2016;**42**(1):56-66

[3] Roe D, Yanos PT, Lysaker PH. Coping with psychosis: An integrative developmental framework. Journal of Nervous and Mental Disease. 2006;**194**(12):917-924

[4] Chadwick PK. Schizophrenia: The Positive Perspective. London: Routledge; 1997

[5] Torrey FE. Surviving Schizophrenia. New York: Harper Collins; 2001

[6] Ronen D. Schizophrenia: The coping with psychosis and schizophrenia. In: Self Help Handbook. Seattle, WA: Amazon; 2011

[7] Deleuze G, Guattari F. Anti-Oedipus, Capitalism and Schizophrenia. Minneapolis: University of Minnesota Press; 1983

[8] Plath S. In: Ted H, editor. The Collected Poems. NY, New York: Harper Perennial Modern Classics; 2008

[9] Wiesel E. Night. NY, New York: Hill and Wang; 2006. p. 31

[10] Yeiser B. Mind Estranged: My Journey from Schizophrenia and Homelessness to Recovery. Seattle, WA: Amazon; 2014. p. 69

[11] Heinssen RK. Person-centered psychiatric care: A tribute to Wayne Fenton. Schizophrenia Bulletin. 2007;**33**(5):149-150

# 6

# Impact of Social Media on Social Anxiety

Anca Dobrean and Costina-Ruxandra Păsărelu

**Abstract**

**Introduction**: Online social networking sites are being used all around the world. However, only recently researchers have started to investigate their relationship with mental health. Evidence coming from literature suggests that they have both advantages and disadvantages for individuals. The aim of this study is to critically review the existent research conducted on the relationship between online social networking and social anxiety.

**Method:** According to PRISMA guidelines, comprehensive systematic searches of electronic databases were conducted (PsychInfo, Cochrane, PubMed, Scopus, Web of Science). Terms related to online social networking were combined with social anxiety terms. After identifying relevant papers, the relationship between social media networking and social anxiety as well as limitations of each study were presented. All of the papers included were cross-sectional, relying on self-report assessments.

**Conclusion:** There are several papers published on the relationship between social media and social anxiety; however, more research needs to be done in order to clarify the influence of one variable over the other. Rigorous experimental studies need to be conducted with different time-point assessments, and bidirectionality should be investigated. Important mediators and moderators have to be considered in order to explain the relationship between social media networking and social anxiety.

**Keywords:** social media, social anxiety, online social networking, Facebook

# 1. Introduction

Social networking sites have become part of twenty-first century people's lives. From all online social networking sites, Facebook is the most widely used. According to a recent report published by Facebook regarding data for the second quarter of 2016, there is a considerable increase (17% in comparison with last year) in the number of both daily and monthly active users, with 1.13 billion daily active Facebook users for June 2016 and approximately 1.71 billion monthly active Facebook users for 30 June 2016 [1].

# 2. Online social networking

## 2.1. Benefits of online social networking

Online social networking sites may have a useful role in mental health research (for a comprehensive review of the use of Facebook in social science see Ref. [2]). For instance, Facebook, the most widespread form of online social networking site, can easily be used as a great clinical research tool, as it can provide the recruitment of patients and involve them in programmes [3]. Also, it can be used to guide interventions and in treatment monitoring (e.g. in physical activity or overweight programs [4, 5]). So far, several studies have investigated the role of social media in people with serious illness, and research shows that it is a promising approach in patients with schizophrenia [6].

Social media is a valuable resource for receiving peer-to-peer support. Facebook, Twitter or YouTube can be used by people with several conditions in order to find support or advice from others and to share personal experiences. Naslund et al. [7] proposed a model that illustrated potential benefits for people with serious mental illness, which they can have in an online community on online social networking sites (overcome stigma, seek professional help, receive adequate treatment).

Regarding mental health interventions delivered via Facebook, research is only starting to emerge. In an online randomized controlled experiment, a depression awareness campaign delivered via Facebook for adults was associated with enhanced mental health literacy [8]. Facebook allows for establishing and maintaining connections with others, and studies show that there is a positive relation between Facebook use and social capital, with greater advantages for people with low self-esteem and life satisfaction [9]. According to a review on the applications of social media in medicine and healthcare services, it seems that social networking is a promising approach. However, much uncertainty exists in terms of ethics and safety [10]. Furthermore, social media seemed to be an effective method to promote health-related behaviours [11].

There are studies showing that online social networking sites are important factors in youths' social lives, as in a large sample ($N = 3.068$) of adolescents (aged 11–14), there were significant positive associations between the use of online social networking sites and several friendship-related variables (friendship quality, face-to-face interaction, bridging/bonding social capital) [12].

Online social networking sites can have benefits in terms of cognitive abilities for older healthy adults [13], as it was shown in a study involving older adults (mean age comprised between 78 and 80), in which participants were randomly assigned into three groups: Facebook training, online diary website and waiting list. The Facebook intervention was delivered over 8 weeks and older adults received weekly training in how to use Facebook.

### 2.2. Disadvantages of online social networking

Recent research has associated social media networking with several negative outcomes, both in adolescent populations and in adults.

#### *2.2.1. Adolescent literature*

According to a report published by the Pew Research Center, adolescents are avid users of online social networking sites, with approximately 71% of them using more than one online social networking site [14] in 2015, and the most widely used online social networking site was Facebook (41%). Frequency of using social networking sites expressed as the amount of time spent on online social networking sites was associated with mental health problems in children and adolescents [15]. Namely, the same study shows that spending more than 2 h per day on online social networking sites is associated with higher psychological distress, poor self-rated mental health, suicidal ideation and an unmet need for mental health support. In another study conducted on a large sample of adolescents ($N$ = 5.126), there were significant positive associations between the use of online social networking sites, psychological distress, suicide ideation and suicide attempts [16]. In this study, cyberbullying victimization served as a full mediator in the relationship between the use of online social networking sites and psychological distress/suicide attempts and acted as a partial mediator in the relationship between the use of online social networking sites and suicidal ideation.

"Facebook depression" [17] is a term introduced in a report of the American Academy of Pediatrics to describe the impact of social media on youths' mental health, according to which depression arises as a consequence of youths spending a large amount of time on social media [18]. When it comes to mechanisms explaining why the use of online social networking sites is associated with negative mental health outcomes, one study shows that negative comparison on Facebook is related with adolescents' life satisfaction [19]; negative comparison on Facebook predicts life satisfaction, but the opposite relationship is also significant.

Research regarding problematic online social networking sites in adolescents is scarce, and very few studies have investigated the relationship between Facebook addiction and youths' mental health problems. In a study conducted with adolescents, both personality traits and social influence processes emerged as significant predictors of problematic Facebook use and Facebook use frequency. Problematic Facebook use was predicted by emotional stability, extraversion, conscientiousness and norms, while the frequency of Facebook use was predicted by gender, group norms and social identity [20].

#### 2.2.2. *Adult studies*

With the rapid emergence of technology, the term "iDisorders" was introduced to define mental health problems related to technology usage. In a meta-analysis including eighteen papers on the relationship between Facebook use and loneliness, it resulted that the two variables were significantly associated and that loneliness predicted Facebook use and not the other way around [21]. Facebook use had a significant contribution to mental health, with Facebook use, impression management and friends predicting mood disorders, with different contributions across disorders (having more friends is negatively associated with major depression and dysthymia, while positively predicting mania) [22]. Social media, operationalized as the total time spent per day, visits per day and global frequency of visits on social media, was associated with depression in a large sample of U.S. young adults [23]. Facebook intrusiveness was correlated with obsessive-compulsive disorder severity and with obsessive beliefs in a sample of young adults (aged 18–24) [24].

There is ample literature on the role of online social networking sites, and Facebook in particular, in mental health outcomes. However, there is high heterogeneity in what online social networking sites and Facebook mean. Facebook is conceptualized and measured differently across studies, given that while several studies investigate Facebook use, others investigate either the number of friends, Facebook disclosure, Facebook activities, Facebook motives or Facebook addiction/intrusiveness/problematic use.

Despite the fact that no diagnostic manual recognizes Facebook addiction as a diagnostic category, more and more research focuses on pathological uses of online social networking sites, and Facebook in particular (see Ref. [25] for a complex review of online social networking sites addiction). Online social networking sites addiction is related to deficits in emotion regulation and susceptibility to drug and alcohol addictions [26], somatic symptoms, anxiety, insomnia, social dysfunction and depression [27].

## 3. Social media and social anxiety

Online social networking sites, and Facebook in particular, can offer great opportunities, in terms of interaction with others, for individuals with social anxiety. Two different hypotheses have been proposed in order to explain why socially anxious individuals use computers [28], which can easily be applicable to online social networking sites. The first hypothesis proposed is the social *compensation hypothesis* [29], according to which individuals use online social networking sites in order to compensate for deficits in social skills or discomfort in face-to-face situations. The second theory, opposed to the first, is called the social enhancement hypothesis. According to this hypothesis, socially skilled individuals use online social networking sites to find additional opportunities to interact with others. In the existent literature on the relationship between online social networking sites and social anxiety, there is mixed evidence regarding the two hypotheses, as both have received support.

In an experimental study, Rauch et al. [30] investigated whether previous exposure to Facebook attenuates or augments physiological arousal during face-to-face interaction in a sample composed exclusively of adult female students. Participants were randomly assigned to four groups: Facebook exposure only, face-to-face exposure only, Facebook exposure first plus face-to-face exposure second and face-to-face exposure first plus Facebook exposure second. The results indicated that participants who only had seen the stimulus on Facebook had less physiological arousal than participants who had seen the stimulus face-to-face. However, regarding the combined conditions, physiological arousal was higher when seeing the person face-to-face when this preceded seeing the person on Facebook. Social anxiety moderated the relationship between physiological arousal and Facebook exposure so that exposing an individual to a stimulus person on Facebook is related with increased arousal in a face-to-face meeting with that person, and this, moreover, appears in highly social anxious persons.

No systematic approach has been conducted so far investigating the relationship between social anxiety and online social networking sites, or Facebook in particular, despite growing evidence on how socially individuals use online social networking sites. Therefore, the main aim of the current paper is to offer a comprehensive review of the state of the art of existent studies on the relationship between online social networking sites and social anxiety.

## 4. Methods

The current systematic review has been conducted in accordance with the Preferred Reporting Items for Systematic Reviews and Meta-Analyses (PRISMA) statement [31].

### 4.1. Inclusion and exclusion criteria

In order to be included, studies had to:

**(a)** involve participants with social anxiety symptoms/disorder;

**(b)** include online social networking assessments;

**(c)** include social anxiety assessments;

**(d)** be published in peer-reviewed journals;

**(e)** be published in English.

There were no age constraint criteria applied and no year of publication limitation.

Studies were excluded if there was no assessment of social networking and social anxiety, and they were not published in English.

### 4.2. Search strategy

Electronic databases (PsychInfo, PubMed, Scopus, Web of Science) were consulted by two independent assessors up to 20th June 2016. Several terms related to social networking were combined with terms related to social anxiety. No additional records were identified through the manual search in the references of the articles published and meta-analyses related to the subject. The reference lists of relevant papers and meta-analyses related to the subject were screened in order to identify potentially relevant articles. We repeated the search on 25th July 2016 to double-check and identify whether new articles had been published since the first search. The search terms were as follows:

**1.** Social network* OR Facebook OR LinkedIn OR Tweeter OR Instagram OR Youtube* OR Myspace OR Social Network Sites OR social media*

**2.** Social phobia OR social anx* OR social phobi* OR social* anxious* OR generalised social anx* OR generalized social anx*

**3.** 1 AND 2

## 5. Results

### 5.1. Literature search

The flowchart describing the inclusion of studies is described in **Figure 1**. The literature search yielded 673 articles, of which 98 were duplicates. After removing duplicates, the titles and abstracts of 575 articles were screened. Thirty-eight relevant papers were selected for full-text reading. Of these papers, 18 were excluded based on the following reasons: no social anxiety assessments ($n$ = 20), not peer-reviewed articles ($n$ = 2), not published in English ($n$ = 1), no measure on social networking ($n$ = 1), and theoretical reviews or meta-analyses ($n$ = 2). This left a total number of 20 articles to be included in the systematic review.

### 5.2. Information extracted

The following information was extracted from each of the studies included:

**(a)** authors and year of publication;

**(b)** sample characteristics (number of participants, mean age, age range, proportion of female participants, type of sample);

**(c)** amount of time spent using social networking sites per day;

**(d)** online social networking conceptualization;

**(e)** concepts assessed in the study;

**(f)** information regarding the association between online social networking and social anxiety.

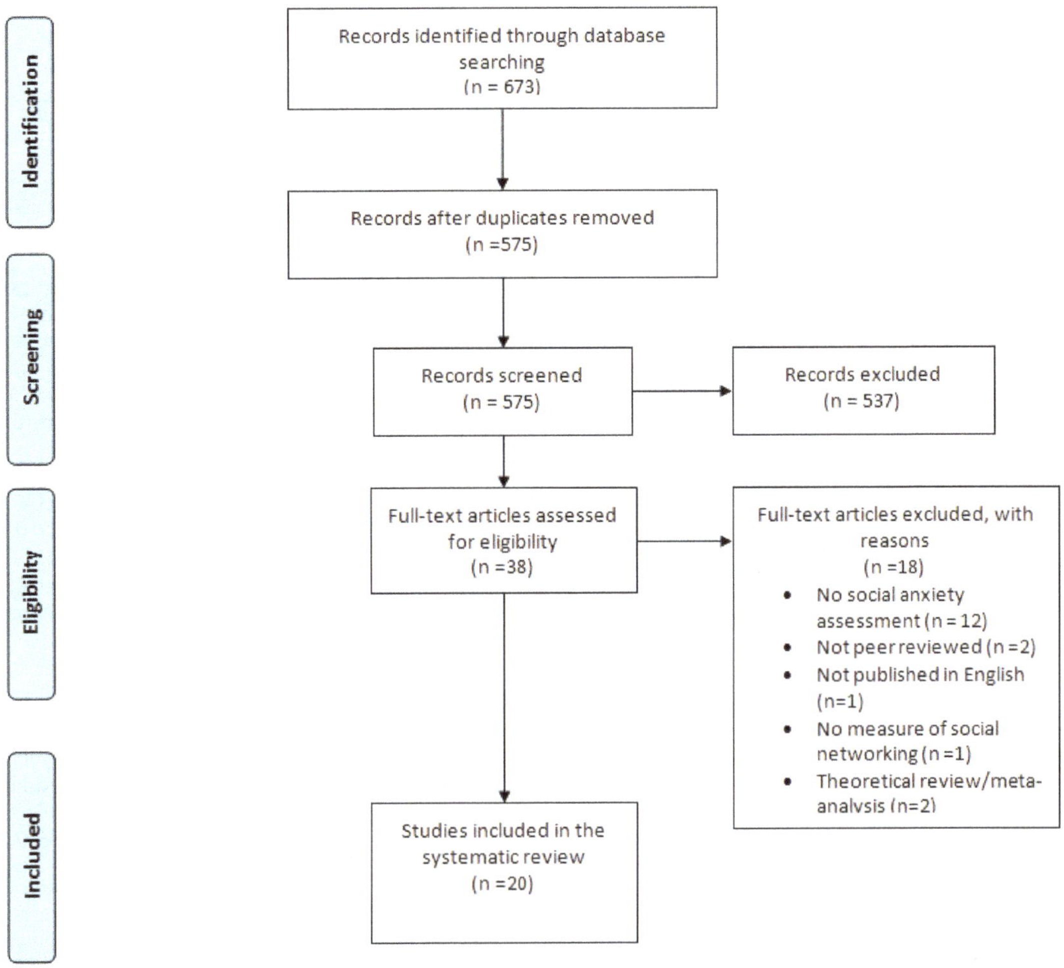


**Figure 1.** Flow diagram of study selection process.

## 5.3. Characteristics of the studies included

A summary of the characteristics of the studies included (number of participants, age, online social networking sites conceptualization, primary results) is described in **Table 1**.

| Study name | *N* (% F) | $M_{age}$ (SD) Age range | Sample | Time spent in social media per day (SD) | SNSs construct | Measures | Primary results |
|---|---|---|---|---|---|---|---|
| Aladwani and Almarzouq [45] | 407 (54%) | 20.04 (1.16) | Students | 1.86 h (0.99) | Compulsive SM use | Interaction anxiousness<br>Self-esteem<br>Problematic learning<br>Media complementarity | Significant positive associations between compulsive SM use and SA<br>$r = 0.26, p < 0.05$ |
| Antheunis et al. [12] | 3.068 (53.7%) | 13.46 (0.56) 11–14 | Adolescents | 7.27 h (8.54) | SNSs use intensity | Social anxiety<br>Quality of friendships | Significant negative associations between SNS and SA |

| Study name | N (% F) | $M_{age}$ (SD) Age range | Sample | Time spent in social media per day (SD) | SNSs construct | Measures | Primary results |
|---|---|---|---|---|---|---|---|
| | | | | | | Bridging social capital<br>Bonding social capital<br>Offline interaction with friends | $r = -0.08$, $p < 0.001$ |
| Bodroža and Jovanović [32] | 804<br>1st phase 445 (79.1%)<br>2nd phase 359 (79.4%) | 26.95 (6.35) 15–62<br>21.29 (2.96) 18–44 | Students and general population | Combined sample: ½ of the sample uses FB 1–3 h/day, 27% <1 h, 15% 3–5 h and 8% >5 h<br>Student sample: FB 1–3 h/day, 35% <1 h, 11% 3–5 h, 3% >5 h a day. | Psycho-social aspects of Facebook use (PSAFU):<br>Compensation<br>Self-presentation<br>Socialization<br>FB addiction<br>Virtual self | Social anxiety personality<br>Sensation seeking | Significant positive associations between FB and SA<br>$r$ between 0.11 and 0.58, $p < 0.001$ and 0.05 in both samples<br>Significant positive associations between FBA and SA<br>$r = 0.19$, $p < 0.001$ (FB users sample)<br>$r = 0.17$, $p < 0.001$ (Student sample) |
| Casale and Fioravanti [46] | 400 (51.8%) | 22.45 (2.09) | Students | Not reported | Generalized problematic Internet use | Social anxiety<br>Satisfaction with the needs through SNS:<br>-The need to belong-The need for self-presentation<br>-The need for assertiveness | Significant positive associations between problematic Internet use and SA<br>$r = 0.22$, $p < 0.001$ |
| Clayton et al. [39] | 229 (74.3%) | 18.19 (0.43) 18–21 | Students | 30 min to 1 h | Emotional connectedness to FB<br>Facebook connection strategies | Anxiousness-social anxiety subscale<br>loneliness<br>Alcohol use<br>Marijuana use | Significant positive associations between emotional connectedness to Facebook and anxiousness<br>$r = 0.18$, $p < 0.001$<br>Significant positive associations between Facebook connection strategies and anxiousness<br>$r = 0.23$, $p < 0.001$ |
| Davidson and Farquhar [49] | 336 (70%) | Not reported | Students | Not reported | Facebook intensity<br>Facebook anxiety | Social anxiety<br>number of unique groups<br>Role conflict<br>Self-monitoring<br>Religious activities | Non-significant positive associations between FB Intensity and SA<br>$r = 0.05$, $p =$ ns<br>Significant positive associations between FB anxiety and SA<br>$r = 0.66$, $p < 0.001$ |
| Fernandez et al. [29] | 62 (63%) | 19 (1.05) | Students | Not reported | Facebook usage | Social anxiety<br>Depression<br>Personality | Significant negative associations between FB friends and SA<br>$r = -0.45$, $p < 0.001$ |

| Study name | N (% F) | $M_{age}$ (SD) Age range | Sample | Time spent in social media per day (SD) | SNSs construct | Measures | Primary results |
|---|---|---|---|---|---|---|---|
| | | | | | | | Significant positive associations between FB usage and SA<br>$r$ between 0.27 and 0.50, $p < 0.001$ (i.e., number of lines in about me, number of TV shows, number of music interests)<br>Non-significant associations between SA and number of activities, self-reported time spent on FB, No. of status updates, No. of posts by friends, and no of posts by self. |
| Green et al. [43] | 306 (65.69%) | 20.52 (1.45) | Online participants from all around the world | 2.44 h (2.82)/day | FB self-disclosure (public and private) | Social anxiety<br>Controllability<br>Reduced cues<br>Disinhibition<br>Offline self-disclosure | Non-significant associations between FB self-disclosure public and SA<br>$r = 0.05$, $p = ns$<br>Non-significant associations between FB self-disclosure private and SA<br>$r = 0.00$, $p = ns$<br>Non-significant associations between time spent on FB and SA<br>$b = 0.11$, $p = ns$ |
| große Deters et al. [33] | 1st study 153 (60.78%)<br>2nd study 209 (88.52%) | 1st study 20.18 (3.24)<br>2nd study 23.50 (3.24) | 1st study Students<br>2nd study General population | Not reported | Status updates, No. of likes received per status update<br>No. of individual commenters per status update | Social anxiety personality (extraversion) | SA did not predict no. status updates, No. of likes received per status update, No. of individual commenters per status update<br>$p = ns$ |
| Hong et al. [40] | 230 (31.7%) | Not reported | Students | 34.3% spent < 1 h; 30.9% spent 1–2 h; 17.4% 2–4 h; 17.4% >4 h | Continuance intention to interact with others on FB<br>Online social anxiety | General social anxiety<br>Belief in dangerous virtual communities | Significant negative associations between FB continuance intention and SA<br>$r = -0.48$, $p < 0.001$<br>Significant positive associations between OSA and SA<br>$r = 0.38$, $p < 0.001$ |
| Indian and Grieve [41] | 299 (85.95%) | 28.35 (10.88) | Recruited from Facebook | 30–60 min, 14% with daily usage >3 h | Facebook social support items | Social anxiety<br>Offline social support<br>Subjective well-being | No difference in perceptions of Facebook social support in high and low socially anxious, $t(297) = 0.14$, $p = 0.89$<br>FB social support explained a significant amount of additional |

| Study name | N (% F) | $M_{age}$ (SD) Age range | Sample | Time spent in social media per day (SD) | SNSs construct | Measures | Primary results |
|---|---|---|---|---|---|---|---|
| | | | | | | | variance in subjective well-being over and above offline social support for the high social anxiety group |
| Landoll et al. [34] | 1st study: 216 (63%) 2nd study: 214 (54%) | 19.06 (1.28) 15.72 (1.22) | Adolescents and young adults | Not reported | Aversive social networking peer experiences | Social anxiety Internet use Social Peer victimization Depression | Significant positive associations between negative SNSs experiences and SA $r = 0.37, p < 0.001$ |
| Lee [47] | 304 (56%) | 22.45 (6.10) 17–55 | College students | Not reported | Facebook addiction | Social anxiety Smartphone addiction Personality traits Multitasking | Significant positive associations between FBA and SA $r = 0.25, p < 0.01$ |
| Lee-Won [35] | 243 (71.6%) | 19.69 (1.12) | College students | Assessed but not reported | Amount of FB use Problematic Facebook use | Social anxiety Personality Need for social assurance | Non-significant negative associations between FB use and SA $r = -0.03, p =$ ns Significant positive associations between FBA and SA $r = 0.45, p < 0.001$ |
| Liu et al. [44] | 780 (50.9%) | 13.94 (0.90) 13–18 | Adolescents | Not reported | Personally identifiable information (PII) disclosure | Social anxiety Privacy concern Parental mediation Narcissism | Non-significant negative associations between PII and SA $r = -0.07, p =$ ns SA indirectly decreases PII disclosure by increasing privacy concern. |
| McCord et al. [38] | 216 (85.64 %) | 32.2 (12.43) 18–69 | 31.5% undergraduate students, 12.0% graduate students, and 55.6% were not students | Not reported | FB use FB social interaction anxiety | Social anxiety | Non-significant associations between FB use and SA $r = 0.01, p =$ ns Significant positive associations between FB SA and SA $r = 0.64, p < 0.001$ |
| Ramirez et al. [42] | 244 (51%) | 34.59 (11.19) | Facebook users | Not reported | FB reconnection | Social anxiety Information seeking Uncertainty predicted outcome value Sociability | Marginal significant negative associations between SA and FB reconnect $b = 0.14, p = 0.05$ |
| Rizvi [48] | 150 (75%) | 18–27 | Different educational institution | 46% <30 min 32.7% 30 min to 1 h 11.3% 1–2 h 10% > 2 h | Excessive FB use (log in) | Social anxiety Personality | Non-significant negative associations between excessive FB use and SA $r = -0.02, p =$ ns |
| Shaw et al. [36] | 75 (55.2%) | 19.2 (1.27) | Students | 2.04 (1.13) Range 1–5 | FB time passive FB use | Rumination | Significant positive associations between |

| Study name | N (% F) | $M_{age}$ (SD) Age range | Sample | Time spent in social media per day (SD) | SNSs construct | Measures | Primary results |
|---|---|---|---|---|---|---|---|
| | | | | | FB content production<br>Interactive FB communication | Depressive symptoms<br>Mood and anxiety symptoms<br>Content production<br>Interactive communication<br>Social anxiety | time spent on FB and SA<br>$r = 0.33, p < 0.01$<br>Significant positive associations between passive FB use and SA<br>$r = 0.32, p < 0.01$<br>Non-significant associations between content production on FB<br>$r = 0.23, p = \text{ns}$<br>Non-significant associations between interactive FB communication and SA<br>$r = 0.21, p = \text{ns}$ |
| Weidman and Levinson [37] | 77 (77%) | 18.91 (1.05) | Students | Not reported | Facebook profile (no. friends, no. photographs, no. videos, photo albums, relationship status, people in profile picture, status update, quote)<br>Social activity<br>Social inactivity<br>Close relationship quality<br>Self-disclosure | Social interaction anxiety | Significant negative associations between no. friends and SA<br>$r = -0.21, p < 0.05$<br>Significant negative associations between FB quote length and SA<br>$r = -0.38, p < 0.05$ |

Note: $N$ = number of participants; $\%F$ = percentage of female participants; $M_{age}$ = mean age; SD = standard deviation; SNSs = social networking site; SM = social media; SA= Social anxiety; FB= Facebook; FBA= Facebook addiction; OSA = online social anxiety; ns= non-significant; no. = number; h = hours; min = minutes.

**Table 1.** Characteristics of the included studies.

We included 20 papers in the systematic review, of which three papers [32–34] consisted of two studies/phases each. Most of the studies included were conducted with adults ($n = 14$), recruited either from university (students), or from the general populations, while several papers were conducted with adolescents ($n = 3$), and some studies did not report the age of the participants ($n = 2$). Nine of the papers included reported the time spent on Facebook; one study also assessed this indicator but did not report it, and the rest of the studies did not include reports on the time spent on Facebook. Social media was operationalized differently in the papers included and while few studies reported social media variables, most of the papers included referred specifically to Facebook.

With respect to the manner in which online social networking sites or Facebook were conceptualized in these studies, we have encountered several approaches:

- *Facebook use* ($n$ = 7), which in turn can be conceptualized as the amount of time spent on online social networking sites, passive use of Facebook or using interactive Facebook features (updates, comments, likes);
- *Psychosocial aspects of Facebook use* ($n$ = 6), which can also mean Facebook connection strategies, Facebook continuance intention, Facebook reconnection decision, Facebook social support, aversive Facebook experiences or cybervictimization;
- *Personal disclosure on Facebook* ($n$ = 3), which can also mean private or public disclosure, personal identifiable information (profile information and privacy settings) and status/quote update/length;
- *Problematic use of online social networking sites* ($n$ = 6), which can be found as Internet addiction, compulsive social media use, Facebook addiction or Facebook intrusiveness;
- *Facebook anxiety* ($n$ = 3), with different terms such as Facebook-specific anxiety, Facebook interaction anxiety or online anxiety.

Most of the papers included found a significant association between social networking (Facebook) and social anxiety ($n$ = 16), while the rest of the studies included found no significant relationship between social media and social anxiety.

## 5.4. Online social networking and social anxiety

### *5.4.1. Usage of online social networking sites and social anxiety*

There are mixed findings regarding the relationship between online social networking and social anxiety. On the one hand, there are studies reporting significant associations between the two variables. For example, Antheunis et al. [12] showed that Facebook use was negatively associated with social anxiety in a large sample of adolescents. Lee-Won [35] found evidence that Facebook use, defined as the amount of time participants spend on Facebook on an average day, was associated with social anxiety. Shaw et al. [36] found a significant relationship between the time spent on Facebook and social anxiety in a sample of undergraduate students. The same study found a significant association between passive Facebook use, defined as passive content consumption (e.g. passively viewing one's Facebook profile) and social anxiety. The relationship between passive Facebook use and social anxiety was significant even after checking for depressive and anxiety symptoms. Weidman and Levinson [37] considered both offline (self-reported indicators) and online indicators (using the profiles of coders for Facebook) of social anxiety. Results on self-reported social anxiety and objective Facebook use indicated significant negative relationships between the two variables, with number of friends, number of photographs and quotes length being negatively related to social anxiety. Regarding the rated social anxiety symptoms observed and objective Facebook signs, there were significant negative associations between social activity composite (number of friends, photographs, videos, photo albums), the number of people in profile pictures and social anxiety.

On the other hand, there are several research papers that show no association between Facebook use and social anxiety. große Deters et al. [33] found no significant relationship between social anxiety and different parameters of Facebook use (status updates, number of likes or individual commenters per like), and none of the prediction models investigated, in which social anxiety was used as a predictor and Facebook as a criterion, were significant. McCord et al. [38] found no significant relationship between general Facebook use, defined as the frequency of using the socially interactive features of Facebook (sending messages, using chat, writing on events/friends walls, sending friend requests, posting comments, updating status) and social anxiety. Fernandez et al. [29] did not find a positive association between the frequency of Facebook usage, operationalized as time spent on Facebook, status updates, number of posts by friends/self and social anxiety, in a sample of students. In this study, several independent coders rated each participant's level of social anxiety based on viewing their Facebook profiles and associated it with participants' self-rated social anxiety symptoms. Social anxiety was not associated with an increased frequency of Facebook use, either based on self-report data or based on coders' reports. However, there were positive associations between profile information sections and social anxiety. The number of activities was not associated with social anxiety. Using multiple regression, the results indicated that social anxiety had a unique contribution, apart from depression and neuroticism, to profile information (excepting the number of movies and activities).

### *5.4.2. Psychosocial aspects of Facebook use and social anxiety*

Bodroža and Jovanović [32] constructed a scale in order to measure several psychosocial aspects of Facebook use. Five factors emerged for the structure of the scale, namely: compensation (use Facebook in order to compensate for personal insecurity/inadequacy), self-presentation (concern related to impression on others), socialization (striving to acquaint new friends/intimate partners), Facebook addiction and virtual self (Facebook adequately represents one's personality). Social anxiety had positive associations with each of these factors. Clayton et al. [39] found a positive relationship between anxiousness (public and private self-consciousness, social anxiety), emotional connectedness to Facebook (integration of Facebook in one's daily life) and Facebook connection strategies (reasons to use Facebook, use Facebook to learn more information about people, to maintain current relationships). Anxiousness was a significant predictor of both emotional connectedness to Facebook and Facebook connection strategies. Hong et al. [40] investigated the relationship between the continuance intention to interact with other people on Facebook and social anxiety and found a significant negative relationship between them. Social anxiety predicted the continuance intention to interact with other people on Facebook and, together with online social anxiety, accounted for 44% of the continuance intention. Indian and Grieve [41] found no differences between low and high socially anxious individuals in Facebook social support. There were significant association in both groups between Facebook social support and subjective well-being, as well as between Facebook social support and offline social support. Finally, Facebook social support was a significant individual predictor of subjective well-being for highly social anxious individuals. Landoll et al. [34] developed an instrument that assesses negative peer experiences on social networking sites. There were significant associations between negative online peer experiences and social anxiety and depression. Ramirez et al. [42] investigated factors related to the decision to reconnect on Facebook with a past contact in a sample group of adult participants. Using hierarchical logistic regression, they found several predictors that accounted for almost 40% of the variance of the decision to reconnect on Facebook, in which social anxiety was also included and has a marginally negative contribution to it. There were other factors (e.g. relational factors and information seeking factors) that have a greater contribution to the decision to reconnect than social anxiety.

#### *5.4.3. Personal disclosure on Facebook and social anxiety*

There was no significant evidence stemming from the papers included of an association between Facebook disclosure and social anxiety. Green et al. [43] found no relationship between Facebook self-disclosure (public and private) and social anxiety. Two hypothesized pathways from social anxiety to Facebook self-disclosure considered online attributes (reduced cues, controllability) and feelings of disinhibition. Results showed that the model accounted for 23% of the variance in Facebook private self-disclosure and 7% of the variance in Facebook public self-disclosure. Liu et al. [44] did not find any relationship between Facebook disclosure and social anxiety in a sample group of adolescents aged between 13 and 18. Disclosure in this study referred to personally identifiable information, a composite score computed by adding a measure for attitudinal information disclosure (profile information on Facebook page and personal photographs) and a scale assessing behavioural information disclosure (items actually posted on Facebook and privacy regarding photographs). There was only an indirect relationship between social anxiety and Facebook disclosure through the role of privacy concern, defined as concern related to the security of the personal information presented online. Namely, by increasing privacy concern, social anxiety indirectly decreases disclosure. Using a path analysis approach, parental mediation had only an indirect effect on disclosure through privacy concern, and no direct effect. Self-disclosure, defined as the presence or absence of status update/quote and length of status update/quote, was also considered in Weidman and Levinson [37] as a measure of social inactivity. Status update was unrelated to social anxiety in both self-reported and observer-rated social anxiety and objective Facebook signs, while the length of the quote was related to social anxiety only in self-reported and not in observer-rated social anxiety.

#### *5.4.4. Problematic social media use/Facebook addiction and social anxiety*

Most of the papers included sustained the relationship between problematic use of online social networking sites or online social networking sites addiction and social anxiety. For instance, Aladwani and Almarzouq [45] found a significant positive association between interaction anxiousness and compulsive social media used, which finally has a significant effect on learning outcomes. Bodroža and Jovanović [32] found a significant relationship between social addiction and social anxiety both in a sample of Facebook users recruited online and in a sample of students. Casale and Fioravanti [46] considered the Self-Determination Theory in the context of Facebook use and proposed that the satisfaction for unmet needs through social networking sites should be a viable candidate in the development of problematic use of Internet communicative services. Results showed that social anxiety had a significant effect on generally problematic Internet use for both women and men, in a sample group of undergraduate students. They also considered several needs for using social networking sites, such as the need to belong, self-presentation and assertiveness. Problematic use of Internet communicative services was significantly associated with all the three needs considered. However, only the need for self-presentation was a significant mediator in the relationship between social anxiety and problematic Internet use only in the case of males. Lee [47] investigated the relationship between Facebook addiction and social anxiety in a sample group of African American students and found a significant positive relationship between the two variables. Using hierarchical multiple regression, the results showed that approximately 19% of the variance of Facebook addiction was explained by eight predictors, of which age, social interaction anxiety and multitasking were the most related to Facebook addiction. Finally, Facebook addiction was significantly associated with smartphone addiction. Lee-Won [35] found a significant association between problematic Facebook use and social anxiety, with the latter being a noteworthy predictor for problematic Facebook use. Furthermore, the results indicated that a significant moderator in the relationship between problematic Facebook use and social anxiety was the need for social assurance. Rizi [48] found no relationship between social anxiety and excessive Facebook use in a sample of 150 young adults; there were no differences in Facebook use according to high vs. low social anxiety levels. However, the majority of the participants from this study logged on to their Facebook accounts few times a day (47%) and spent less than 30 min on Facebook (46%). The only parameter regarding Facebook usage that was considered in this study for the association with social anxiety was the frequency with which participants log onto Facebook, with no other variables considered.

### *5.4.5. Facebook anxiety and social anxiety*

Three of the studies included that assessed online social networking sites anxiety indicated significant positive relationships with social anxiety. Davidson and Farquhar [49] investigated the relationship between social anxiety, religion and Facebook. They developed a Facebook-specific anxiety scale, an adaptation of a social anxiety scale related to Facebook and found a strong association with social anxiety. Online social anxiety and social anxiety were positively associated in Hong et al. [40], with general social anxiety being a significant predictor of online social anxiety. McCord et al. [38] used a Facebook social interaction scale and found a significant association with social anxiety in an adult sample group. Using multiple regression results indicated that social anxiety and anxiety on Facebook predicted Facebook social use. There was a significant interaction between social anxiety and Facebook social anxiety, which is in line with the social compensation theory. According to this theory, highly socially anxious individuals tend to use Facebook in order to compensate for the discomfort associated with face-to-face communication. A second regression model was also significant, with anxiety on Facebook and social Facebook use predicting social anxiety; again, there was a significant interaction between the two predictors.

## 6. Discussion

Online social networking sites are widespread means through which people can interact with others. There are many advantages of online social networking sites; however, recent research focuses mainly on the negative impact they have on mental health. Terms like "iDisorders", "Facebook depression" and "Facebook addiction" abound in the literature on online social networking sites and mental health, proposing new disorders that are determined by the use of online social networking sites/Facebook. Moreover, their particularities in terms of manifestations make some advocate their inclusion in current diagnostic nosologies.

The present review aims to synthetically present the existing literature on the relationship between social anxiety and social networking. Twenty studies met our inclusion criteria. Most of these studies referred to a particular online social networking site, Facebook, and assessed different related parameters. Overall, most of the papers reported significant associations between online social networking and social anxiety, with four papers reporting no relationship between the two variables. There were mixed results on the relationship between Facebook use and social anxiety, as there were both studies sustaining a significant positive association between the two variables and those that found no association. Several psychosocial aspects of Facebook use were significantly related, both positively and negatively, to social anxiety. There was no relationship between Facebook disclosure and social anxiety in any of the papers included that assessed this construct. With one exception, there was a significant positive relationship between online social networking sites addiction/ problematic use and social anxiety. There was evidence of a significant association between Facebook anxiety and social anxiety.

This results should be interpreted in the light of the fact that there was a high heterogeneity of Facebook conceptualizations, as in several studies, the amount of time spent on Facebook was assessed, while other studies assessed Facebook/ Internet/ social networking problematic use/intrusiveness/addiction, or psychosocial aspects related to Facebook use, or Facebook disclosure, and in fewer studies, Facebook anxiety was considered. Therefore, one cannot conclude that online social networking sites have a negative or a positive effect on social anxiety without carefully taking into consideration what they mean. An important limitation of the current review was the fact that although we aimed to investigate the relationship between social media and social anxiety, most of the papers included referred only to social networking sites such as Facebook and we cannot generate findings pertaining to other social networking sites, such as Instagram, Tweeter, Youtube, LinkedIn or Myspace. Future studies should also investigate the role of these other social networking sites in mental health problems and in social anxiety per se. Another limitation of this paper refers to the sample groups. As most of the participants included were students, this does not enable us to extend our to other populations. Involving more heterogeneous samples of participants, adolescents, young and older adults can help us to find significant moderators in the relationship between social networking and social anxiety. As all the studies included were cross-sectional, we cannot conclude that there is causality between social networking media, namely Facebook, and social anxiety. Does social media (time spent, pathological use, number of friends, activities) contribute to social anxiety symptomatology or do socially anxious individuals tend to use more social media? According to what we currently know, no directionality can be assumed. However, much like in the meta-analysis on Facebook and loneliness [21], in this case, social anxiety can predict social media use rather than the other way around.

Future experimental studies manipulating independent variables would be useful in order to draw more conclusions on the relationship between social networking and social anxiety. Longitudinal studies would allow us to test bidirectional relationships between the two variables and investigate time-related patterns in social networking use and social anxiety. Up to this moment, it remains unclear whether social anxiety leads to more online social networking use, or whether the relationship is opposite, with more use of online social networking predicting social anxiety. Bidirectionality between the variables could also be an important aspect to investigate, as there is preliminary evidence for both directions.

The findings of the current review have important clinical implications regarding social networking use for individuals with social anxiety. The benefits/advantages of online social networking sites should be used and investigated in order to overcome existing barriers in clinical practice. Testing interventions delivered over social networking sites in randomized controlled trials would have great implications on the development of evidence-based remote interventions.

## Acknowledgements

Funding for this study was provided by a grant from the Romanian Executive Unit for Financing Education Higher Research, Development and Innovation (the "Effectiveness of an empirically based web platform for anxiety in youths", grant number PN-II-PT-PCCA-2011-3.1-1500, 81/2012) awarded to Dr. Anca Dobrean.

## Author details

Anca Dobrean[1*] and Costina-Ruxandra Păsărelu[2]

*Address all correspondence to: anca.dobrean@ubbcluj.ro

1 Department of Clinical Psychology and Psychotherapy, Babeş-Bolyai University, Cluj-Napoca, Romania

2 Doctoral School Evidence-Based Assessment and Psychological Interventions, Babeş-Bolyai University, Cluj-Napoca, Romania

## References


[1] Facebook Reports Second Quarter. 2016. Available from: https://investor.Facebook.com/investor-news/press-release-details/2016/Facebook-Reports-Second-Quarter-2016-Results/default.aspx [Accessed 4 August 2016].

[2] Kosinski M, Matz SC, Gosling SD, et al. Facebook as a research tool for the social sciences: opportunities, challenges, ethical considerations, and practical guidelines. Am Psychol 2015; 70: 543–556.

[3] Ryan GS. Online social networks for patient involvement and recruitment in clinical research. Nurse Res 2013; 21: 35–39.

[4] Merchant G, Weibel N, Patrick K, et al. Click 'like' to change your behavior: a mixed methods study of college students' exposure to and engagement with Facebook content designed for weight loss. J Med Internet Res 2014; 16: e158.

[5] Ruotsalainen H, Kyngäs H, Tammelin T, et al. Effectiveness of Facebook-delivered lifestyle counselling and physical activity self-monitoring on physical activity and body mass index in overweight and obese adolescents: a randomized controlled trial. Nurs Res Pract 2015; 2015: 159205.

[6] Torous J, Keshavan M. The role of social media in schizophrenia: evaluating risks, benefits, and potential. Curr Opin Psychiatry 2016; 29: 190–195.

[7] Naslund JA, Aschbrenner KA, Marsch LA, et al. The future of mental health care: peer-to-peer support and social media. Epidemiol Psychiatr Sci 2016; 25: 113–122.

[8] Hui A, Wong PW-C, Fu K-W. Evaluation of an online campaign for promoting help-seeking attitudes for depression using a Facebook advertisement: an online randomized controlled experiment. JMIR Ment Health 2015; 2: e5.

[9] Ellison NB, Steinfield C, Lampe C. The benefits of Facebook 'Friends:' social capital and college students' use of online social network sites. J Comput-Mediat Comm 2007; 12: 1143–1168.

[10] Grajales FJ, Sheps S, Ho K, et al. Social media: a review and tutorial of applications in medicine and health care. J Med Internet Res 2014; 16: e13.

[11] Laranjo L, Arguel A, Neves AL, et al. The influence of social networking sites on health behavior change: a systematic review and meta-analysis. J Am Med Inform Assoc 2015; 22: 243–256

[12] Antheunis ML, Schouten AP, Krahmer E. The role of social networking sites in early adolescents' social lives. J Early Adolesc 2016; 36: 348–371.

[13] Myhre JW, Mehl MR, Glisky EL. Cognitive benefits of online social networking for healthy older adults. J Gerontol B Psychol Sci Soc Sci. Epub ahead of print 16 March 2016. DOI: 10.1093/geronb/gbw025.

[14] Lenhart A. Teens, social media & technology overview 2015. Pew Research Center: Internet, Science & Tech. 2015. Available from: http://www.pewinternet.org/2015/04/09/teens-social-media-technology-2015 [Accessed 4 August 2016].

[15] Sampasa-Kanyinga H, Lewis RF. Frequent use of social networking sites is associated with poor psychological functioning among children and adolescents. Cyberpsychol Behav Soc Netw 2015; 18: 380–385.

[16] Sampasa-Kanyinga H, Hamilton HA. Social networking sites and mental health problems in adolescents: the mediating role of cyberbullying victimization. Eur Psychiatry 2015; 30: 1021–1027.

[17] Jelenchick LA, Eickhoff JC, Moreno MA. 'Facebook depression?' Social networking site use and depression in older adolescents. J Adolesc Health 2013; 52: 128–130.

[18] O'Keeffe GS, Clarke-Pearson K, Mulligan DA, et al. Clinical report – The impact of social media on children, adolescents, and families. Pediatrics 2011; 127: 800–804.

[19] Frison E, Eggermont S. 'Harder, Better, Faster, Stronger': negative comparison on Facebook and adolescents' life satisfaction are reciprocally related. Cyberpsychol Behav Soc Netw 2016; 19: 158–164.

[20] Marino C, Vieno A, Pastore M, et al. Modeling the contribution of personality, social identity and social norms to problematic Facebook use in adolescents. Addict Behav 2016; 63: 51–56.

[21] Song H, Zmyslinski-Seelig A, Kim J, et al. Does Facebook make you lonely? A meta analysis. Comput Human Behav 2014; 36: 446–452.

[22] Rosen LD, Whaling K, Rab S, et al. Is Facebook creating 'iDisorders'? The link between clinical symptoms of psychiatric disorders and technology use, attitudes and anxiety. Comput Human Behav 2013; 29: 1243–1254.

[23] Lin LY, Sidani JE, Shensa A, et al. Association between social media use and depression among U.S. young adults. Depress Anxiety 2016; 33: 323–331.

[24] Soon-Li Lee, Miriam Sang-Ah Park, Cai-Lian Tam. The relationship between Facebook attachment and obsessive-compulsive disorder severity. Cyberpsychology 2015; 9: 39–47.

[25] Andreassen CS. Online social network site addiction: a comprehensive review. Curr Addict Rep 2015; 2: 175–184.

[26] Hormes JM, Kearns B, Timko CA. Craving Facebook? Behavioral addiction to online social networking and its association with emotion regulation deficits. Addiction 2014; 109: 2079–2088.

[27] Koc M, Gulyagci S. Facebook addiction among Turkish college students: the role of psychological health, demographic, and usage characteristics. Cyberpsychol Behav Soc Netw 2013; 16: 279–284.

[28] Desjarlais M, Willoughby T. A longitudinal study of the relation between adolescent boys and girls' computer use with friends and friendship quality: support for the social compensation or the rich-get-richer hypothesis? Comput Human Behav 2010; 26: 896–905.

[29] Fernandez KC, Levinson CA, Rodebaugh TL. Profiling predicting social anxiety from Facebook profiles. Soc Psychol Personal Sci 2012; 3: 706–713.

[30] Rauch SM, Strobel C, Bella M, et al. Face to face versus Facebook: does exposure to social networking web sites augment or attenuate physiological arousal among the socially anxious? Cyberpsychol Behav Soc Netw 2014; 17: 187–190.

[31] Moher D, Liberati A, Tetzlaff J, et al. Preferred reporting items for systematic reviews and meta-analyses: the PRISMA statement. Ann Intern Med 2009; 151: 264–269, W64.

[32] Bodroža B, Jovanović T. Validation of the new scale for measuring behaviors of Facebook users: psycho-social aspects of Facebook use (PSAFU). Computers in Human Behavior 2016; 54: 425–435.

[33] große Deters F, Mehl MR, Eid M. Social responses to Facebook status updates: the role of extraversion and social anxiety. Comput Human Behav 2016; 61: 1–13.

[34] Landoll RR, La Greca AM, Lai BS. Aversive Peer Experiences on Social Networking Sites: Development of the Social Networking-Peer Experiences Questionnaire (SN-PEQ). *J Res Adolesc* 2013; 23: 695–705.

[35] Lee-Won RJ, Herzog L, Park SG. Hooked on Facebook: The role of social anxiety and need for social assurance in problematic use of Facebook. Cyberpsychol Behav Soc Netw 2015; 18: 567–574.

[36] Shaw AM, Timpano KR, Tran TB, et al. Correlates of Facebook usage patterns: the relationship between passive Facebook use, social anxiety symptoms, and brooding. Comput Human Behav 2015; 48: 575–580.

[37] Weidman AC, Levinson CA. I'm still socially anxious online: offline relationship impairment characterizing social anxiety manifests and is accurately perceived in online social networking profiles. Comput Human Behav 2015; 49: 12–19.

[38] McCord B, Rodebaugh TL, Levinson CA. Facebook: social uses and anxiety. Computers in Human Behavior 2014; 34: 23–27.

[39] Clayton RB, Osborne RE, Miller BK, et al. Loneliness, anxiousness, and substance use as predictors of Facebook use. Comput Human Behav 2013; 29: 687–693.

[40] Hong J-C, Hwang M-Y, Hsu C-H, et al. Belief in dangerous virtual communities as a predictor of continuance intention mediated by general and online social anxiety: the Facebook perspective. Comput Human Behav 2015; 48: 663–670.

[41] Indian M, Grieve R. When Facebook is easier than face-to-face: social support derived from Facebook in socially anxious individuals. Pers Individ Dif 2014; 59: 102–106.

[42] Ramirez A, Sumner EM, Hayes J. Reconnect on Facebook: The Role of Information Seeking Behavior and Individual- and Relationship-Level Factors. *Cyberpsychology, Behavior, and Social Networking* 2016; 19: 494–501.

[43] Green T, Wilhelmsen T, Wilmots E, et al. Social anxiety, attributes of online communication and self-disclosure across private and public Facebook communication. Comput Human Behav 2016; 58: 206–213.

[44] Liu C, Ang RP, Lwin MO. Cognitive, personality, and social factors associated with adolescents' online personal information disclosure. J Adolesc 2013; 36: 629–638.

[45] Aladwani AM, Almarzouq M. Understanding compulsive social media use: the premise of complementing self-conceptions mismatch with technology. Comput Human Behav 2016; 60: 575–581.

[46] Casale S, Fioravanti G. Satisfying needs through social networking sites: a pathway towards problematic Internet use for socially anxious people? Addict Behav Rep 2015; 1: 34–39.

[47] Lee EB. Too much information heavy smartphone and Facebook utilization by African American young adults. J Black Stud 2015; 46: 44–61.

[48] Rizvi AZ. Personality, social anxiety and excessive use of Facebook. Int J Psychol Behav Sci 2016; 6: 119–127.

[49] Davidson T, Farquhar LK. Correlates of social anxiety, religion, and Facebook. J Media Religion 2014; 13: 208–225.

7

# Epigenetic and Schizophrenia

Ariel Cariaga-Martinez and Raúl Alelú-Paz

**Abstract**

Schizophrenia is a complex psychiatric disorder characterised by the presence of positive, negative and cognitive symptoms that lack a unifying neuropathology. The absence of consistently replicated genetic effects, together with evidence for lasting changes in gene expression after environmental exposures, suggests a role of epigenetic mechanisms. In this chapter, we will focus on these mechanisms, such as DNA methylation, hydroxymethylation, histone modifications or non-coding RNA, as key mechanisms through which environmental factors interact with individual's genetic constitution which affect the risk of psychotic conditions throughout life. Due to the advances experienced in recent years, it is to be expected that in the next decades, an increasing amount of data will provide us with a more complete landscape of the contribution of epigenetics to the development of mental disorders such as schizophrenia.

**Keywords:** schizophrenia, epigenetic, DNA methylation, histone modifications, human brain

## 1. Introduction

Schizophrenia is a complex illness characterised by different types of positive, negative and cognitive symptoms that affect all aspects of mental activity. This disorder has a world prevalence of 1%, but it is higher in first-degree relatives as well as in monozygotic twins.

Although one of the main repository of scientific publications (the US National Library of Medicine, accessible from www.pubmed.com website) compiles, on average, more than 6000 original research papers per year, we only have fragmented knowledge about the aetiology, development and accurate diagnosis of schizophrenia.

What are the causes of schizophrenia? Does the genetic background of the individuals play a role in predisposition, onset and progression of this disorder? Or are the environment and its different types of pressures (stress, nutrition, diseases, etc.) responsible for the development of this disorder? For decades, the nature versus nurture debate absorbed efforts from scientist either from biological sciences to psychiatry professionals. However, recent advances indicate that this debate could be finally overcome. In fact, nature and nurture interact in different ways, and we can imagine this situation as a cycle. In a dynamically changing environment, stimuli should enter the cell where this information is 'interpreted' and a plethora of biological mechanisms are able to produce a molecular response. Usually, this molecular response implies expression of genes that, in due course, will generate an organic response to confront the initial stimuli. And the cycle begins again (**Figure 1**), allowing to the cell to maintain its homeostasis.

Currently, we can see the intimacy of this interaction at a molecular level and we can understand how a single cell (whether an epithelial cell or a neuron) is able to adapt to an environment that is in a constant change, whether they be minimum changes (for example, a new cellular interaction) or significant changes (from a pH change to microbe attacks or environmental catastrophes).

Certainly, cells do not carry a gene for every possible response against environmental stimuli; we therefore need another 'way of reading' the genetic information or, even more, another layer of information. In fact, genetic information tends to be rigid: it is hard to change it, and when it happens (what we usually know as mutations) it biological meaning is comprised from cell death to cell survival, through a wide range of decisions that clash with the dynamics of environment changes. Although this rigidity is key to passing all this information from generation to generation, it does not seem to be useful when the cell needs a quick, dynamic response to its medium.

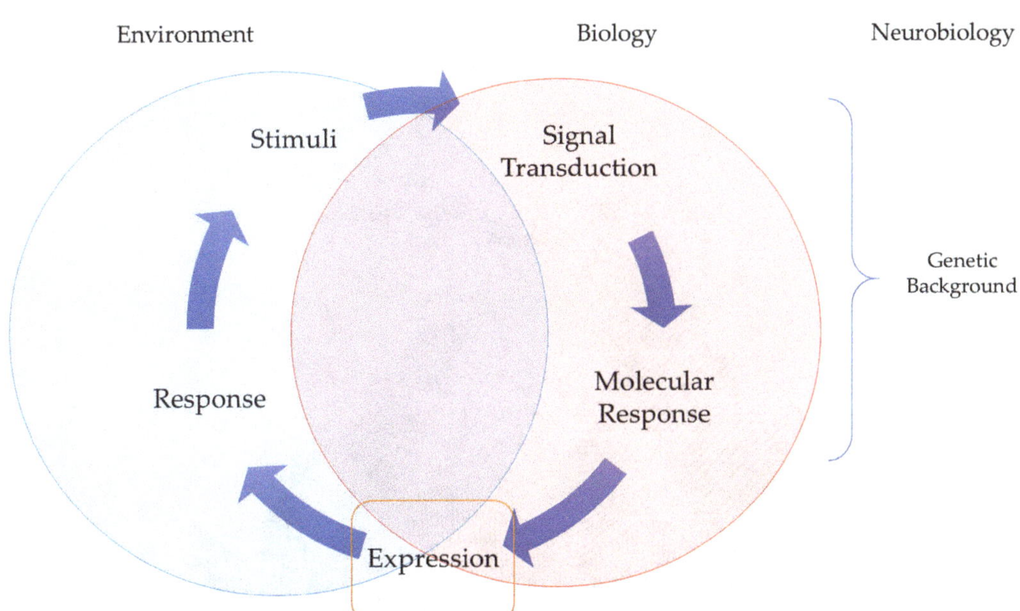


**Figure 1.** Interactions nature-nurture. Genetic and environment constantly interact to assure the maintaining of a constant internal medium for every cell, despite facing several types of stimuli.

In 1942, Conrad Waddington coined the term 'Epigenetic' to name the plasticity of genomes when facing environmental changes through his metaphor of marbles (representing cells in its developmental process) rolling down a hill, through valleys and forks (representing the environment) that affect the cellular fate (**Figure 2**) [1].

Since 1942, we have developed a more precise definition of epigenetic:

> *Epigenetic comprises all the molecular mechanisms that affect gene expression without changing the DNA sequence.*

As we will see throughout this chapter, epigenetics is both a new layer of information and a new way of reading the genetic information, leading to a gain in actual plasticity of the rigid genetic information.

In this sense, epigenetics could shed some light on elusive points of the aetiology, and general pathology of mental disorders, especially in schizophrenia, where interactions nature-nurture seems to be key to its onset [2].

### 1.1. Is epigenetic that important? A new layer of information

We can imagine epigenetic as a new layer of information that regulates the differential reading of genetic information, or the access to it. In turn, this regulation of reading or access to the genetic information is also regulated, as is common in living cells, by epigenetic mechanisms, too. Therefore, we can distinguish:

**a.** Mechanisms implied in differential reading of the genetic information: these mechanisms are responsible to selectively guiding the genetic expression according to minor (and sharply defined) atomic modifications of DNA. When these modifications are located in the right places along the DNA sequence, all the genetic expression can increase or decrease, thereby allowing the cells to response when facing dynamic changes. In this category, we could indicate the DNA methylation and hydroxymethylation.

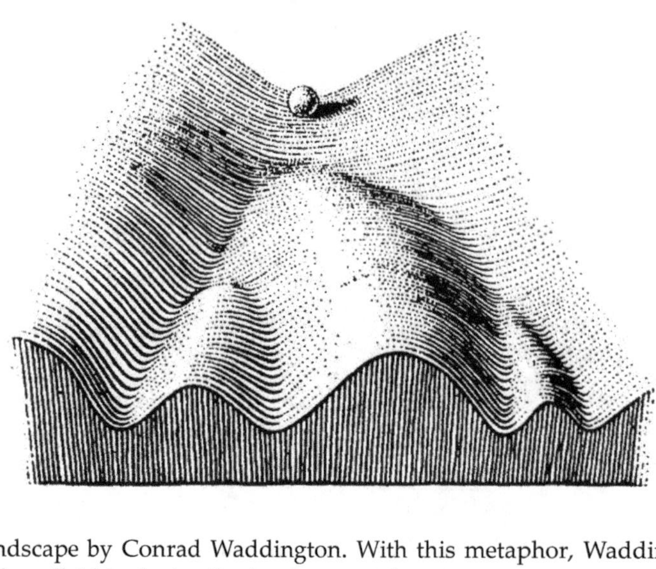

**Figure 2.** The epigenetic landscape by Conrad Waddington. With this metaphor, Waddington tries to illustrate how environment can influence the cells' fate during its developmental process.

**b.** Mechanisms implies in allowing (or avoiding) access to the genetic information: these subtle mechanisms encompass molecular changes that physically allow or avoid the access to DNA sequences or specific regions. In this category, we could indicate the post-translational histone modifications and the role of chromatin remodelling complexes.

**c.** Mechanisms that regulate epigenetic changes: the presence of feedback loops is common in living cells and epigenetic changes are also regulated in this way. There are several types of molecules (in particular, some types of RNA as we will see later in this chapter) that can regulate the epigenetic landscape in a healthy cell or be affected in an unhealthy cell.

The role of genetic background has been widely demonstrated in relation to the onset of schizophrenia. However, this factor is not unique as a causal one, and the individual needs to be in contact with several kinds of environmental factors to develop this mental disorder. In other words, the genetic information should interact with an environment to generate a schizophrenic phenotype, which may position epigenetic changes as key to understanding the molecular basis of this pathology.

As we can see, epigenetic changes could be subtle (such as specific atomic changes on a DNA base, or molecular changes in its associated proteins), or they can imply an actual remodelling of huge portions of chromatin, but always differently depending on the tissue, even more, depending on cell type. However, to understand how epigenetic mechanisms could trigger a mental disorder, we need to understand all the epigenetic changes as a whole, generating a framework instead of interpreting fragmented data. We call this framework the neuroepigenome. This new field implies efforts from several branches of Science in order to get a complete view of the epigenetic modifications of the nervous system which, in due course, will leads to a better understanding of pathological conditions.

Throughout the next sections, we will discuss the neuroepigenome from simpler modifications (such as DNA methylation) to the more extensive changes (such as the remodelling of chromatin), focusing on its role and recent advances regarding molecular pathology of schizophrenia. Given this field is still under frantic research, we will try to offer the most established (and replicated) facts, while leaving open doors to new developments and knowledge.

## 2. Differential reading of genetic information: DNA methylation and hydroxymethylation

The existence of DNA methylation was firstly proposed by Hotchkiss in 1948. More precisely, in those experiments, Hotchkiss was able to separate a modified cytosine by using chromatography. It was called 5-methylcytosine (5mc) and it was hypothesised that this form could be commonly present in nature. However, its role in regulation of genetic expression was not unveiled until the decade of the 1980s [3].

What is currently known as 'DNA methylation' is, in fact, cytosine methylation, and it consists of the transferring of a methyl group to 5′ carbon of cytosine, to generate 5mc. This modification is extremely active during embryo development, but it is relatively slower in differentiated cells, and generates a characteristic pattern of methylation distributed along the genome. This pattern is not part of a random distribution but a tightly regulated distribution.

DNA methylation is frequently observed in cytosines adjacent to guanines, in the so-called CpG sites. This dinucleotide is mainly enriched at promoter sequences where it is repeated and grouped generating what is known as 'CpG island'. These 'islands' comprise around 1000 base pairs of the promoter region, with a high degree of conservation between species, becoming clear hotspots for methylation. Given the role of gene promoters, it was proposed that methylation acts as a regulator of genetic expression and this was the more replicated finding throughout research in life sciences. However, methylation was also observed in gene bodies, introns and intergenic sequences, with other functions that still remain elusive. On the other hand, it was also described methylation of non-CpG sites in murine cellular models or human stem cells, however its role is currently unclear, and it is under extensive research [4].

DNA methylation is a tightly regulated process and we can distinguish several types of enzymes that catalyse the necessary steps either to write or to erase this addition. The DNA methyltransferase (DNMT) catalysed the addition of methyl groups to cytosines. Three members of this DNMT family were described (DNMT1, DNMT3a and DNMT3b) and, despite its similarities, they have unique functions. DNMT1 catalyses the addition of methyl groups to the nascent DNA chain during replication, maintaining the methylation pattern of the cell lineage. However, DNMT3a and DNMT3b do not show specificity for hemimethylated sequences, so it was proposed that these enzymes are responsible for *de novo* methylation. However, how these enzymes target specific DNA regions or sequences are still unknown. There is also described a third isoform, called DNMT3L, that lacks its catalytic domain and it is mainly expressed during early development and in germinal cells. Although without its own catalytic function, this isoform could be associated to DNMT3a and DNMT3b to promote their methyltransferase activity.

On the other hand, the erasing of DNA methylation patterns could be a passive or active process. In mammals, DNA methylation in the form of 5mC can be actively reversed to unmodified cytosine (C) through TET dioxygenase-mediated oxidation of 5mC to 5-hydroxymethylcytosine (5hmC), 5-formylcytosine (5fC) and 5-carboxylcytosine (5caC), followed by replication-dependent dilution or thymine DNA glycosylase (TDG)-dependent base excision repair [5]. Instead, as a passive process, it was proposed that several chemical changes (deamination, oxidation) could generate a modified cytosine that activates the base excision repair (BER) system that eventually replaces that cytosine.

However, 5hmc it is also a modification that may have more biological function, different from an intermediary product of demethylation. In fact, high expression of this modification is found in brain tissue and during embryogenesis as well as in stem cells. It was proposed that this modification could influence the genome structuration during early phases of development. In fact, it was described that oxidation of 5mc to 5-hmc only takes place in paternal (but not in maternal) pronucleous [6, 7]. Regarding brain tissue, Wang et al. [8] reported a positive correlation between 5-hmc levels and cerebellum development in humans. Given that the previous methods to interrogate 5mc were unable to distinguish from 5hmc, this modification has only recently been assessed as an actual epigenetic marker. Therefore, many of its biological functions are currently under research.

## 2.1. DNA methylation as a research tool: main findings in schizophrenia

The development of methylation-specific polymerase chain reaction (MSP) allowed us to interrogate specific DNA sequences to assess its methylation status. In this technique, DNA is treated with sodium bisulfite that deaminates unmethylated cytosines to generate thymine (uracil). This conversion does not occur when there is a methyl group at the 5′ position of cytosine, which remains as a cytosine. This change allows researchers to generate specific primers for PCR amplification, in order to discriminate methylated from unmethylated alleles. This technique was a useful tool to understand the pattern of methylation in different gene regions. However, it was mainly applied to research promoter sequences trying to find correlations with gene expressions. In general, it was accepted that high levels of promoter's methylation mean decreased expression, whereas lower levels mean increased genetic expression. Of course, this is just a general rule and it is not applied to all genes. However, with this general idea, brain tissue of schizophrenic patients was evaluated. Although interesting, the main results are controversial. The base of this controversy relies on the usage of MSP, that only allows to interrogate some selected CpG sites, which leads to a fragmented information if we want to extrapolate (and correlate) to genetic expression. Keeping this situation in mind will facilitate us to understand some controversial findings in the next paragraphs.

Initial reports try to shed some light on the molecular mechanism of schizophrenia by using MSP and focused on the methylation changes of single genes. In this sense, in schizophrenic brain tissue, a higher level of methylation of GABA promoter regions that leads to lower levels of GABA mRNA was observed [9]. A similar finding was observed regarding *RELN* gene, that codifies reelin, a secreted protein involved in neurodevelopment with putative roles in schizophrenia onset [10].

Several other genes also showed changes of methylation pattern in schizophrenia, as those related to glutamate and serotonin signalling. For instance, hypermethylation of glutamate transporter genes or serotonin receptor genes (leading to a lower protein expression) was observed in schizophrenic brain [11, 12], but not in other studies [13].

On the other hand, specific changes of gene methylation carried out in specific anatomical regions could represent a more concrete regulatory event. For instance, hypomethylation of *COMT* gene (that leads to higher levels of COMT mRNA) may contribute to dopamine degradation in frontal lobes of schizophrenic patients [14], although it is a result that has not been replicated in other studies [13].

Finally, in a recent study, Alelú-Paz et al. [15] compared the DNA methylation pattern across the human genome in several normal and schizophrenic brain areas that have previously been linked to neuropathological features of schizophrenia, such as dorsolateral prefrontal cortex (DLPFC), hippocampus and the anterior cingulate cortex (ACC), reported several genes associated with cognitive impairment characteristic of schizophrenia, such as *LIF*, *PRKCE* or *CNTNAP2*.

We may indicate several studies related to single-gene changes in brain samples. However, currently scientists are more interested in understanding the epigenetic changes as a whole and, in fact, the recent development of Epigenetic-Wide Association Studies (EWAS) allow researchers to interrogate several thousand methylated sequences in a single chip. Even more, this technique is not restricted to gene promoter but to all genome, including gene bodies, introns and intergenic regions, leading to a more complete scenario of methylation changes. It is relatively easy to assess around 450,000 selected sequences in a single chip. And the number of interrogated regions is rapidly increasing. In fact, by using this technique with schizophrenic brain tissues, it was demonstrated that changes in methylation occur along several portions of genes of glutamate transporters as well as dopamine and serotonin receptors, among others. In blood cells, this technique was also applied to study discordant monozygotic twins, where researchers observed several differentially methylated regions (DMR) between twins, in genes related to cell death, survival and cell movement [16].

By using EWAS technique, researchers are able to find several candidates as predisposition marks or putative biomarkers but, despite its higher resolution, EWAS generates a huge amount of information and the limits of its usage in diagnosis, treatment or prognosis of schizophrenia remains still elusive. It is still a novel field of investigation and its findings will need several years to clearly reveal molecular aspects of schizophrenia. In this sense, EWAS confounding factors are still under research. For instance, antipsychotics (as clozapine or sulpiride), smoking, age and several other environmental factors may also affect methylation and be detected by applying this approach.

An additional problem for using this technique is sample selection. Unfortunately, several EWAS were (and still are) carried out in peripheral blood or even in saliva samples [17]. More than a decade ago, it was completely demonstrated that epigenetic patterns are cell specific, so findings from tissues other than brain are controversial in their correlation to schizophrenia [17]. Even more, different anatomical zones (or cells) of brain may contain its specific epigenetic signature, leading to complications in the interpretation of results [15, 18]. Also, statistical analysis is key to ensure validity of results, therefore scientist need to be aware of these points to trust the technique and its results.

## 3. Accessing to the genetic information: histone modifications

If we were able to extend all the DNA molecule that lies in the nucleus, we would have a line measuring 2 m. In addition, all this information should be packed into a space measuring around 5 μm (1 μm is the millionth part of the meter). DNA condensation is key to ensure that all the genetic information is protected while is not in use, but it also need to assure that the required information could be accessible according to cells' needs. This condensation is achieved via several highly regulated steps, which begin with the formation of a DNA:protein complex. In doing this, a group of proteins called 'histones' are the key. Five histones have been described: H1, H2a, H2b, H3 and H4. Two molecules of every histone (except H1) are grouped to form a kind of flattened disk around which DNA is spun (approximately) two turns: this complex of protein and DNA is known as 'nucleosome' and it is the minimal structure implicated in DNA condensation. Histone H1 is located 'under' every nucleosome to keep them in place, and around 50 base pairs ahead another nucleosome is formed [19]. This sequence is repeated along the DNA molecule. In successive steps, groups of nucleosomes are gathered to form a highly condensed molecule. Finally, the mitotic chromosome represents the higher level of condensation of a DNA molecule.

This condensation is necessary to pack the DNA in the limited space of nuclei, but also to 'hide' genetic information, that may not be potentially necessary for the homeostasis of cells. Being more precise, it is well-known that a part of genetic information should not be physically accessible (for instance, the condensation of one chromosome X in males): this part of the genome constitutes what is called heterochromatin.

However, another part of genetic information should be accessible according to cell's needs which constitute what is called euchromatin. Although accessible, euchromatin information is still packed, so how this information is reached in a condensed molecule? As we previously indicate, eight molecules of histones form the protein core of nucleosome. As with every protein, histones have an N-terminal portion that is called the 'histones' tails' and are subject of different kinds of modifications: the post-translational modifications of histones. When a post-translational modification occurs, it implies a structural modification that is communicated as a nucleosome's opening or closing. Under these circumstances, genetic information is more accessible (or not) to transcription factors, which eventually promotes the gene expression.

Among these modifications we can find methylation, acetylation, phosphorylation, ubiquitination and others. These modifications can occur on many different residues, some of them harbouring more than one type of modification (i.e., residues can be either acetylated or methylated). Likewise, we can find different types of modifications on different amino acid residues. To complicate this picture, each modification carries implicit information that may indicate an opening (or closing) of nucleosomes, affecting the access of transcription factors to genetic information. Even more, modifications are different (and independent) in every tail of every histone. In the next paragraphs, we will describe some of the better-established histone modifications and indicate the most replicated role in regulation of gene expression. However, we need to take into account that the 'final conclusion' of all these modifications is, in fact, a balance between 'opening' and 'closing' signals, that eventually will lead to allow (or not) transcription factors to generate a mRNA.

### 3.1. Histone acetylation

One of the best-studied histone modifications is acetylation. It consists in the transfer of an acetyl group from acetyl coenzyme A to a specific histone lysine. This action is modulated by two enzymes, histone acetyltransferases (HATs) and histone deacetylases (HDACs): increases in former activity promote acetylation and the corresponding increase in gene transcription and increases in HDAC activity, which involves removing the acetyl group from histones, results in a repression of gene expression.

### 3.2. Histone phosphorylation

Histone phosphorylation is restricted to tyrosine (Y), serine (S) and threonine (T) residues. It has been described eight characterised phosphorylation sites on histones H2A, H2B, H3 and H4, which have been linked to specific cognate kinases. Although we still do not know in depth the role of histone phosphorylation, probably is important in the interpretation of combinatorial post-translational modifications which together regulate various biological processes, including gene transcription and DNA repair.

### 3.3. Histone methylation

Acting S-adenosyl-l-methionine as the methyl donor, the methylation of histones is carried out, mainly, by lysine methyltransferases (KMTs) and, to a lesser extent, by protein arginine (R) methyltransferases (PRMTs). More than 50 different histone methyltransferases have been described in humans, including SET1, MLL, SMYD3, ESET, G9a, SETDB or EZH2, that catalyse methylation of H3 at K4, K9 and K27 in mammalian cells.

On the contrary, histone demethylation, that is, the removal of methyl groups via histone lysine demethylases (KDMs) is, at the very least, a controversial topic. The discovery of KDMs suggests that this mechanism is not a permanent modification. To date, two classes of enzymes have been described: the amine oxidase-type lysine-specific demethylases 1 and 2 (KDM1A and KDM1B) and the Jumonji C (JmjC) domain-containing histone demethylases.

### 3.4. Histone ubiquitination

Clearly, the less well studied post-translational modifications. We know this mechanism acts by the addition of ubiquitin molecule to specific lysine residues on histone tails, which requires the sequential activities of ubiquitin-activating enzymes (E1), ubiquitin-conjugating enzymes (E2) and ubiquitin ligase enzymes (E3). It is important to note that histones are the most abundantly monoubiquitinated conjugates in the nucleus of mammalian cells, including ubiquitination at K119 on histone H2A, K34 and K120 on histone H2B, all of them associated with the transcriptional control of gene expression and the DNA damage response, including transcriptional reprogramming and DNA repair.

A summary of the aforementioned modification is shown in **Figure 3**.

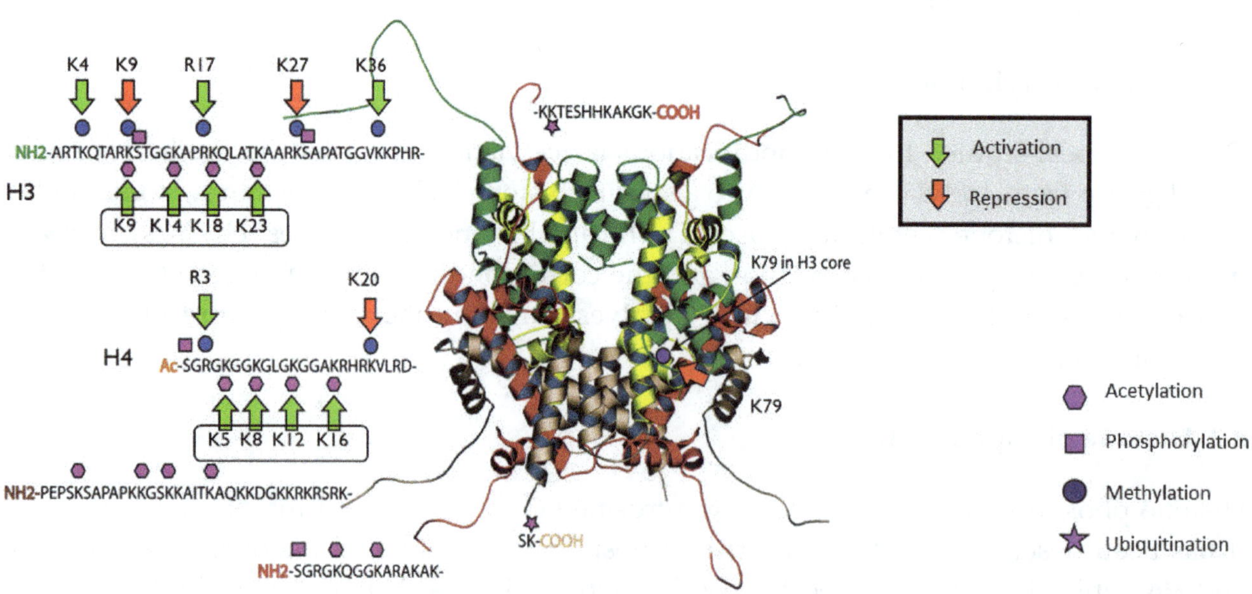


**Figure 3.** Main histone modifications and their roles regarding gene expression. The complexity of this information may facilitate gene expression or repression according to environmental (and internal) signals. The final combination of every modification will generate the proper response.

### 3.5. Histone modifications and molecular pathology of schizophrenia

Given their complexity, histone modifications were mainly studied in pathologies with well-characterised cellular and animal models. Unfortunately, the role of histone modifications is not clear for the development of mental disorders, although we find some post-mortem brain tissue studies that can be established as an interesting starting point.

Huang and Akbarian reported shifts in the prefrontal cortex chromatin surrounding GAD1 promoter accompanied by a decrease in GAD1 mRNA [20], whilst the latter author suggested a correlation between methylation of histone H3 at arginine 17 and down-regulation of several metabolic genes in schizophrenia [21].

Chase et al. [22] employed fresh-frozen parietal cortex post-mortem tissue, found significant increased levels of H3K9me2 in parietal cortical samples from patients with schizophrenia when compared to healthy controls, suggesting that initial inactivation of gene promoter activity at various schizophrenia candidate genes can result in gradual entrenchment of the heterochromatin state as a result of disease chronicity and disuse.

Other authors, focused on the role of interneurons in the pathophysiology of the disorders, suggested that acetylation of H3K9K14 correlated with gene expression levels for several schizophrenia-related genes, including GAD1, considered to be among the most frequently replicated findings in schizophrenia post-mortem brain [23].

Kurita and colleagues found a relationship between long treatment with antipsychotics and down-regulation of GRM2, a metabotropic glutamate 2 receptor, through decreased histone acetylation at its promoter region in the human frontal cortex, which could represent a promising new target for schizophrenia treatment [24].

Finally, in a recent paper, Schroeder et al. [25] reported decreased HDAC2 transcript in the dorsolateral prefrontal cortex of schizophrenia patients which represents a set of targets with demonstrated therapeutic relevance.

It is easy to see that we still need to understand more in depth the dynamic changes of histones during the development of mental disorders. Maybe, the main obstacle is not having proper models either animal or cellular. In this sense, the rapid development of techniques that implies stem cells (and induced pluripotent stem cells) may represent an option in the next years.

## 4. Regulation of genetic information by RNA molecules

A few decades ago, the huge amount of apparently useless DNA sequences lead scientist to coin the term 'junk sequences'. Nowadays, we know that a clear majority of the genome is transcribed, but only 2% generates proteins. So, a third epigenetic mechanism includes several activities carried out by different types of RNA molecules that were called 'non-coding RNA' (ncRNA) to differentiate from coding RNA that generates proteins.

The ncRNAs are classified according to their length: short non-coding RNAs (sncRNA) (length < 30 nucleotides and <200 nucleotides in general) and long non-coding RNAs (lncRNA) (length > 200 nucleotides). Among sncRNA we can find the so-called short interfering RNA (siRNA), microRNAs (miRNA) and Piwi-interacting RNA (piRNA).

Short non-coding RNAs are widely known, as well as the processes carried out to generate them. For a more extensive review of these molecular aspects, see Ref. [26]. In general, their functions are related to protein silencing by interfering the mRNA processing. Long non-coding RNA, as the name indicates, do not generates proteins, although their processing may be closer (or similar) to the normal mRNA. Furthermore, the length could easily reach more than 2000 nucleotides, they could be distributed either at nucleus or cytoplasm and their origins belong to introns or to transposable elements. Recently, it was observed a new type of lncRNA, which has its origin at the intergenic regions. This molecule was called long intergenic non-coding RNA (lincRNA).

In general, both types of transcripts are generated as a response to face environmental changes or as intermediary in other cellular processes. Even more, DNA methylation or histone modifications are targets of (or responsible for) their actions. For instance, some sncRNA are transcribed according to the methylation pattern of the specific gene (either at promoters or bodies), generating a siRNA that silence a target protein. On the other hand, the X chromosome silencing is mainly mediated by a 17 kb lncRNA that acts as an intermediary of histone methylations that generates 'repressive' marks (H3K27me3).

Although interesting and powerful, these mechanisms are poorly understood with regard to mental disorders and there is a clear lack of information. Regarding schizophrenia, there are relatively few reports that describe a general landscape or putative functions of non-coding RNA in development, onset, prognosis or diagnosis of this mental disorder. This is partly because this area is currently under active research (but mainly in oncology where ncRNA roles are better established). This also leads to generate only fragmented data with regard to other diseases that are different from cancer. Given this picture, we can summary some findings:

- Some miRNA showed association with schizophrenia risk in Chinese populations [27] although some controversy during its replication was generated [28].
- miRNAs were proposed as biomarkers of schizophrenia by assessing them in blood samples [29].
- Furthermore, miRNA seem to be dysregulated even in progenitor cells from schizophrenic patients [30].
- By using microarrays, lncRNAs were assessed in blood cells of schizophrenic patients and researchers found that downregulation of two lncRNA (from 40,000 tested lncRNA) were associated to better treatment outcomes and symptoms when patients were evaluated by using the Positive and Negative Syndrome Scale (PANSS) [31].
- A recent report proposed to lncRNAs as key elements in the dynamic of neurostructure and, in consequence, may have putative roles in schizophrenia development [32].

As we previously indicate, this are only selected items, and we hope that we will soon get a more complete view of the role of RNA molecules in schizophrenia development.

## 5. Epigenetics in the development of treatments: feasibility and challenges

Throughout this chapter, we summarised the main epigenetic findings focused on schizophrenic patients. Do these findings open any door to treatment development? Certainly, it is hard to predict the actual utility of epigenetic findings in drugs or treatment development and we may need to observe what happens in another pathology, mainly cancer. Nervi et al. [33], provide us with a more concrete point of view of clinical trials of epigenetic treatments for solid tumours.

With regard to schizophrenia, HDACs inhibitors are promising drug targets. In this sense, it was observed that HDACs expression may be associated to schizophrenia-like phenotypes [34] and that also their mRNA could be differentially expressed (and reduced) in prefrontal cortex of schizophrenic patients [25]. Valproic acid is a well-characterised HDAC inhibitor and it may be used in combination with clozapine (a demethylating agent) in order to promote chromatin remodelling, and eventually, to correct genetic expression deficits [35]. On the other hand, the role of HDACs isoform-specific inhibitors is still under frantic research. For instance, it was proposed that HDAC2 inhibition may help to treat symptoms in schizophrenia [24, 36]. Finally, methylating and demethylating agents lack specificity and its usage is restricted to research in cell models.

Despite the aforementioned, we must keep in mind that the possibility of treatment development arises from an extensive knowledge of the related epigenetic mechanisms about the pathology. In other words, firstly, we need the knowledge of basic processes and then we can develop successful treatments. Unfortunately, this could take time, and, in schizophrenia, we are at the beginning of a new research era, and still lack information about the epigenetic mechanisms triggered along its onset and progression. Therefore, in the next decade we will see an increase in our knowledge. The success of this approach will rely on sample selection, statistical accuracy and generated hypotheses by responsible and committed scientist aimed to obtain reliable results instead adding 'noise' to research in mental disorders [37].

## 6. Conclusions

Epigenetic mechanisms add a new layer of information that improves the cell plasticity against environmental changes. These processes are key to maintaining cellular health while frequently also being disorganised during the development of illness. Although there is no change to DNA sequence, these mechanisms play several roles in reading or providing access to the genetic information. Given this feature, epigenetic mechanisms were proposed as new targets to understand how a genetic background interacts with an environment to develop schizophrenia. The first results obtained were promising, showing changes in methylation pattern of specific genes. However, this was only a piece of information and scientists are currently working in the development and application of more powerful techniques, such as Epigenetic-wide association studies. On the other hand, there is still an almost unexplored field regarding of role of histone modifications in the development of mental disorders. Great efforts are being made to unravel their role, although there is still a clear lack of information. We could indicate the same regarding other mechanisms as chromatin remodelling, therefore it is to be expected that in the next decades, an increasing amount of data will provide us with a more complete landscape of the contribution of epigenetics to the development of mental disorders as schizophrenia.

## Author details

Ariel Cariaga-Martinez and Raúl Alelú-Paz*

*Address all correspondence to: ralelu@canismajoris.es

Laboratory for Neuroscience of Mental Disorders Elena Pessino, Madrid, Spain

## References

[1] Noble D. Conrad Waddington and the origin of epigenetics. The Journal of Experimental Biology. 2015;**218**:816-818. DOI: 10.1242/jeb.120071

[2] Urdinguio R, Sanchez-Mut J, Esteller M. Epigenetic mechanisms in neurological diseases: Genes, syndromes, and therapies. Lancet Neurology. 2009;**8**(11):1056-1072. DOI: 10.1016/S1474-4422(09)70262-5

[3] Moore L, Le T, Fan G. DNA methylation and its basic function. Neuropsychopharmacology. 2013;**38**(1):23-38. DOI: 10.1038/npp.2012.112

[4] He Y, Ecker JR. Non-CG methylation in the human genome. Annual Review of Genomics and Human Genetics. 2015;**16**:55-77. DOI: 10.1146/annurev-genom-090413-025437

[5] Wu X, Zhang Y. TET-mediated active DNA demethylation: Mechanism, function and beyond. Nature Reviews. Genetics. 2017;**18**(9):517-534. DOI: 10.1038/nrg.2017.33

[6] Iqbal K, Jin S, Pfeifer G, Szabó PE. Reprogramming of the paternal genome upon fertilization involves genome-wide oxidation of 5-methylcytosine. Proceedings of the National Academy of Sciences of the United States of America. 2011;**108**(9):3642-3647. DOI: 10.1073/pnas.1014033108

[7] Wossidlo M, Arand J, Sebastiano V, Lepikhov K, Boiani M, Reinhardt R, Schöler H, Walter J. Dynamic link of DNA demethylation, DNA strand breaks and repair in mouse zygotes. The EMBO Journal. 2010;**29**(11):1877-1888. DOI: 10.1038/emboj.2010.80

[8] Wang T, Pan Q, Lin L, Szulwach K, Song C, He C, Wu H, Warren S, Jin P, Duan R, Li X. Genome-wide DNA hydroxymethylation changes are associated with neurodevelopmental genes in the developing human cerebellum. Human Molecular Genetics. 2012;**21**(26):5500-5510. DOI: 10.1093/hmg/dds394

[9] Ruzicka W, Zhubi A, Veldic M, Grayson D, Costa E, Guidotti A. Selective epigenetic alteration of layer I GABAergic neurons isolated from prefrontal cortex of schizophrenia patients using laser-assisted microdissection. Molecular Psychiatry. 2007;**12**(4):385-397

[10] Grayson D, Jia X, Chen Y, Sharma R, Mitchell CP, Guidotti A, Costa E. Reelin promoter hypermethylation in schizophrenia. Proceedings of the National Academy of Sciences of the United States of America. 2005;**102**(26):9341-9346

[11] Mill J, Tang T, Kaminsky Z, Khare T, Yazdanpanah S, Bouchard L, Jia P, Assadzadeh A, Flanagan J, Schumacher A, Wang SC, Petronis A. Epigenomic profiling reveals DNA-methylation changes associated with major psychosis. American Journal of Human Genetics. 2008;**82**(3):696-711. DOI: 10.1016/j.ajhg.2008.01.008

[12] Abdolmaleky H, Yaqubi S, Papageorgis P, Lambert AW, Ozturk S, Sivaraman V, Thiagalingam S. Epigenetic dysregulation of HTR2A in the brain of patients with schizophrenia and bipolar disorder. Schizophrenia Research. 2011;**129**(2-3):183-190. DOI: 10.1016/j.schres.2011.04.007

[13] Alelú-Paz R, González-Corpas A, Ashour N, Escanilla A, Monje A, Guerrero Márquez C, Algora Weber M, Ropero S. DNA methylation pattern of gene promoters of major neurotransmitter systems in older patients with schizophrenia with severe and mild cognitive impairment. International Journal of Geriatric Psychiatry. 2015;**30**(6):558-565. DOI: 10.1002/gps.4182

[14] Abdolmaleky H, Cheng K, Faraone S, Wilcox M, Glatt S, Gao F, Smith C, Shafa R, Aeali B, Carnevale J, Pan H, Papageorgis P, Ponte J, Sivaraman V, Tsuang M, Thiagalingam S. Hypomethylation of MB-COMT promoter is a major risk factor for schizophrenia and bipolar disorder. Human Molecular Genetics. 2006;**15**(21):3132-3145

[15] Alelú-Paz R, Carmona F, Sanchez-Mut J, Cariaga-Martínez A, González-Corpas A, Ashour N, Orea M, Escanilla A, Monje A, Guerrero Márquez C, Saiz-Ruiz J, Esteller M, Ropero S. Epigenetics in schizophrenia: A pilot study of global DNA methylation in different brain regions associated with higher cognitive functions. Frontiers in Psychology. 2016;**7**(1496). DOI: 10.3389/fpsyg.2016.01496

[16] Castellani C, Laufer B, Melka M, Diehl E, O'Reilly R, Singh SMDNA. Methylation differences in monozygotic twin pairs discordant for schizophrenia identifies psychosis related genes and networks. BMC Medical Genomics. 2015;**8**:17. DOI: 10.1186/s12920-015-0093-1

[17] Cariaga-Martinez AE, Alelú-Paz R. False data, positive results in neurobiology: Moving beyond the epigenetics of blood and saliva samples in mental disorders. Journal of Negative Results in BioMedicine. 2016;**15**:21. DOI: 10.1186/s12952-016-0064-x

[18] Ladd-Acosta C, Pevsner J, Sabunciyan S, Yolken R, Webster MJ, Dinkins T, Callinan P, Fan J, Potash J, Feinberg APDNA. Methylation signatures within the human brain. American Journal of Human Genetics. 2007;**21**(6):1304-1315

[19] Portela A, Esteller M. Epigenetic modifications and human disease. Nature Biotechnology. 2010;**28**(10):1057-1068. DOI: 10.1038/nbt.1685

[20] Huang HS, Akbarian S. GAD1 mRNA expression and DNA methylation in prefrontal cortex of subjects with schizophrenia. PLoS One. 2007:**2**(8):e809. DOI: 10.1371/journal.pone.0000809

[21] Akbarian S, Ruehl M, Bliven E, Luiz L, Peranelli A, Baker S, Roberts R, Bunney W, Conley R, Jones E, Tamminga C, Guo Y. Chromatin alterations associated with down-regulated metabolic gene expression in the prefrontal cortex of subjects with schizophrenia. Archives of General Psychiatry. 2005;**62**:829-840. DOI: 10.1001/archpsyc.62.8.829

[22] Chase K, Gavin D, Guidotti A, Sharma R. Histone methylation at H3K9: Evidence for a restrictive epigenome in schizophrenia. Schizophrenia Research. 2013;**149**:15-20

[23] Tang B, Dean B, Thomas E. Disease- and age-related changes in histone acetylation at gene promoters in psychiatric disorders. Translational Psychiatry. 2011;**1**(12):e64. DOI: 10.1038/tp.2011.61

[24] Kurita M, Holloway T, Garcia-Bea A, Kozlenkov A, Friedman A, Moreno J, Heshmati M, Golden S, Kennedy P, Takahashi N, Dietz D, Mocci G, Gabilondo A, Hanks J, Umali A, Callado L, Gallitano A, Neve R, Shen L, Buxbaum J, Han M, Nestler E, Meana J, Russo S, Gonzalez-Maeso J. HDAC2 regulates atypical antipsychotic responses through the modulation of mGlu2 promoter activity. Nature Neuroscience. 2012;**15**:1245-1254. DOI: 10.1038/nn.3181

[25] Schroeder F, Gilbert T, Feng N, Taillon B, Volkow N, Innis R, Hooker J, Lipska B. Expression of HDAC2 but not HDAC1 transcript is reduced in dorsolateral prefrontal cortex of patients with schizophrenia. ACS Chemical Neuroscience. 2017;**8**(3):662-668. DOI: 10.1021/acschemneuro.6b00372

[26] Qureshi I, Mehler M. Emerging roles of non-coding RNAs in brain evolution, development, plasticity and disease. Nature Reviews. Neuroscience. 2012;**13**(8):528-541. DOI: 10.1038/nrn3234

[27] Ou M, Liu G, Xiao D, Zhang B, Guo C, Ye X, Liu Y, Zhang N, Wang M, Han Y, Ye X, Jing C, Yang G. Association between miR-137 polymorphism and risk of schizophrenia: A meta-analysis. Genetics and Molecular Research. 2016;**15**(3). DOI: 10.4238/gmr.15038703

[28] Yuan J, Cheng Z, Zhang F, Zhou Z, Yu S, Jin C. Lack of association between microRNA-137 SNP rs1625579 and schizophrenia in a replication study of Han Chinese. Molecular Genetics and Genomics. 2015;**290**(1):297-301. DOI: 10.1007/s00438-014-0924-3

[29] Liu S, Zhang F, Wang X, Shugart Y, Zhao Y, Li X, Liu Z, Sun N, Yang C, Zhang K, Yue W, Yu X, Diagnostic XY. Value of blood-derived microRNAs for schizophrenia: Results of a meta-analysis and validation. Scientific Reports. 2017;**7**(1):15328. DOI: 10.1038/s41598-017-15751-5

[30] Topol A, Zhu S, Hartley B, English J, Hauberg M, Tran N, Rittenhouse C, Simone A, Ruderfer D, Johnson J, Readhead B, Hadas Y, Gochman P, Wang Y, Shah H, Cagney G, Rapoport J, Gage F, Dudley J, Sklar P, Mattheisen M, Cotter D, Fang G, Brennand K. Dysregulation of miRNA-9 in a subset of schizophrenia patient-derived neural progenitor cells. Cell Reports. 2016;**15**(5):1024-1036. DOI: 10.1016/j.celrep.2016.03.090

[31] Chen S, Sun X, Niu W, Kong L, He M, Li W, Zhong A, Lu J, Zhang L. Aberrant expression of long non-coding RNAs in schizophrenia patients. Medical Science Monitor. 2016; **22**:3340-3351

[32] Merelo V, Durand D, Lescallette A, Vrana K, Hong L, Faghihi M, Bellon A. Associating schizophrenia, long non-coding RNAs and neurostructural dynamic. Frontiers in Molecular Neuroscience. 2015;**8**:57. DOI: 10.3389/fnmol.2015.00057

[33] Nervi E, Codacci-Pisanelli G. Epigenetic treatment of solid tumours: A review of clinical trials. Clinical Epigenetics. 2015;**7**:127. DOI: https://doi.org/10.1186/s13148-015-0157-2

[34] Bahari-Javan S, Varbanov H, Halder R, Benito E, Kaurani L, Burkhardt S, Anderson-Schmidt H, Anghelescu I, Budde M, Stilling RM, Costa J, Medina J, Dietrich DE, Figge C, Folkerts H, Gade K, Heilbronner U, Koller M, Konrad C, Nussbeck SY, Scherk H, Spitzer C, Stierl S, Stöckel J, Thiel A, von Hagen M, Zimmermann J, Zitzelsberger A, Schulz S, Schmitt A, Delalle I, Falkai P, Schulze TG, Dityatev A, Sananbenesi F, Fischer A. HDAC1 links early life stress to schizophrenia-like phenotypes. Proceedings of the National Academy of Sciences of the United States of America. 2017;**114**(23):E4686-E4694. DOI: 10.1073/pnas.1613842114

[35] Guidotti A, Grayson DDNA. Methylation and demethylation as targets for antipsychotic therapy. Dialogues in Clinical Neuroscience. 2014;**16**(3):419-429

[36] Hyman SE. Target practice: HDAC inhibitors for schizophrenia. Nature Neuroscience. 2012;**15**(9):1180-1181. DOI: 10.1038/nn.3200

[37] Maj M. Understanding the pathophysiology of schizophrenia: Are we on the wrong or on the right track? Schizophrenia Research. 2011;**127**(1-3):20-21. DOI: 10.1016/j.schres.2011.01.002

8

# Comorbid Anxiety in Schizophrenia and Schizoaffective Disorder

Delia M. Podea, Aurora I. Sabau and Karol J. Wild

### Abstract

There is some evidence that antipsychotic medication (Quetiapine) is somewhat efficient in reducing anxiety in schizophrenic patients.

This study compared the efficacy of Olanzapine and Quetiapine versus Risperidone, Aripiprazole, and Haloperidolum in reducing the anxiety symptoms in patients diagnosed with schizophrenia and schizoaffective disorder hospitalized in the Psychiatry Department of Arad between 2013–2014.

Considering the treatment, 63 subjects were divided in two groups: T1 (treated with Olanzapine and Quetiapine) and T2 (treated with Haloperidolum, Risperidone, and Aripiprazol).

Anxiety is frequent in the course of schizophrenia and schizoaffective disorder with significant differences among the two groups. After treatment, the level of anxiety reduced with significant improvement of total score of PANSS; the effect is higher in group T2 compared to T1. Before treatment, anxiety is positively correlated with scores of PANSSN ($r=.285$; $p=0.010$), PANSST ($r=.260$; $p=0.040$), and HAM-D ($r=.455$; $p<0.0001$).YMRS is negatively correlated with negative items of PANSSN scale ($r=-.321$; $p=0.010$). IQ (intelligence quotient) was decreased posttreatment for both treatments, but T1 had had a higher effect on it.

Some antipsychotics have been reported to be successful in reducing the anxiety level in psychotic patients: in group T2 the treatment has a higher effect on anxiety and lower size effect on intelligence.

**Keywords:** Anxiety, Schizophrenia, Schizoaffective Disorder, Antipsychotics

## 1. Introduction

Anxiety disorders are serious, debilitating conditions, with wide discrepancies being found in the reports of the prevalence rates, in clinical and epidemiological studies.

Based on the literature, the rate of prevalence of anxiety disorder in patients with schizophrenia or schizoaffective disorder remains uncertain due to limiting factors: the definitions of the disorders themselves the sample size, the study procedures and the utilization of different measures and clinical assessments.

A meta-analysis by Achim et al., in 2011, found a prevalence rate for anxiety disorder of 38.3% in the schizophrenic population, compared with 28.8% reported for the general population [1].

Seedat et al., in 2007, in a study of hospitalized schizophrenic patients, found that 25% suffered from anxiety disorder [2]. In 2007, using a sample of inpatients, Ciapparelli et al. found anxiety disorders in 74% of the subjects [3].

In a study conducted by Braga et al., in 2004, 42% of schizophrenic outpatients presented anxiety disorders [4].

In schizoaffective disorder, the rates of anxiety disorders range from 32% in outpatients [3] to 45% in inpatients [5].

Schizophrenia is a common, chronic and severe mental illness defined by the presence of delusions, hallucinations, and disorganized behavior (positive symptoms); by the presence of apathy, social withdrawal, and involution (negative symptoms); and by cognitive disorganization [6].

It has long been known that anxiety has an important role in the psychopathology of schizophrenia. However, the nature of the development of anxiety disorder in psychosis is not well understood.

The presence of the comorbidity of anxiety in major psychotic disorders (schizophrenia, schizoaffective disorder) results in reduced cognitive functioning, increases the severity of comorbid medical conditions, increases the risk of reoccurrence, adds to internalized stigma, reduces functioning, and has a negative impact on the overall outcome for the patient.

Comorbid anxiety in schizophrenia and schizoaffective disorder is associated with the more positive symptoms: extrapyramidal symptoms suggesting more severe medication side effects [6], an increase in drug/alcohol abuse, a worsening of social and professional functioning, and in the quality of life [7].

Anxiety is common among patients with schizophrenia or schizoafective disorder, and it may also manifest itself as a symptom during an acute psychotic episode [8], as a result of the side effects of medication or as a symptom of a comorbid anxiety disorder. Patients are generally discharged as soon as their psychotic episode is resolved, with little recognition of the presence of an anxiety disorder [9].

It is difficult to evaluate the relation of anxiety to psychotic symptoms since it is not clear which anxiety symptoms the disorder is associated with. Furthermore, the operational criteria developed for the assessment of the level of anxiety found in the nonpsychotic population (Hamilton Anxiety Rating Scale, Yale Brown Obsession Compulsion Rating) may themselves be problematic. Extrapyramidal symptoms which develop secondary to neuroleptic treatment may coincide with anxiety symptoms [7].

Progress in understanding the etiology of comorbid anxiety in major psychotic disorders such as schizophrenia or schizoaffective disorder has been made. For example, in the field of genetics, two basic genetic strategies have been developed, enabling a better understanding of the etiology of anxiety: the linkage approach and the polymorphism or susceptibility allele, which associates different genes (e.g., dysbindin, the gene for the dystrobrevin-binding protein 1, located within the linkage peak on chromosome 6 p; or chromosomal regions, e.g., 6p22.3) with traits or illness [10].

Generally, anxiety disorders are relatively responsive to treatment so greater awareness should be paid to their comorbidity with psychosis in order to obtain clinical benefits.

Comorbid anxiety may have implications for treatment choice. Generally, anxiety is considered to be secondary to the psychotic condition and it is expected to improve simultaneous with an improvement in the schizophrenic symptoms. There is some evidence that antipsychotic medication (such as Quetiapine) has some degree of efficacy in reducing anxiety in schizophrenic patients [11].

The treatment for acute schizophrenia involves one of the newer generation antipsychotic drugs which is well-tolerated and can be used for maintenance therapy. In particular, it is desirable to use drugs with little sedative effect in order to optimize functioning and to preserve the quality of life [12,13]. However, lack of compliance with antipsychotics must be taken in consideration as it is known that nonadherence plays a significant role in psychotic relapse. In these cases, long-acting injectable antipsychotics (administered at two to four week intervals) are preferable as they may result in a lower risk of dose-related adverse effects (because of lower peak antipsychotic plasma levels) and lower rates of hospitalization due to acute exacerbations. These factors contribute to improving the individual quality of life.

A personalized treatment approach is necessary in the management of comorbid anxiety with schizophrenia which should be based on the pathogeneses and the clinical assessments.

In clinical practice, in those patients with significant agitation and anxiety, drugs with low sedative potential are not sufficient for the reduction of these symptoms. In these patients, anxiety may interfere with compliance to medication. So, benzodiazepines or sedative neuroleptics (levomepromazine) are often incorporated into the antipsychotic treatment [13].

In practice, two strategies are available to satisfactorily manage the severe anxiety associated with acute psychotic episodes: the use of sedative antipsychotic drugs (thioridazine, pipamperone, melperone, cyamemazine, a-flupenthixol, and levomepromazine) [14, 15, 16] or the use of adjuvant benzodiazepines therapy [17, 18, 19]. These sedative antipsychotics have been shown to have anxiolytic effects at low doses both in nonpsychotic patients and during acute psychotic episodes [18].

In order to prevent the risk of benzodiazepine dependence and rebound anxiety on the cessation of treatment, the use of benzodiazepines should be for as short a period as possible. Benzodiazepines should be prescribed in combination with nonsedative disinhibitory atypical antipsychotics.

Benzodiazepines used in psychotic episodes are drugs with potent anxiolytic action, a low propensity for pharmacokinetic drug interactions, and a long half-life to ensure uninterrupted cover [19, 20].

After the patient reaches a position where the symptoms are well-controlled, the treatment can be switched to a nonsedative antipsychotic for maintenance therapy.

Some atypical antipsychotics rely on the serotonin (5-HT) neurotransmitter system. The antagonism of 5-HT receptors permits the atypical antipsychotics to have a lower propensity to cause extrapyramidal symptoms and tardive dyskinesia.

The 5-HT actions may also result in improvements in the negative or cognitive symptoms of schizophrenia.

It has been proposed that the antagonism of 5-HT receptors and/or partial antagonism of 5-HT receptors and antihistaminic properties may play a role in the antianxiety effect of some atypical antipsychotics.

The literature indicates that Olanzapine and Quetiapine have a degree of efficacy in reducing anxiety in schizophrenic and schizoaffective patients [11, 19].

In order to explore the efficacy of atypical antipsychotics in reducing comorbid anxiety in schizophrenic and schizoaffective patients, we performed a study in our clinic.

We aimed to measure the efficacy of various antipsychotics in reducing anxiety levels in patients diagnosed with schizophrenia and schizoaffective disorder, who had been hospitalized in Arad between 2013-2014.

## 2. Methodology

### 2.1. Objectives

The aims of this study are: (a) to determine the relationship between anxiety and schizophrenia/ schizoaffective disorder, (b) to determine if the anxiety level is reduced under pharmacological treatment and to compare the efficacy in the two groups (T1- Olanzapine, Quetiapine; and T2- Haloperidolum, Risperidone, Aripiprazol), and (c) to estimate the effect of antipsychotic treatment on cognitive ability (intelligence level, IQ).

### 2.2. Sample

Sixty three patients diagnosed with schizophrenia, schizoaffective disorder, and anxiety were evaluated on admission and after 28 days of antipsychotic treatment. The patients were hospitalized in the Psychiatry Ward of The County Clinical Emergency Hospital in Arad, between 2013–2014. The patients were divided in two groups: T1, who receieved anthypsichotic treatment with Olanzapine or Quetiapine; and group T2, who received treatment with typical and atypical antipsychotics (Haloperidolum, Risperidone, and Aripiprazol).

The diagnoses of schizophrenia, schizoaffective disorder and anxiety disorders were established according to the ICD-10[21][and DSM-V-TM[22]] criteria.

| | | | | |
|---|---|---|---|---|
| **GENDER** | Females:54% | Mean: 43.27 | | |
| **AGE** | Mean:43.27 | SD: 7.5 | | |
| **EDUCATION** | Secondary school: 9% | High school: 33.3% | Professional school: 46% | University: 7% |
| **MARITAL STATUS** | Never married: 7.9% | Married: 20.6% | Divorced: 20.6% | In a relationship: 7.9% |
| **ALCHOL USE** | 6.3% | | | |

**Table 1.** Sample characteristics

The sample (Table 1) presented the following socio-demographic characteristics: (a) gender: 54% females, 46% males; (b) age: mean = 43.27, SD = 7.5; (c) education: 9% secondary school, 33.3% high school, 46% professional school and 7% university; (d) marital status: 7.9% never married, 20.6% married, 20.6% divorced, and 7.9% in a relationship; and (e) 6.3% alcohol use.

### 2.3. Measures

All subjects were evaluated using the following measures:

a. **The Hamilton Anxiety Scale** (HAM-A; Hamilton, 1959) [23] is a rating scale used to quantify the severity of anxiety symptomatology. It consists of 14 items, each defined by a series of symptoms. Each item is rated on a 5-point scale, ranging from 0 (not present) to 4 (severe).

b. **Positive and Negative Syndrome Scale** (PANSS; Kay SR, Fiszbein A, Opler LA. 1987) [24] is a semistructured clinical interview scale comprising 30 items and a seven point severity rating. There are seven psychiatric parameters belonging to a positive symptoms subscale, seven parameters belonging to a negative symptoms subscale and 16 parameters belonging to a general psychopathology subscale. The interitem correlations for PANSS were significant with a Cronbach's alpha between.71 to.83.

c. **The Hamilton Depression Rating Scale** (HAMD - 17 items; Hamilton M. A Rating Scale for Depression 1960) [25] is a scale that measures the symptoms of depression experienced over the previous week, and was originally developed for hospital inpatients. One limitation of the HAMD is that atypical symptoms of depression (e.g., hypersomnia, hyperphagia) are not assessed. A score of 0–7 is generally accepted to be within the normal range (or in clinical remission), while a score of 20 or higher (indicating at least moderate severity) is usually required for entry into a clinical trial. HAMD have good internal consistency, between 0.77 to 0.91.

d. **YoungMania Rating Scale (YMRS)** [26] is a rating scale used to evaluate manic symptoms in individuals with mania. The scale has 11 items and is based on the patient's subjective report of his or her clinical condition over the previous 48 hours. The studies regarding the psychometric characteristics of YMRS report a high degree of internal consistency ($\alpha$ = 0.91).

e. **Raven's Progressive Matrices** [27] is a nonverbal multiple choice measure of general intelligence; in each test item, the subject is asked to identify the missing element that completes a pattern. On the Romanian sample of 2755 subjects, RPM reported a high internal consistency ($\alpha$ =.91).

### 2.4. Procedure and design

The participants of this study filled in the tests package presented at the section work instruments. For the protection of the participants, they only noted a code on the answer papers. We shall use the variance analysis (ANOVA factorial) considering that we shall observe the simultaneous influence of two interdependent variables on the dependent variable.

We have structured our research into three studies as follows:

a. a correlation study—for which we have used Pearson correlation "r," in order to establish the relationship between all measurements in the pretreatment phase.

b. a comparative study—between pre- and postintervention, respectively, between the two treatments on the dependent variables (anxiety, mania, depression, and positive versus negative psychotic symptoms); we have calculated **ANOVA 2 x 2 - General Lineal Model for Repeated Measurements** for the cases in which there was no initial (pretreatment) difference between the dependent variables means (e.g., HAMA, YMRS, PANSS-N).

ANOVA 2 x 2 as a statistical indicator is helpful to observe as well the evolution in time, as well the effect on the dependent variables of the interaction between treatment condition and evolution in time as independent variables.

We have calculated **ANCOVA - General Lineal Model Univariate Analysis of Variance** for the cases in which we have observed an initial difference between the dependent variables means (e.g., PANSS-P, PANSS-G, PANSS-T, HAMD).

ANCOVA as a statistic indicator helps to eliminate the initial difference (preintervention) from the end-results (postintervention) in order to see if at the end the difference is significant as a result of intervention and to estimate which would be the end-results means if we wouldn't had initial differences.

c. a comparative study—on effect of the treatment on IQ as a dependent variable, for this propose we have used ANCOVA - Univariate Analysis of Variance, because we have observed a initial difference between the two groups regarding the IQ level.

# 3. Results

## 3.1. Correlations

Before treatment, anxiety is positively correlated with the total score of negative items on the PANSS scale (PANSSN: r =.285; p = 0.010); anxiety is also positively correlated with the total score on PANSS (PANSST: r =.260; p = 0.040) and the total score for depression assessed according to the Hamilton Depression Scale (HAM-D: r =.455; p<0.0001).

The score on the YMRS is negatively correlated with negative items on the PANSSN scale (r = -.321; p = 0.010). In general, it is to be expected that a subject with negative symptoms will have a lower level of mania.

The IQ was positive correlated with the total score on the PANSS scale (PANSST: r =.261; p = 0.036) suggesting, in our study, that a higher level of intelligence represents possible a risk in the development of psychotic symptoms. The observed positive correlation between PANSST and IQ accounts for approximately 9% of the variation.

| Pearson | IQ | PANSSP | PANSSN | PANSSG | PANSST | HAMA | YMRS | HAMD | No. Relapse | Age |
|---|---|---|---|---|---|---|---|---|---|---|
| IQ initial | 1 | .044 | .162 | .233 | **.261*** | .108 | -.015 | .241 | -.035 | -.003 |
| **PANSS-P** | | 1 | **.272*** | -.052 | **.403**** | .114 | -.018 | .053 | .055 | .082 |
| **PANSS-N** | | | 1 | .174 | **.688**** | .057 | **-.321*** | .217 | **.286*** | **.352**** |
| **PANSS-G** | | | | 1 | **.769**** | **.285*** | .003 | **.304*** | .027 | .062 |
| **PANSS-T** | | | | | 1 | **.260*** | -.155 | **.332**** | .171 | .242 |
| **HAMA** | | | | | | 1 | .001 | **.455**** | .133 | .240 |
| **Sample N** | 63 | 63 | 63 | 63 | 63 | 63 | 63 | 63 | 63 | 63 |

PANSS-P = positive items of PANSS scale; PANSS-N = negative items of PANSS scale; PANNS-G = general items of PANSS scale; PANSS-T = total score of PANSS scale; HAMA = Hamilton anxiety scale; YMRS = Young Mania Rating scale; HAMD = Hamilton Depression scale; *. Significant at the 0.05 level (2-tailed). **. Significant at the 0.01 level (2-tailed).

**Table 2.** Preintervention correlations between all measurements

Based on these results, there is a possibility that IQ can be a risk factor in 9% of the cases to stimulate the productivity of psychotic symptoms. Given this fact, we need to exercise a degree of caution with regard to the afore mentioned conclusion.

## 3.2. Comparing treatments

To assess the level of the anxiety disorders in both groups before and after 28 days of antipsychotic treatment, we used an ANOVA 2 x 2 design.

Because we expected that there would be initial differences between the two groups (T1 and T2), we also performed a t-test for independent samples (table 2) for the pretreatment values, in order to eliminate, if necessary, any initial differences from the postintervention results by calculating ANCOVA in such cases.

We obtained statistically significant difference for the PANSS-P, PANSS-G, PANSS-T, and HAM-D. To compare the efficacy of the treatment for these dependent variables between the two groups we used ANCOVA.

| **Pre-intervention measurments** | | *t-test for Equality of Means* | | | | | | |
|---|---|---|---|---|---|---|---|---|
| | | **.t.** | **df** | **Sig. (2-tailed)** | **Mean Difference** | **Std. Error Difference** | **95% Confidence Interval of the Difference** | |
| | | | | | | | **Lower** | **Upper** |
| PANSS-P | Equal variances assumed | **-2.800** | **61** | **.007** | -1.8589 | .6638 | -3.1862 | -.5315 |
| PANSS-N | Equal variances assumed | .578 | 61 | .566 | .6310 | 1.0926 | -1.5538 | 2.8159 |
| PANSS-G | Equal variances assumed | **4.302** | **61** | **.000** | 6.1028 | 1.4187 | 3.2659 | 8.9397 |
| PANSS-T | Equal variances assumed | **2.206** | **61** | **.031** | 4.8468 | 2.1966 | .4543 | 9.2392 |
| HAMA | Equal variances assumed | 1.025 | 61 | .310 | 1.2319 | 1.2023 | -1.1723 | 3.6360 |
| YOUNG MANIA | Equal variances assumed | .181 | 61 | .857 | .3992 | 2.2024 | -4.0047 | 4.8031 |
| HAMD | Equal variances assumed | **3.208** | **61** | **.002** | 3.4980 | 1.0903 | 1.3179 | 5.6781 |

PANSS-P = positive items of PANSS scale; PANSS-N = negative items of PANSS scale; PANNS-G = general items of PANSS scale; PANSS-T = total items of PANSS scale; HAMA = Hamilton anxiety rating scale; YMRS = Young Mania Rating SCALE; HAMD = hamilton depression rating scale;

**Table 3.** Preintervention differences between the two groups (in order to see if it is necessary to use ANCOVA

As the main goal of this study was to evaluate the efficacy of antipsychotic treatment for anxiety, we compared the level of anxiety pre and postintervention, by using ANOVA because there were no initial differences observed (see table 3).

Results showed that there were differences in the level of anxiety reduction between the two groups: in group T2, the efficacy of the treatment was significantly higher than that of group T1. The result obtained was confirmed by the t-test for independent samples applied postintervention at T1 and T2 ($t = 3.018$; $p =.004$).

| General Lineal Model – for Repeated Measurements for Anxiety | | | | | |
|---|---|---|---|---|---|
| **Source** | **Sum of Squares** | **df** | **Mean Square** | **F** | **Sig.** |
| Time (pre – post) | 574.777 | 1 | 574.777 | 211.821 | .000 |
| **Time * Treatments (T1 vs T2)** | 22.904 | 1 | 22.904 | 8.441 | .005 |
| Error (Time) | 165.524 | 61 | 2.714 | | |

**Table 4.** Comparing the level of anxiety pre and postintervention and between groups

The difference in anxiety reduction between the two groups (see table 4) was also measured, by comparing T2 with T1 with Cohen's D = 0, 7583; r = 0.3545.

Using the t-test for paired samples *t* (T1) = -4.901, p<0.0001 and *t* (T2) = -9.043, p<0.001, the results obtained in our preliminary study revealed that both types of treatments are effective in significantly reducing the intensity of anxiety both for schizophrenic and schizoaffective patients.

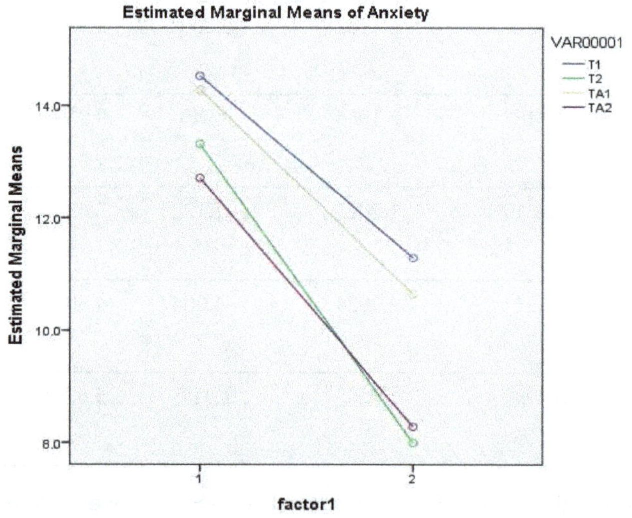


TS1= schizophrenic patients in T1 group

TA1 = schizoaffective patients in T1 group

TS2= schizophrenic patients in T2 group

TA2 = schizoaffective patients in T2 group

**Figure 1.** Pretreatment and posttreatment level of anxiety for both groups T1 (TS1 and TA1) and T2 (TS2 and TA2)

For both groups(Figure1), the results showed that with regard to the efficacy of the treatments for the patients diagnosed with schizoaffective disorder compared to schizophrenic patients, there was no difference, *t* (T1) = -3.94, p = 0.697 and *t* (T2) = 0.212, p = 0.933.

### 3.3. Comparing IQ

To eliminate the initial preintervention IQ differences between groups (*t*=5,162; p<.0001) we applied ANCOVA. In both groups of patients, antipsychotic treatment has a negative effect on cognitive functioning reducing IQ level, but the cognitive dysfunction was higher in group T1.

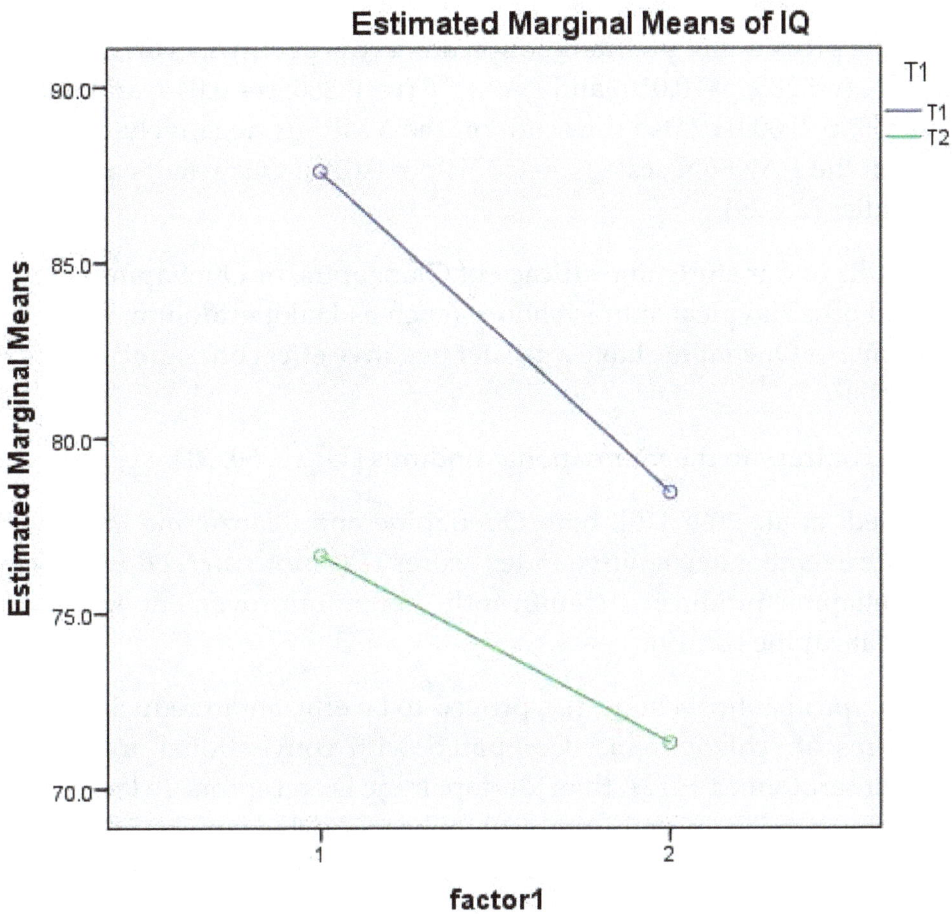


**Figure 2.** Evolution of the IQ levels in T1 and T2 group

The results obtained showed that in posttreatment (Figure 2) there were no statistically significant differences between the two groups, ANCOVA F = 1.085, p = 0.302. A possible explanation for these results is that the T1 treatment had a greater effect on cognitive functioning when compared with the T2 treatment, so that even if the T2 group initially had a lower intelligence level, after 28 days the difference was no longer significant (see Table 5).

**Dependent Variable: IQ in evolution**

| Pre-Post | Mean | Std. Error | 95% Confidence Interval | |
|---|---|---|---|---|
| | | | Lower Bound | Upper Bound |
| T1 treatment | **74.07**[a] | .93 | 72.21 | 75.93 |
| T2 treatment | **75.551** | .91 | 73.72 | 77.37 |

Note: a.Covariates appearing in the model are evaluated at the following values: IQ initial = 82.048.

**Table 5.** Estimated marginal means after eliminating the covariance of the Initial IQ

## 4. Discussions and conclusions

The study's results proved that preintervention anxiety is positively correlated with the total score on PANSSN ($r = .285$; $p = 0.010$) and PANSST ($r = 0.260$; $p = 0.040$) and the total score on HAM-D ($r = 0.455$; $p<0.0001$). Also the score on the YMRS is negatively correlated with the negative items on the PANSSN scale ($r = -0.321$; $p = 0.010$). Our results are corroborated by international studies [28, 29].

Based on the results of our study, the efficacy of Olanzapine or Quetiapine is lower than that of the typical and other atypical antipsychotics (such as Haloperidolum, Risperidone, Aripiprazol). Olanzapine or Quetiapine have a greater negative effect on cognitive functioning than other antipsychotics.

These results are contrary to the international findings [11, 19, 30, 31].

In a study by Riedl et al., 2007 [19], both Quetiapine and Olanzapine improved cognition; however, the improvement in cognitive index scores was more marked in patients receiving Quetiapine. Quetiapine produce a significantly better improvement in reaction quality/attention than Olanzapine [11, 19].

Olanzapine, an atypical antipsychotic, has proved to be efficient in reducing the positive and negative symptoms of schizophrenia. Compared with conventional antipsychotics, it has greater affinity for serotonin 5-HT2A than for dopamine D2 receptors. In large, well-controlled trials involving patients diagnosed with schizophrenia, Olanzapine (5 to 20 mg/day) was superior to Haloperidol (5 to 20 mg/day) in the treatment of depressive and negative symptoms, comparable with effects on positive psychotic symptoms [28]. Contrary to these findings, in our study patients treated with haloperidol, Risperidone, and Aripiprazol (group T2) showed a greater reduction of symptomatology.

The 1-year risk of relapse of rehospitalisation was significantly lower with Olanzapine than with Haloperidol treatment [35].

In the first double-blind comparative study [28, 29, 33]) of Olanzapine 10 to 20 mg/day and Risperidone 4 to 12 mg/day, Olanzapine proved to be significantly more effective than Risperidone in the treatment of negative and depressive symptoms but not for overall psychopathological symptoms.

In contrast, preliminary results from an 8-week controlled study [34] suggested that Risperidone 2 to 6 mg/day was superior to Olanzapine 5 to 20 mg/day in the treatment of positive and anxiety/depressive symptoms, and that both agents demonstrated similar efficacy on overall psychopathology. These results are similar to our findings (Risperidone was superior to Olanzapine in reducing anxiety symptoms as confirmed by t-test for independent samples applied postintervention at T1 and T2: $t = 3.018$; $p = 0.004$).

However, preliminary results from an 8-week trial showed comparable cognitive enhancing effects for Olanzapine and Risperidone in patients with schizophrenia or schizoaffective disorder [30]. In our study, in both groups of patients, (T1, T2), antipsychotic treatment has a negative effect on cognition with a larger effect on group T1 treated with Olanzapine and Quetiapine.

Olanzapine demonstrated superior antipsychotic efficacy when compared to Haloperidol in the treatment of acute phase schizophrenia, and in the treatment of some patients with first-episode or treatment-resistant schizophrenia [35].

The reduced risk of adverse events and the therapeutic superiority, compared with Haloperidol and Risperidone, in the treatment of negative and depressive symptoms support the choice of Olanzapine as a first-line option in the management of schizophrenia in the acute and maintenance phase of treatment response [36].

Aripiprazole, a 5-H1A partial agonist was found to have a considerable antianxiety effect which may concur with procognitive and mood-ameliorating effects [32, 37, 38]. These are similar to our results: when comparing T2 with T1 using effect size based on differences between means (Cohen's D = 0.7583; r = 0.3545), Aripiprazol is superior to Olanzapine and Quetiapine in reducing anxiety in schizophrenic and schizoaffective disorder patients. Regarding the cognitive dysfunction, posttreatment, in both groups of patients, we noticed a negative effect on cognition, although there was no statistically significant differences between the groups as determined by analysis of covariance (ANOVA F = 1.085; p = 0.302).

One hypothesis could be that this agonism of Aripiprazole is a mechanism contributing to antianxiety effects. Case reports and studies on the antipsychotic augmentation by Aripiprazole in partial responders to Clozapine found a considerable antianxiety effect [32].

However, this could be due to external factors or to the natural evolution of the illness. A randomized controlled study is required to evaluate the efficacy of the Clozapine-Aripiprazole combination in cases of treatment-resistant schizophrenia with a predominance of anxiety [39].

Risperidone's antianxiety action was demonstrated in the study by Blider et al. in 2002 [30], conducted on 62 patients hospitalized for acute exacerbations of schizophrenia, randomly assigned to receive Risperidone (a mean dose, 7.4 mg/day), Haloperidol (7.6 mg/day), or Methotrimeprazine (100 mg/day) for 4 weeks. The antianxiety effects were significantly greater in the Risperidone patients than the Methotrimeprazine patients. The difference between Haloperidol and Methotrimeprazine was not significant.

It is concluded that Risperidone is an effective antipsychotic and anxiolytic agent in schizophrenic patients. These result are confirmed by our findings in group T2 (t = 3.018; p = 0.004).

## New Drug Perspectives

It is generally agreed upon that anxiety is a frequently occurring symptom of schizophrenia, strongly associated with an increased risk of relapse and more severe symptomatology. The effects of antipsychotics in reducing anxiety in psychotic patients remain controversial and the practice of prescribing adjuvants (benzodiazepines) is unsatisfactory [17, 18].

The next clinical trials for schizophrenia with comorbid anxiety perhaps will show the efficacy of some new compounds (the anticonvulsant/anxiolytic pregabalin and the atypical antipsychotic Quetiapine) [40].

Consequently, we think there is a need for more research in order to obtain a clear perspective of the efficacy of Olanzapine or Quetiapine. It should also be pointed out that our findings suffer from certain limitations: such as (a) the lack of a control group, (b) the small sample size, (c) the short treatment time, and (d) the lack of a follow-up evaluation after three and six months, and after one year. Our results can serve as a guide to future studies regarding the efficacy of psychopharmacological treatment on comorbid anxiety.

### Limitations

The methodological limitations of this study will be addressed in a follow-up study: this was a preliminary study with a small sample size, lacking follow up evaluations at 3 months, 6 months and 1 year. Given that some of these patients will be inevitably lost to the follow up, a large sample size will need to be used in order to ensure that sufficient numbers are available to obtain meaningful repeat measures.

## Acknowledgements

This paper is partly supported by the Sectorial Operational Programme Human Resources Development (SOPHRD), financed by the European Social Fund and the Romanian Government under contract number POSDRU 141531.

## Author details

Delia M. Podea[1*], Aurora I. Sabau[1] and Karol J. Wild[1]

*Address all correspondence to: deliapodea@yahoo.com

1 "Vasile Goldis" Western University of Arad, County ClinicalEmergency Hospital of Arad, Psychiatry Department, Arad, Romania

"Vasile Goldis" Western University of Arad, Psychology Department, Arad, Romania

## References

[1] Achim A. M., Maziade M., Raymound E., Olivier D., Merette C., Roy M.A.: How prevalent are anxiety disorders in schizophrenia? A meta-analysis and critical review on a significant association. Schizophrenia Bulletin, 2011, 37:811-821.

[2] Seedat S., Fritelli V., Oosthuizen P., Emsley R. A., Stein D. J.: Measuring anxiety in patients with schizophrenia. Journal of Nervous Mental Disease. 2007; 1995 : 320-324.

[3] Ciapparelli A., Paggini R., Marazitti D., Carmassi C., Bianchi M., Taponecco C., Consoli G., Lombardi V., Massimetti G., Dell'Osso L.: Comorbidity with axis 1 anxiety disorders in remitted psychotic patients 1 year after hospitalization. CNNS Spectr 2007; 12:913-919.

[4] Braga R. J., Petrides G., Figuueira I.: Anxiety disorders in schizophrenia. Compr Psychiatry 2004; 45:460-468.

[5] Cosoff S.J., Hafner R.J.: The prevalence of comorbid anxiety in schizophrenia, schizoafective disorder and bipolar disorder. Aust NZJ Psychiatry 1998;32:67-72.

[6] American Psychiatric Association: The Diagnostic and Statistical Manual of Mental Disorders, 5th edition, Washington, DC. 2013.

[7] Tibbo P., Swainson J., Chue P., LeMelledo J.M.: Prevalence and relationship to delusion and hallucinations of anxiety disorders in schizophrenia. Depress Anxiety 2003;17:65-72. DOI:10.1002/da.10083.

[8] Argyle N., et al.: Panic attacks in chronic schizophrenia. Br J Psychiatry 1990;430–433.DOI: 10.1192/bjp.157.3.430.

[9] Blanchard Jack J., Mueser Kim T., Bellack Alan S.: Anhedonia, positive and negative affect, and social functioning in schizophrenia. Schizophrenia Bulletin 1998;24.3:413-424.

[10] Schwab S.G., Albus M., Hallmayer J., Honig S., Borrmann M., Lichtermann D., Ebstein R.P., Ackenheil M., Lerer B., Risch N., Maier W., Wildenauer D.B.: Evaluation of a susceptibility gene for schizophrenia on chromosome 6p by multipoint affected sib-pair linkage analysis. Nature Genetics. 1995; 11:325-327.doi:10.1038/ng1195-325.

[11] Cutler Andrew J., Quetiapine, Evidence in reducing Anxiety: Clinical Evidence may suggest the atypical antipsychotic (quetiapine fumarate) tablets, is effective in reducing anxiety in patients with schizophrenia. Presented at the American Psychiatric Association annual meeting, May 5 - 10 2001; New Orleans, Louisiana 2001.

[12] Garay RP., d'Alche-Birée, Cyamémazine F.: Profil neuroleptique ou anxiolytique? L'Information Psychiatrique Lille 1995;71: 969-971.

[13] Goodwin R.D., Amador X.F., Malaspina D., Yale S.A., Goetz R.R., Gorman J.M.: Anxiety and substance use comorbidity among inpatients with schizophrenia. Schizophr Res 2003 May 1; 61(1): 89-95.

[14] Squelart P., Saravia J.: Pipamperone (Dipiperon), a useful sedative neuroleptic drug in troublesome chronic psychotic patients. Acta Psychiatr Belg. 1977;77:284-293.

[15] Meltzer H.Y., Sumiyoshi T., Jayathilake K.: Melperone in the treatment of neuroleptic-resistant schizophrenia. Psychiatry Res. 2001;105:201-209.

[16] Poldinger W. J.: Melperone in low doses in anxious neurotic patients. A double-blind placebo-controlled clinical study. Neuropsychobiology. 1984;11:181-186.

[17] Barbee J.G., Mancuso D.M., Freed C.R., Todorov A.A.: Alprazolam as a neuroleptic adjunct in the emergency treatment of schizophrenia. Am J Psychiatry 1992;149:506-510.

[18] Wolkowitz O.M., Pickar D.: Benzodiazepines in the treatment of schizophrenia: a review and reappraisal. Am J Psychiatry. 1991;148:714-726.

[19] Riedel M, Muller N, Spellmann I, Engel RR.: Efficacy of Olanzapine versus Quetiapine on cognitive dysfunction in patients with an acute episode of schizophrenia. Arch. Psychiatry Clin Neurosa 2007;402-412.

[20] Lingjaerde O.: Benzodiazepines in the treatment of schizophrenia: an updated survey. Acta Psychiatr Scand. 1991;84:453-459.

[21] World Health Organization: The ICD-10 classification of mental and behavioural disorders: Clinical descriptions and diagnostic guidelines. 1992. Geneva: World Health Organization.

[22] American Psychiatric Association: Diagnostic and statistical manual of mental disorders (4th ed., text rev.). Washington, DC: APA.2000.

[23] Hamilton M.: The assessment of anxiety states by rating. Br. J Med Psychol 195932:50-55.

[24] Kay S.R., Fiszbein A., Opler L.A.: The positive and negative syndrome scale (PANSS) for schizophrenia. Schizophrenia Bulletin 1987 ;13261-275.

[25] Hamilton M.: A rating scale for depression. J Neurol Neurosurg Psychiatry 1960; Hamilton Depression Rating Scale (HDRS).

[26] Young R.C., Biggs J.T., Ziegler V. E., Meyer D. A.: Young Mania Rating Scale. In: Handbook of Psychiatric Measures. Washington, DC: American Psychiatric Association; 2000: 540-542.

[27] Raven J.: Raven's Progressive Matrices. Journal of Psychoeducational Assessment 1998; 17,354-361. doi: 10.1177/0013164498058003002.

[28] Bhana N., Foster R.H., Olney R.: Olanzapine: an updated review of its use in the management of schizophrenia. Drugs 2011;61(1):111-161.

[29] Gao K., Muzina D., Gajwani P., Calabrese J. P.: Efficacy of typical and atypical antipsychotics for primary and comorbid anxiety symptoms or disorders: a review. Journal of Clinical Psychiatry 2006 ;67(9):1327–1340.

[30] Bilder R.M., Goldman R.S., Volavka J., Czobor P., Hoptman M., Sheitman B., Lindenmayer J.P., Citrome L., McEvoy J., Kunz M., Chakos M., Cooper T.B., Horowitz T.L., Lieberman J.A.: Neurocognitive effects of Clozapine, Olanzapine, Risperidone, and Haloperidol in patients with chronic schizophrenia or schizoaffective disorder. Am. J. Psychiatry2002;159:1018–1028.

[31] Schirmbeck F., Esslinger C., Rausch F., Englisch S., Meyer-Lindenberg A., Zink M.: Antiserotonergic antipsychotics are associated with obsessive-compulsive symptoms in schizophrenia. Psychol Med 2011;41(11):236.

[32] Chanachev A. et al.: Case Reports in Psychiatry Volume 2011. Article ID 846489, 3 pages.

[33] Moore N. A., Tye N.C., Axton M.S., Risius F.C.: The behavioral pharmacology of Olanzapine, a novel "atypical" antipsychotic agent. Journal of Pharmacology and Experimental Therapeutics1992; 262(2): 545–551.

[34] Kim S.W., Shin I.S., Kim J.M., Youn T., Yang S.J., Hwang M.Y., Yoon J.S.S.O.: The 5-HT2 receptor profiles of antipsychotics in the pathogenesis of obsessive-compulsive symptoms in schizophrenia. Clin Neuropharmacol 2009; 32(4):224.

[35] Csernansky J.G., Schuchart E.K.: Relapse and rehospitalisation rates in patients with schizophrenia: effects of second generation antipsychotics. CNS Drugs2002;16:473–484.

[36] TollefsonG.D., Sanger T.M., Lieberman J.A.: Olanzapine versus Haloperidol in the treatment of first episode psychosis. Schizophrenia Research 1997; 24.doi: 10.4103/2279-042X.128142

[37] Paton C., Whittington C., Barnes T.R.: Augmentation with a second antipsychotic in patients with schizophrenia who partially respond to Clozapine. a meta analysis. J Clin Psychopharmacol 2007; 27:198-204.

[38] Swainston Harrison T., Perry C.M.: Aripiprazole: a review of its use in schizophrenia and schizoaffective disorder Drugs 2004;64(15):1715-1736.

[39] Karunakaran K., Tungaraza T.E., Harborn G.C.: Is Clozapine-Aripiprazole combination a useful regime in the management of treatment-resistant schizophrenia? Journal of Psychopharmacology 2007; 21(4):453–456. doi: 10.1093/schbul/sbn018.

[40] Garay R.P., Samalin L., Hameg A., Llorca P. M.: Investigational drugs for anxiety in patients with schizophrenia. [Internet]. 2014, November 25. Available from http://informahealthcare.com/doi/abs/10.1517/13543784.2014.987339.[Accesed:2014-12-20].

9

# Genetics and Epigenetics of Schizophrenia

Esmaeil Shahsavand Ananloo

**Abstract**

Schizophrenia (SCZ) is a complex mental disorder, with a longstanding history of neurobiological investigation. It is more common in those persons who are genetically predisposed to the disorder. Since Kraepelin, psychiatrists were aware that the SCZ tended to run in families. Its heritability is up to 85%. Although the etiology of SCZ is unknown, it is now thought to be multifactorial, with multiple susceptibility genes interacting with environmental and developmental factors. There is a huge amount of genetic studies, including polymorphisms, expression, methylation, microRNAs, and epigenomics. However, identifying genes for SCZ using traditional genetic approaches has thus far proven quite difficult. Reasons for this include the complexity, heterogeneity, and comorbidity of this disorder, and also the poor definition of the clinical phenotype. Important approaches to find the relation between genotype and phenotype and may be causal genetic factors are endophenotypes and pathway analysis. However, genetic researchers need to consider carefully the models of causality they choose. There is a pathophysiological pathway that extends from genes, through proteins, neurons, neural circuits, neural regions, mental functions, external behaviors, and symptoms of SCZ. In this chapter, the genetics and epigenetics of SCZ are briefly discussed.

**Keywords:** schizophrenia, genetic, epigenetic, etiology, pathophysiology, endophenotype, pathway analysis

## 1. Introduction

Schizophrenia is a serious, disabling, and complex mental disorder, with a longstanding history of neurobiological investigation [1]. It may be one of the most disabling disorders known to human. Schizophrenia can affect anyone at any point in his or her life. It is more common in those persons who are genetically predisposed to the disorder. The first psychotic episode generally occurs in late adolescence or early adulthood and often appears earlier in men than in women. Schizophrenia, as a common disorder, has a worldwide prevalence of around 0.3–1.0% [2]. Clinically, it is characterized by a combination of positive and negative symptoms, cognitive impairments, and disorganized behaviors.

There are 130,024 citations (110,613 papers, 17,847 reviews, and 1564 meta-analysis) related to "schizophrenia," 12,038 citations (9666 papers, 2134 reviews, and 238 meta-analysis) related to "schizophrenia gene," 1317 citations (1060 papers, 178 reviews, and 79 meta-analysis) related to "schizophrenia genome-wide association study," and 234 citations (216 papers, 11 reviews, and 7 meta-analysis) related to "schizophrenia gene enrichment" in PubMed (accessed on January 29, 2018).

Since Kraepelin delineated the disorder dementia praecox in 1899, psychiatrists were aware that the SCZ tended to run in families. Until now, there are several family studies in SCZ [3, 4]. While, the probability of developing SCZ in general population is 1%, the probability of its developing as the offspring of one parent with the disorder is approximately 17%, and the offspring of both parents with the disorder is approximately 46% [5].

A vulnerability-stress model, in which SCZ is thought to be multifactorial, with multiple susceptibility genes is interacting with environmental and developmental factors. For example, the immune response to a wide variety of bacterial or viral pathogens may be the link between prenatal infection and postnatal brain pathologies, including SCZ [6]. Additionally, intrauterine or postnatal complications with a negative impact on fetal brain development, nutritional deficiencies with effects on neurotransmitter systems, or maternal exposure to stressors are among the other important factors [7]. Identifying genes for psychiatric disorders using traditional genetic approaches has thus far proven quite difficult. Reasons for this include the complexity, heterogeneity, and comorbidity of these disorders and also the poor definition of the clinical phenotype [8]. Different studies, including MicroRNAs [9, 10], genetic polymorphisms [11, 12], gene expression [13, 14], methylation [15], and epigenomics [16, 17] are the most important genetic studies in SCZ.

## 2. Genetics of schizophrenia

### 2.1. An overview

Evidence including genetic findings shows that the early neurodevelopmental events have been implicated in the pathogenesis of disorder (**Table 1**) [1]. Traditionally, the most genetic researches on SCZ have concentrated on chromosomes and genes. These include cytogenetics, linkage, association, gene expression, and whole genome and exome scans. Although these studies have identified a number of genomic regions of interest, these have not produced any confirmed causations.

There are reasons as to why genetic approaches have met with little success in SCZ. First is that, there are no specific biological markers. Diagnostic systems, including diagnostic and statistical manuals of mental disorders (DSMs) and international classifications of diseases (ICDs), are categorical classifications and are based on interview and self-reporting of the patients. So, they are not optimal in genetic research on complex disorders. Second is the problem of

| Traditional structural genetic studies | Newer structural genetic studies | Traditional functional genetic studies (gene encoding studies) | Newer functional genetic studies | Epigenetic studies |
|---|---|---|---|---|
| Cytogenetic studies | Genome-wide association studies (GWASs) | mRNA studies | microRNA studies | DNA modification studies |
| Linkage studies | Whole exome studies | Protein studies | Long noncoding RNA studies | Histone modification studies |
| Candidate gene association studies | | | Other noncoding RNA studies | |
| | | | Genome-wide expression studies | |

**Table 1.** An overview to the genetic and epigenetic studies of schizophrenia.

genotype-phenotype relationship. After a century ago, when Wilhelm Johannsen proposed the terms "genotype" and "phenotype," our knowledge about the genetics, phenotype, and the concept of causality has evolved dramatically [18]. For example, genotype heterogeneity means that there are many genotypes that produce the same phenotype. In addition, phenotype heterogeneity means that the same genotype may produce different phenotypes. The alternate approach to find the relationship between genotype and phenotype may be endophenotypes that will be useful in detecting genes contributing to SCZ [19, 20]. However, the studies of endophenotypes (characteristics that are intermediate between the genotype and a phenotype of interest) associated with SCZ are not yet enough. Another approach may be the path analysis to identify causal variables that produce phenotypes [21, 22]. However, the chosen models of causality are very important [18]. Third is the genetic hypothesis being tested. The problems are the number of gene variants involved, the heterogeneous mechanism of the disorder, and the understanding of their interactions with the environmental and developmental factors to predisposition to SCZ. So, there is a long pathophysiological chain that extends from genes, through proteins, neurons, neural circuits, neural pools, neural regions, mental functions, external behaviors, and symptoms construct of SCZ.

By using high-throughput technologies, a huge amount of studies, including genome-wide association studies (GWASs) have reported that genetic variants, such as copy number variations (CNVs) or single nucleotide polymorphisms (SNPs) play significant roles in the pathogenesis of SCZ. In recent years, and based on the emergence of international consortia to achieve larger sample sizes, clinical, and statistically expertise and also replicable genetic findings [23], our understanding of the genetic architecture of SCZ, the number of risk variants, and their frequencies and effect sizes have been transformed. Genome-wide association studies of genetic variants have approximately tripled the number of candidate genetic loci [24]. The Schizophrenia Working Group of the Psychiatric Genomics Consortium (PGC) used GWAS arrays to identify 128 independent associations spanning 108 regions. These findings demonstrate the involvement of biological processes of the brain. For example, there are associations among gene expression patterns in tissues with some roles in the immune system, providing support for the link between the immune system and SCZ [23].

### 2.2. Heritability

The heritability is a statistic that estimates the degree of variation in a phenotypic trait or disorder in a population that is due to genetic variation between individuals [25]. Schizophrenia is highly heritable [26] and its genetic architecture is complex and heterogeneous. Its heritability has been estimated from 81% [26] up to 85% [27], showing a non-Mendelian inheritance pattern [28]. Reported concordance rate of SCZ in monozygotic twins is about 50%; from 41–65% [27, 29], while siblings and dizygotic twins show proband concordance rates as high as 28% [27]. The risk of the general population developing the SCZ is about 0.3–1.0% worldwide [2, 30].

Evidence shows the heritability of different aspects of SCZ, such as brain region volumes [31, 32] and cognitive disabilities [33]. Thus, the combination of genetics and brain imaging (imaging-genetics approach) will be a useful strategy to assess the effects of risk genetic variants on anatomical and functional connectivities [32]. For example, the heritability in subcortical and limbic volumes ranged from 0.45 in the right hippocampus to 0.84 in the left putamen [31]. General cognitive disabilities in SCZ have also genetic contributors. By using the genome-wide complex-trait analysis (GCTA) approach, to estimate the total heritability captured by common DNA markers on genotyping arrays [34], it was shown that individuals at ultra-high risk for the disorder, relatives of the patients with SCZ spectrum disorders, and children with antecedents of SCZ may have cognitive impairments as well [33].

### 2.3. Candidate gene association studies

The candidate gene association study has been a major approach to discover the causative genetic factors of complex traits or disorders. Prior to the GWAS era, candidate studies were a major approach in SCZ genetics [35] and have been a pioneer in the field of genetic association studies to identify risk genetic variants associated with a particular trait or disorder [36]. These studies, including case-control and family studies, directly test the effects of genetic variants, usually CNVs or SNPs of potentially contributing genes. The candidate gene studies are relatively cheap and quick to perform, but are limited by how much is known about the biology of the disorder being investigated [37]. With the advent of rapidly changing technology, there has been an explosion of *in silico* tools available to researchers, giving them fast, efficient resources, and reliable strategies to find casual genetic variants for candidate study or GWAS [36]. Population stratification is also a major confounding factor for population-based case-control association studies and can result in false positive associations [38]. This may be solved by considering a replication study using an independent and random cohort of test and control populations or through a family study. These approaches may reduce the chance of occurrence of a similar admixture showing similar patterns of variations [39]. Prior to the advances brought about by the Human Genome Project [40], the International HapMap Project [41], and then, 1000 Genomes Project [42], it was difficult and expensive to genotype a comprehensive list of genetic variants in a genomic region. Investigators thus tended to genotype a few genetic markers in a candidate gene selected based on prevailing theories of the etiopathology of SCZ or positional candidate genes from linkage or cytogenetic studies.

The more popular hypothesis, the common disease—common variant hypothesis suggests that SCZ is associated primarily with common genetic variants [43]. Based on this hypothesis, most of the genetic association studies have focused on these variations in SCZ. This hypothesis constitutes the rationale of GWASs, in which millions of variants, including SNPs were assessed in thousands of individuals [44, 45]. Copy number variations are sections of the genome that are repeated and the number of repeats in the genome varies between individuals [46]. Structural variations of DNA, such as CNVs, have contribution to normal genomic variability and to risk for human diseases [47]. Many studies have demonstrated that CNVs play important roles in susceptibility to SCZ [47–49].

The SZGene database (obtained 11/2017) listed 1727 candidate gene papers investigating over 1008 genes and 8788 polymorphisms. Based on published genetic association studies of SCZ, it has been reported that across 118 meta-analyses, 16 genes, including *APOE, COMT, DAO, DRD1, DRD2, DRD4, DTNBP1, GABRB2, GRIN2B, HP, IL1B, MTHFR, PLXNA2, SLC6A4, TP53,* and *TPH1* showed significant effects [50]. By using a translational convergent functional genomics approach, using candidate genetic studies, and a poly evidence scoring and pathway analyses, many genes, including *DISC1, TCF4, MBP, MOBP, NCAM1, NRCAM, NDUFV2, RAB18, ADCYAP1, BDNF, CNR1, COMT, DRD2, DTNBP1, GAD1, GRIA1, GRIN2B, HTR2A, NRG1, RELN, SNAP-25, TNIK,* and a few top genes, including *DISC1, HSPA1B, MBP,* and *TCF4* were identified [51]. Across meta-analyses, candidate genes, including *APOE, COMT, DAO, DRD1, DRD2, DRD4, DTNBP1, GABRB2, GRIN2B, HP, IL1B, MTHFR, PLXNA2, SLC6A4, TP53, TPH1, RELN, MnSOD, GSTM1, ZNF804A, CACNA1C, AN K3, BDNF, GRIN3A, FAAH, DNMT1, MYO18B, CFB, GRM7, GRM8, miR-137, MPC2,* and *CSMD1* showed nominally significant effects [11, 50, 52]. However, some of them have been questioned [35, 53–55]. A likely reason why candidate gene studies did not achieve their primary aims is inadequate statistical power. However, the considerable efforts embodied in early studies unquestionably set the stage for current successes in genomic approaches to SCZ [35].

### 2.4. Genome-wide association studies

A GWAS or whole genome association study (WGAS) is an approach that involves rapidly scanning genetic variants across the genomes of many people to find variations associated with a particular trait or disease. By using this approach, researchers can use the information to develop better hypotheses to detect, treat, and prevent the diseases. Such studies are particularly useful in finding genetic variations that contribute to mental disorders. Genome-wide association study searches the genome for a genome-wide set of genetic variants in different individuals to see if any variant is associated with a normal trait or a disease. This is a hypothesis-free strategy, and typically searches the genome for SNPs, or CNVs that occur more frequently in people with a particular disease than in people without the disease. Genome-wide significance is $P < 5.0 \times 10^{(-8)}$. Meta-analyses of GWAS data have begun to lead to promising new discoveries for SCZ [56]. Within the last few years, large-scale GWASs of SCZ have identified multiple risk variants with significant association with the disorder. However, these variants could explain only a small proportion of the heritability of SCZ and their effect sizes are relatively small, suggesting that more risk variants may be detected when increasing sample size in analysis [57, 58].

By the analysis of an European ancestry sample GWAS and then through a replication study, Ripke et al. [45] found significant associations for seven loci, including 1p21.3, 2q32.3, 6p21.32-p22.1, 8p23.2, 8q21.3, 10q24.32-q24.33, and 18q21.2 with SCZ. The strongest finding was with a miRNA-137 SNP, a known regulator of neuronal development. In a meta-analysis of 18 GWASs and a replication study, Aberg et al. [3] found significant effect with SCZ for *TCF4, NOTCH4, POM121L2, AS3MT, CNNM2,* and *NT5C2* genes. By carrying out a GWAS meta-analysis, Sleiman et al. [59] found 40 SNPs in six significant loci, including *SDCCAG8, ITIH1,* major histocompatibility complex (*MHC*), *MAD1L1, CSMD1,* and *TSNARE1* genes. By analyzing two genome-wide association data sets of European-American patients with SCZ, significant associations between negative symptoms of SCZ and *BCL9, TMEM245, RNF144B, CTNNA3,* and *ZNF385D* genes have been detected [60]. The largest published GWAS meta-analysis of SCZ is of 34,000 patients in a meta-analysis of 52 GWASs from the Psychiatric Genomics Consortium (PGC) which identified 108 genome-wide significant loci [61]. Through large GWAS, an intronic SNP within *CSMD1* gene, rs10503253, one of the top risk SNPs for SCZ in Europeans discovered [11]. It may be concluded that the risk "A" allele is relevant to brain structure and neurocognitive functioning and these effects may be a part of the mechanism by which the *CSMD1* mediates risk for SCZ [62, 63]. By combining two SCZ cohort studies, Luo et al. [58] reported a genome-wide significant risk locus at 22q13.1. In their meta-analysis, seven SNPs on chromosome 22q13.1 reached the genome-wide significant effect, and most significant association was with SNP rs6001946 ($P = 2.04 \times 10[^{-8}]$). All seven SNPs are located in the *MKL1* gene.

It has been reported that a rare risk variation at *AKAP9* and a protective variation at *NRXN1* are in susceptibility to SCZ [64]. By doing a meta-analysis of data from the PGC and additional SCZ family sample, SNP rs4765905 in *CACNA1C* showed a strong effect [65]. Through the meta-analysis of a UK case/control study and GWAS data from the PGC, a significant effect of two *SLC30A3* gene SNPs (rs11126936 and rs11126929) was found in female subjects [66]. Chang et al. [67] in a GWAS study in Europeans (but not in Asians) found a significant effect with SCZ for *VRK2* gene SNP rs2312147. In their GWAS meta-analysis, it has been reported that rs10489202 in *MPC2* gene is significantly associated with SCZ in Han Chinese samples [68].

### 2.5. Gene expression studies

#### *2.5.1. Gene encoding studies*

It has been postulated that the underlying neuropathology of SCZ, at least, resides in the periodic activation of a defective genes, as a progressive process [69]. Changes in gene expression in brains of patients with SCZ have been hypothesized to reflect possible pathways related to its pathophysiology [70]. Progressive cortical reorganization and gray matter abnormalities may be pathophysiological processes in disorder [71, 72]. These changes are in parallel with changes in symptoms and cognitive impairments [73]. Epidemiological evidence suggests the widespread gene-environment interactions in the etiology of SCZ [74, 75]. So, it may be hypothesized that these interactions can alter the gene expression pattern in the brain of patients. By using the Gene Expression Omnibus Database, Karim et al. [76] showed a total of 527 differentially expressed genes of which 314 are up regulated and 213 are down regulated.

There are differences in pathophysiology of SCZ between male and female patients. It seems that the pattern of genetic architecture is different between two sexes. For example, the upregulation of 59 genes and downregulation of other 105 genes in the peripheral blood mononuclear cells (PBMCs) from patients with SCZ have been reported [77]. By using the PBMC samples, a genome-wide expression analysis showed the alterations of gene expressions, such as *MEF2D, S100A12,* and *AKT1,* with immune system function [77, 78]. Additionally, in their meta-analysis, Qin et al. [13] tested for a sex by diagnosis interaction on gene expression. These authors reported that 23 genes were up regulated and 23 genes were down regulated significantly in the male group. Several of these genes, including *ATP5B, ATP5A1, MRPL23, AFG3L2,* and *ABCG2,* are related to energy metabolism. Four genes, including *BEX1, UBL4A, CD99,* and *MID1,* were located on sex chromosome [13]. By using a large European-wide sample in their meta-analysis, Perez-Becerril et al. [66] found the risk alleles of two *SLC30A3* variants in females, which were associated with gene expression. In a meta-analysis of 41 studies, it has been shown a significant increase in expression of pro-inflammatory genes, including *IL-1β, IL-6,* and *TNF-α* on transcript and protein levels in patients with SCZ [79].

### *2.5.2. Micro-ribonucleic acids (miRNAs) studies*

These RNAs are small noncoding RNA molecules which exert their functions by pairing with messenger RNAs (mRNAs) [80] and are powerful negative regulators of gene expression [81, 82]. They function in cell proliferation and death, patterning of the nervous system, and also as modulators of target mRNA translation and stability [83], RNA silencing and post-transcriptional regulation of gene expression [84]. There are different sets of miRNAs expressed in different cell types and tissues [85] and in many other biological processes, such as insulin secretion, B-cell development [86], hematopoiesis [87], and metabolic biochemistry [81]. Aberrant miRNA expression is implicated in many disorders, such as cancers [88], ischemic heart diseases [82], and mental disorders as well. A huge amount of evidence implicates miRNAs as a class of modulator for human tumor initiation and progression [80]. However, miRNA-based therapies are under investigation. In a meta-analysis, Ma et al. [9] reported that *miR-137* genetic variant rs1625579 is significantly associated with SCZ. Additionally, in another meta-analysis of 52 GWASs completed in 2014, Hauberg et al. [10] showed that the SCZ risk genes were regulated by miRNAs ($P < 2 \times 10[^{-16}]$). The strongest miRNAs were *miR-9-5p, miR485-5p,* and *miR-137* [9].

### *2.5.3. Transcriptome and proteome studies*

Transcriptome is the set of all RNA molecules (transcripts) in one cell, a population of cells or in a given organism. The study of transcriptome examines the expression level of RNAs in a given cell population, often focusing on mRNA, but sometimes including others such as transfer RNAs (tRNAs) and soluble RNAs (sRNAs).

The proteome is the entire set of proteins expressed by a genome in a cell, tissue, or organism at a certain time, under defined conditions. Proteomics is the study of the proteome. Understanding of the implication of genetic variations in mental disorders requires translation into functional effects [70]. New technologies allow the investigation of levels of mRNAs and proteins at the same time [89].

A significant increased expression of *SLC2A3*—glucose transporter, and *DAAM2*—actin assembly factor, and a significant decreased expression of *OMA1*—zinc metallopeptidase,

*NLN1*, and *MYBPC3*—myosin C have been reported in the first onset of SCZ [90]. The peripheral mRNA of these genes may be potential biomarkers in early stages of disorder course [89].

## 3. Epigenetics of schizophrenia

### 3.1. Epigenetics and epigenetics code

The Greek prefix *epi-* ("over") in epigenetics implies features that are "on top of" or "in addition to" the traditional genetic basis for inheritance (**Table 1**). Epigenetics is the study of changes in gene functions, including gene expression that are heritable and that does not entail a change in DNA sequence [91]. Examples of epigenetic mechanisms are DNA methylation and acetylation and also histone modifications. The epigenetic changes are potentially reversible. Epigenetic codes are heritable DNA/histone modifications that specify patterns of gene expression through differentiation and development [92].

### 3.2. Epigenetic study of schizophrenia

Epigenotyping might be integrated along with genotyping and phenotyping as means of implementing advanced precision medicine [93]. Epigenetic mechanisms regulate the key neurobiological and cognitive processes in the brain [94]. Epigenetic drugs, such as histone de-acetylation, and DNA methylation inhibitors have received increased attention for the management of mental disorders [95].

Neuroepigenomics represents an effort to unify the research available on the molecular pathology of mental disorders, such as single DNA methylation, to epigenome-wide association studies, post-translational modifications of histones, or nucleosomal positioning [96]. A huge amount of studies examining the role of epigenome, including epigenetic signaling, such as DNA and histone modifications in the etiology of SCZ was published [97, 98]. Large-scale consortia, such as the PGC and the Common Minds Consortium provide detailed insight into the epigenetic risk architectures of SCZ [99]. However, the absence of consistently replicated genetic effects together with changes in gene expression suggests the role of epigenetic mechanisms in SCZ [16].

Brain development is guided by interactions between the genome and environment, such as early life adversity. Epigenetic mechanisms can mediate these interactions and increase the risk of SCZ [17]. In a mixed model of SCZ risk, abnormal epigenetic states with large effects are superimposed on a polygenic liability to SCZ [100]. It has been reported that several genes related to nucleosome and histone structure are dysregulated in PBMC of patients with SCZ. It may be suggesting a potential epigenetic mechanism underlying the risk factor for the development of SCZ [101].

Genome-scale mapping of epigenetic mechanisms, including chromosomal loopings, and other epigenetic determinants of genome organization help to understand the mechanisms contributing to dysregulated expression of synaptic and metabolic genes in SCZ [102]. Some authors have found methylation differences in different genes, including *COMT*, *RELN*, and in some other genes implicated in dopaminergic, serotoninergic, $\gamma$-aminobutyric acid (GABA)ergic, and glutamatergic pathways [103]. It has been proposed that prenatal stress induces neurodevelopmental alterations in the prefrontal cortex that are expressed as cognitive impairments observed in SCZ [104]. Reelin (*RELN*) is involved in cortical neural connectivity and synaptic plasticity. Downregulation of *RELN* expression due to its hypermethylation has been associated with epigenetic changes in this gene of the prefrontal cortex of patients with SCZ [97].

A significant portion of patients with SCZ shows deficits in glutamate decarboxylase 1 (*GAD1*). This gene encodes a 67 kDa glutamate decarboxylase (*GAD67*) protein in multiple areas of adult cerebral cortex. This event, possibly reflecting molecular defects in subtypes of GABAergic interneurons essential for network synchronization and cognition [105]. Dysfunction of prefrontal cortex in SCZ includes the changes in GABAergic mRNAs, including decreased expression of *GAD1*. It has been demonstrated that the methylation frequency at CpG dinucleotides located at the proximal *GAD1* promoter shows a significant deficit in repressive DNA methylation in patients with SCZ [106]. Adverse life events have been found to control DNA methylation in postmitotic neurons. This phenotype in SCZ was accompanied by a persistent increase in *AVP* gene expression [107].

## 4. Pathway analysis

### 4.1. An overview

The concept of pathway is more complex structure than a cluster. Pathways in biology correspond to series of interactions among different molecules in a cell that lead to a certain product. Pathway-based analysis provides a technique, which allows a comprehensive understanding of the molecular mechanisms underlying complex traits or disorders, such as mental disorders. There are a variety of pathway-based approaches, including SNP/GWAS-derived pathway analysis, which correspond to different research designs and data types [108].

In pathway analysis, data come from high throughput biology. Gene sets corresponding to biological pathways are tested for significant relationships with a phenotype. Genotyping, gene expression arrays, or any data elements that could be mapped to genes or gene products could be used. It may be concluded that the pathway analysis represents a potentially powerful and biologically-oriented bridge between genotypes and phenotypes [109]. Pathway analysis has become the first choice for gaining insight into the underlying biology of differentially expressed genes and proteins, as it reduces complexity and has increased explanatory power [110].

### 4.2. Pathway analysis in schizophrenia

By using the key words of "genome-wide association study" in PubMed database, over 22,000 human GWAS publications have described genetic associations to a wide range of disorders and traits. Additionally, by using the key words of "genome-wide association study and schizophrenia" in PubMed, more than 1190 human GWAS publications have described genetic associations to SCZ. Genome-wide data sets are increasingly viewed as foundations for discovering pathways and networks relevant to phenotypes [111]. However, extending GWAS findings to mechanistic hypotheses about the development of SCZ has been a major ongoing challenge.

Sundararajan et al. [22] have been used the clinically relevant and reported susceptibility genes associated with SCZ and available gene analysis program, and created a molecular profile of the updated SCZ genes. These genes were predominantly expressed in specific brain regions, including the cerebellum, cerebral cortex, medulla oblongata, thalamus, and hypothalamus. Interestingly, by the analysis of major biological pathways and mechanisms associated with SCZ genes, these authors identified glutaminergic, serotonergic, GABAergic, and dopaminergic receptors, calcium-related channels, solute transporters, and neurodevelopmental genes. Biological mechanisms, including synaptic transmission, membrane potential, and transmembrane ion transport regulation were identified as leading molecular functions associated with SCZ genes [22].

Regarding the involvement of neuroinflammation in pathogenesis of SCZ in postmortem brains of patients with SCZ, neuroinflammatory markers and an overall increase in expression of pro-inflammatory genes have been reported [79].

By using a translational convergent functional genomics approach and a poly evidence scoring and pathway analyses, Ayalew et al. [51] identified top genes (e.g., *DISC1, HSPA1B, MBP,* and *TCF4),* brain development, myelination, cell adhesion, glutamate receptor signaling, G-protein coupled receptor signaling, and cAMP-mediated signaling as key to pathophysiology and as targets for therapeutic intervention.

Karim et al. [76] carried out pathway and gene ontology analyses and observed alteration in a few signaling pathways in neurons. These pathways were GABA receptor, immune response, G beta gamma, dopamine and cyclic AMP, complement system, axonal guidance, dendritic cell maturation, *CREB*, and interleukin-1 signaling pathways and networks.

By using the network-based approach for evaluating gene co-expression, Mistry et al. [112] found separate gene co-expression networks. Functional enrichment analysis showed that altered genes expression in SCZ associate with biological processes such as oxidative phosphorylation, myelination, synaptic transmission, and immune function [112].

Differentially expressed genes in PBMC of patients with SCZ have been reported that were involved in pathways such as cell adhesion, neuronal guidance, neurotrophins, oxidative stress, glucose metabolism, apoptosis, and cell-cycle regulation [78].

It has been suggested that the genetic basis of SCZ has a complex evolutionary history. It has been hypothesized that the genetic architecture components of SCZ are attributable to human lineage-specific evolution [113]. It has been shown that the SCZ genes are located near previously identified human accelerated regions (HARs). Additionally, these genes enrich in a GABA-related co-expression module significantly. These genes are differentially regulated in patients with SCZ. It has been concluded that genes located near the HARs are associated with important functional roles in the genetic architecture of SCZ [113].

Cell death is an active process that maintains tissue homeostasis. Three types of distinct cell death are apoptosis, autophagic cell death, and necrosis [114]. The apoptotic pathway will begin with death receptor activation. This activation leads to the formation of death receptor signaling pathways, resulting in the demolition of the cell [115]. It has been hypothesized that an increase in apoptosis may underlie neuropathology of SCZ [116]. There are significant expression changes in death genes receptor signaling pathways in the dorsolateral prefrontal cortex of patients with SCZ, including the *TNFSF13* and *TNFSF13*. It has been concluded that the increased *TNFSF13* expression may be one of the abnormalities that contribute to the brain pathology in SCZ [116].

By using the factor analysis of symptoms of narrowly defined patients with SCZ through the clinician-rated operational criteria checklist items in an Irish family sample, implemented genome-wide association, gene-based, and gene-pathway analyses of these SCZ-based symptom factors, Docherty et al. [117] could find three factors, including: a manic, a depressive, and a positive symptom factor. Gene-based analysis of these factors showed *PTPRG* and *WBP1L* genes. These genes were also implicated by the PGC study of SCZ [45]. It has been suggested that variants in these two genes might also act as modifiers of SCZ symptoms. Gene pathway analysis of the mania factor indicated over-representation of glutamatergic transmission, GABA-A receptor, and cyclic GMP pathways and these pathways may have differential influence on affective symptoms in SCZ [117].

Through the interrogating SCZ genes and their complex interactions at various levels, including transcripts and proteins and also environmental and developmental factors, our knowledge and insight into the disorder processes will increase. This may possibly open the new avenues for more effective therapeutic interventions.

## 5. Future perspective

Although a huge amount of studies has been performed and significant progress has been made in past decades, the high heritability, phenotype heterogeneity, and strong genetic and epigenetic heterogeneity of SCZ still post as major challenges to the genetic dissection of this complex syndrome. Therefore, more studies are needed to explain its missing heritability [118]. It is essential to shift paradigm in understanding the etiopathology of SCZ. A critical question is "What is schizophrenia?" Is it a specific disorder or a heterogeneous syndrome? Changes in brain gene expression of the patients with SCZ may reflect the possible pathways related to pathophysiology of the syndrome.

A few suggestions for the next decade are studying the multiple brain regions in normal people to better understand neural circuitry, genetics and epigenetic patterns of the brain, peripheral biomarker studies, and analyze the other omics data, such as transcriptomics across a developmental series of brains. System biology and computational approaches will be useful to advance from normal brains to a more reliable and valid definition of the SCZ interactome and connectome [70].

Through the better understanding of pathophysiology of SCZ, at the levels of genetic and epigenetic, we could identify new leads for the management of this complex syndrome. However, which gene(s) is causal, how the risk genetic or epigenetic factors alter gene expression, and how they fit into pathology and syndrome pathways [119]. New drugs for SCZ are essential needs for the patients. These drugs have to target pathophysiological alterations that are specific to syndrome. Schizophrenia is a multifactorial and strongly biologically heteroge-neous syndrome. Identification of homogenous subgroups is increasingly necessary for new drugs discovery [120]. So, the above mentioned assays will help the researchers to understand the pathological processes and the development of better treatments [15, 119].

In addition to different approaches to the analysis for genes associated with SCZ, the genetics and epigenetic of specific psychopathology, including cognitive impairments, negative signs, disor-ganized behaviors, etc., need to be addressed. In this regard, neuroimaging genetics approach will be useful. In addition, a psychiatric translational and phenomics approach (genome to mind phenome), understanding the pathology of syndrome in different levels, such as genetics, epi-genetic, proteomics, and other omics data, and also neural circuit abnormalities, and endopheno-types related to psychopathology and clinical phenotypes are another essential steps.

## 6. Conclusion

Schizophrenia is a complex, heterogeneous, and multifactorial syndrome. It has many levels, including genomics, epigenomics, transcriptomics, proteomics, metabolomics, neural circuit, endophenotype, and albeit clinical presentations. It seems that an ideal "multi-level diagnostic system" has to include all of these levels to make a bioprofile. By doing this in the near future, we hope to have a more reliable and valid diagnostic system, better approach to its treatment and also prevention of mental disorders, including SCZ.

## Author details

Esmaeil Shahsavand Ananloo

Address all correspondence to: esmaeilshahsavand@gmail.com

Department of Genomic Psychiatry and Behavioral Genomics (DGPBG), Roozbeh Hospital, School of Medicine, Tehran University of Medical Sciences (TUMS), Tehran, Iran

## References

[1] Birnbaum R, Weinberger DR. Genetic insights into the neurodevelopmental origins of schizophrenia. Nature Reviews. Neuroscience. Dec 2017;**18**(12):727-740. DOI: 10.1038/nrn.2017.125

[2] Vita A, Barlati S, De Peri L, et al. Schizophrenia. Lancet. 2016;**388**(10051):1280. DOI: 10.1016/S0140-6736(16)31674-9

[3] Aberg KA, Liu Y, Bukszár J, et al. A comprehensive family-based replication study of schizophrenia genes. JAMA Psychiatry. Jun 2013;**70**(6):573-581. DOI: 10.1001/jamapsychiatry.2013.288

[4] Pantavou KG, Braliou GG, Kontou PI, et al. A meta-analysis of FZD3 gene polymorphisms and their association with schizophrenia. Psychiatric Genetics. Dec 2016;**26**(6):272-280. DOI: 10.1097/YPG.0000000000000155

[5] Gottesman II, Erlenmeyer-Kimling L. Family and twin strategies as a head start in defining prodromes and endophenotypes for hypothetical early-interventions in schizophrenia. Schizophrenia Research. Aug 1, 2001;**51**(1):93-102. DOI: 10.1016/s0920-9964(01)00245-6

[6] Fatemi SH, Folsom TD, Rooney RJ, et al. The viral theory of schizophrenia revisited: Abnormal placental gene expression and structural changes with lack of evidence for H1N1 viral presence in placentae of infected mice or brains of exposed offspring. Neuropharmacology. Mar 2012;**62**(3):1290-1298. DOI: 10.1016/j.neuropharm.2011.01.011

[7] Meyer U, Feldon J. Epidemiology-driven neurodevelopmental animal models of schizophrenia. Progress in Neurobiology. Mar 2010;**90**(3):285-326. DOI: 10.1016/j.pneurobio.2009.10.018

[8] Niculescu AB. Schizophrenia: From genetics to biology to predictive medicine. The Journal of Clinical Psychiatry. 2014;**75**(Suppl 2):4-7. DOI: 10.4088/JCP.13065su1.01

[9] Ma G, Yin J, Fu J, et al. Association of a miRNA-137 polymorphism with schizophrenia in a southern Chinese Han population. BioMed Research International. 2014;**2014**:751267. DOI: 10.1155/2014/751267

[10] Hauberg ME, Roussos P, Grove J, Børglum AD, Mattheisen M, Schizophrenia Working Group of the Psychiatric Genomics Consortium. Analyzing the role of MicroRNAs in schizophrenia in the context of common genetic risk variants. JAMA Psychiatry. Apr 2016;**73**(4):369-377. DOI: 10.1001/jamapsychiatry.2015.3018

[11] Liu W, Liu F, Xu X, Bai Y. Replicated association between the European GWAS locus rs10503253 at CSMD1 and schizophrenia in Asian population. Neuroscience Letters. Apr 2017;**24**(647):122-128. DOI: 10.1016/j.neulet.2017.03.039

[12] Mostaid MS, Mancuso SG, Liu C, et al. Meta-analysis reveals associations between genetic variation in the 5′ and 3′ regions of Neuregulin-1 and schizophrenia. Translational Psychiatry. Jan 17, 2017;**7**(1):e1004. DOI: 10.1038/tp.2016.279

[13] Qin W, Liu C, Sodhi M, Lu H. Meta-analysis of sex differences in gene expression in schizophrenia. BMC Systems Biology. Jan 11, 2016;**10**(Suppl 1):9. DOI: 10.1186/s12918-015-0250-3

[14] Alizadeh F, Tavakkoly-Bazzaz J, Bozorgmehr A, Azarnezhad A, Tabrizi M, Shahsavand AE. Association of transcription factor 4 (TCF4) gene mRNA level with schizophrenia,

its psychopathology, intelligence and cognitive impairments. Journal of Neurogenetics. Dec 2017;**31**(4):344-351. DOI: 10.1080/01677063.2017.1396330

[15] Hoffmann A, Ziller M, Spengler D. The future is the past: Methylation QTLs in schizophrenia. Genes (Basel). Nov 24, 2016;**7**(12). DOI: 10.3390/genes7120104

[16] Cariaga-Martinez A, Saiz-Ruiz J, Alelú-Paz R. From linkage studies to epigenetics: What we know and what we need to know in the neurobiology of schizophrenia. Frontiers in Neuroscience. May 11, 2016;**10**:202. DOI: 10.3389/fnins.2016.00202

[17] Hoffmann A, Sportelli V, Ziller M, Spengler D. Epigenomics of major depressive disorders and schizophrenia: Early life decides. International Journal of Molecular Sciences. Aug 4, 2017;**18**(8):pii:E1711. DOI: 10.3390/ijms18081711

[18] Fisch GS. Whither the genotype-phenotype relationship? An historical and methodological appraisal. American Journal of Medical Genetics. Part C, Seminars in Medical Genetics. Sep 2017;**175**(3):343-353. DOI: 10.1002/ajmg.c.31571

[19] Owens EM, Bachman P, Glahn DC, Bearden CE. Electrophysiological Endophenotypes for schizophrenia. Harvard Review of Psychiatry. Mar–Apr 2016;**24**(2):129-147. DOI: 10.1097/HRP.0000000000000110

[20] DiLalla LF, McCrary M, Diaz E. A review of endophenotypes in schizophrenia and autism: The next phase for understanding genetic etiologies. American Journal of Medical Genetics. Part C, Seminars in Medical Genetics. Sep 2017;**175**(3):354-361. DOI: 10.1002/ajmg.c.31566

[21] Reble E, Castellani CA, Melka MG, et al. VarScan2 analysis of de novo variants in monozygotic twins discordant for schizophrenia. Psychiatric Genetics. Apr 2017;**27**(2):62-70. DOI: 10.1097/YPG.0000000000000162

[22] Sundararajan T, Manzardo AM, Butler MG. Functional analysis of schizophrenia genes using GeneAnalytics program and integrated databases. Gene. Jan 30, 2018;(641):25-34. DOI: 10.1016/j.gene.2017.10.035

[23] Tansey KE, Owen MJ, O'Donovan MC. Schizophrenia genetics: Building the foundations of the future. Schizophrenia Bulletin. Jan 2015;**41**(1):15-19. DOI: 10.1093/schbul/sbu162

[24] Kotlar AV, Mercer KB, Zwick ME, Mulle JG. New discoveries in schizophrenia genetics reveal neurobiological pathways: A review of recent findings. European Journal of Medical Genetics. Dec 2015;**58**(12):704-714. DOI: 10.1016/j.ejmg.2015.10.008

[25] Wray NR, Goddard ME, Visscher PM. Prediction of individual genetic risk to disease from genome-wide association studies. Genome Research. Oct 2007;**17**(10):1520-1528. DOI: 10.1101/gr.6665407

[26] Sullivan PF, Kendler KS, Neale MC. Schizophrenia as a complex trait: Evidence from a meta-analysis of twin studies. Archives of General Psychiatry. 2003;**60**(12):1187-1192. DOI: 10.1001/archpsyc.60.12.1187

[27] Cardno AG, Gottesman II. Twin studies of schizophrenia: From bow-and-arrow concordances to star wars mx and functional genomics. American Journal of Medical Genetics. 2000 Spring;**97**(1):12-17. DOI: 10.1002/(SICI)1096-8628(200021)97:1<12::AID-AJMG3>3.0.CO;2-U

[28] Lichtenstein P, Yip BH, Björk C, et al. Common genetic determinants of schizophrenia and bipolar disorder in Swedish families: A population-based study. Lancet. Jan 17, 2009;**373**(9659):234-239. DOI: 10.1016/S0140-6736(09)60072-6

[29] Scolnick EM. The path to new therapies for schizophrenia and bipolar illness. The FASEB Journal. Apr 2017;**31**(4):1254-1259. DOI: 10.1096/fj.201700028

[30] Janoutová J, Janácková P, Serý O, et al. Epidemiology and risk factors of schizophrenia. Neuro Endocrinology Letters. 2016;**37**(1):1-8. DOI: 10.1007/s11469-009-9241-1

[31] Roalf DR, Vandekar SN, Almasy L, et al. Heritability of subcortical and limbic brain volume and shape in multiplex-multigenerational families with schizophrenia. Biological Psychiatry. Jan 15, 2015;**77**(2):137-146. DOI: 10.1016/j.biopsych.2014.05.009

[32] Voineskos AN. Genetic underpinnings of white matter 'connectivity': Heritability, risk, and heterogeneity in schizophrenia. Schizophrenia Research. Jan 2015;**161**(1):50-60. DOI: 10.1016/j.schres.2014.03.034

[33] Mark W, Toulopoulou T. Cognitive intermediate phenotype and genetic risk for psychosis. Current Opinion in Neurobiology. Feb 2016;**36**:23-30. DOI: 10.1016/j.conb.2015.08.008

[34] Plomin R, Haworth CM, Meaburn EL, et al. Common DNA markers can account for more than half of the genetic influence on cognitive abilities. Psychological Science. Apr 2013;**24**(4):562-568. DOI: 10.1177/0956797612457952

[35] Farrell MS, Werge P, Sklar MJ, et al. Evaluating historical candidate genes for schizophrenia. Molecular Psychiatry. 2015;**20**(5):555-562. DOI: 10.1038/mp.2015.16

[36] Patnala R, Clements J, Batra J. Candidate gene association studies: A comprehensive guide to useful in silico tools. BMC Genetics. May 9, 2013;**14**:39. DOI: 10.1186/1471-2156-14-39

[37] Kwon JM, Goate AM. The candidate gene approach. Alcohol Research & Health. 2000;**24**(3):164-168

[38] Lee S, Wright FA, Zou F. Control of population stratification by correlation-selected principal components. Biometrics. 2011;**67**:967-974. DOI: 10.1111/j.1541-0420.2010.01520.x

[39] Burdick KE, DeRosse P, Kane JM, et al. Genetic variation in the MET proto-oncogene is associated with schizophrenia and general cognitive ability. The American Journal of Psychiatry. 2010;**167**(4):436-443. DOI: 10.1176/appi.ajp.2009.09050615

[40] Lander ES, Linton LM, Birren B, et al. Initial sequencing and analysis of the human genome. Nature. 2001;**409**(6822):860-921. DOI: 10.1038/35057062

[41] International HapMap Consortium. A haplotype map of the human genome. Nature. 2005;**437**(7063):1299-1320. DOI: 10.1038/nature04226

[42] The 1000 Genomes Project Consortium, Abecasis GR, Auton A, et al. An integrated map of genetic variation from 1,092 human genomes. Nature. 2012;**491**:56-65. DOI: 10.1038/nature11632

[43] Pritchard JK, Cox NJ. The allelic architecture of human disease genes: common disease-common variant or not? Human Molecular Genetics. 2002;**11**:2417-2423. DOI: 10.1093/hmg/11.20.2417

[44] Stefansson H, Ophoff RA, Steinberg S, et al. Common variants conferring risk of schizophrenia. Nature. 2009;**460**:744-747. DOI: 10.1038/nature08186

[45] Ripke S, Sanders AR, Kendler KS, et al. Genome-wide association study identifies five new schizophrenia loci. Nature Genetics. 2011;**43**:969-976. DOI: 10.1038/ng.940

[46] Mccarroll SA, Altshuler DM. Copy number variation and association studies of human diseased. Nature Genetics. 2007;**39**:37-42. DOI: 10.1038/ng2080

[47] Bassett AS, Scherer SW, Brzustowicz LM. Copy number variations in schizophrenia: Critical review and new perspectives on concepts of genetics and disease. The American Journal of Psychiatry. 2010;**167**:899-914. DOI: 10.1176/appi.ajp.2009.09071016

[48] Xu B, Roos JL, Levy S, et al. Strong association of de novo copy number mutations with sporadic schizophrenia. Nature Genetics. Jul, 2008;**40**(7):880-885. DOI: 10.1038/ng.162

[49] Vacic V, McCarthy S, Malhotra D, et al. Duplications of the neuropeptide receptor gene VIPR2 confer significant risk for schizophrenia. Nature. 2011;**471**:499-503. DOI: 10.1038/nature09884

[50] Allen NC, Bagade S, McQueen MB, et al. Systematic meta-analyses and field synopsis of genetic association studies in schizophrenia: The SzGene database. Nature Genetics. 2008;**40**(7):827-834. DOI: 10.1038/ng.171

[51] Ayalew M, Le-Niculescu H, Levey DF, et al. Convergent functional genomics of schizophrenia: From comprehensive understanding to genetic risk prediction. Molecular Psychiatry. 2012;Sep;**17**(9):887-905. DOI: 10.1038/mp.2012.37

[52] Kheirollahi M, Kazemi E, Ashouri S. Brain-derived Neurotrophic factor gene Val66Met polymorphism and risk of schizophrenia: A meta-analysis of case-control studies. Cellular and Molecular Neurobiology. Jan 2016;**36**(1):1-10. DOI: 10.1007/s10571-015-0229-z

[53] González-Castro TB, Hernández-Díaz Y, Juárez-Rojop IE, et al. The role of C957T, TaqI and Ser311Cys polymorphisms of the DRD2 gene in schizophrenia: Systematic review and meta-analysis. Behavioral and Brain Functions. Nov 9, 2016;**12**(1):29. DOI: 10.1186/s12993-016-0114-z

[54] Neale BM, Sham PC. The future of association studies: Gene-based analysis and replication. American Journal of Human Genetics. 2004;**75**(3):353-362. DOI: 10.1086/423901

[55] Sullivan PF. Spurious genetic associations. Biological Psychiatry. 2007;**61**(10):1121-1126. DOI: 10.1016/j.biopsych.2006.11.010

[56] Agrawal A, Edenberg HJ, Gelernter J. Meta-analyses of genome-wide association data hold new promise for addiction genetics. Journal of Studies on Alcohol and Drugs. 2016 Sep;**77**(5):676-680. DOI: 10.15288/jsad.2016.77.676

[57] Lencz T, Knowles E, Davies G, et al. Molecular genetic evidence for overlap between general cognitive ability and risk for schizophrenia: a report from the Cognitive Genomics consorTium (COGENT). Molecular Psychiatry. Feb 2014;**19**(2):168-174. DOI: 10.1038/mp.2013

[58] Luo XJ, Huang L, Oord EJ, et al. Common variants in the MKL1 gene confer risk of schizophrenia. Schizophrenia Bulletin. May 2015;**41**(3):715-727. DOI: 10.1093/schbul/sbu156

[59] Sleiman P, Wang D, Glessner J, et al. GWAS meta analysis identifies TSNARE1 as a novel schizophrenia/bipolar susceptibility locus. Scientific Reports. Oct 29, 2013;**3**:3075. DOI: 10.1038/srep03075

[60] Xu C, Aragam N, Li X, et al. BCL9 and C9orf5 are associated with negative symptoms in schizophrenia: Meta-analysis of two genome-wide association studies. PLoS One. 2013;**8**(1):e51674. DOI: 10.1371/journal.pone.0051674

[61] Schizophrenia Working Group of the Psychiatric Genomics Consortium. Biological insights from 108 schizophrenia-associated genetic loci. Nature. 2014;**511**:421-427. DOI: 10.1038/nature13595

[62] Rose EJ, Morris DW, Hargreaves A, et al. Neural effects of the CSMD1 genome-wide associated schizophrenia risk variant rs10503253. American Journal of Medical Genetics. Part B, Neuropsychiatric Genetics. Sep 2013;**162B**(6):530-537. DOI: 10.1002/ajmg.b.32182

[63] Koiliari E, Roussos P, Pasparakis E, et al. The CSMD1 genome-wide associated schizophrenia risk variant rs10503253 affects general cognitive ability and executive function in healthy males. Schizophrenia Research. Apr 2014;**154**(1-3):42-47. DOI: 10.1016/j.schres.2014.02.017

[64] Suárez-Rama JJ, Arrojo M, Sobrino B, et al. Resequencing and association analysis of coding regions at twenty candidate genes suggest a role for rare risk variation at AKAP9 and protective variation at NRXN1 in schizophrenia susceptibility. Journal of Psychiatric Research. Jul-Aug, 2015;**66-67**:38-44. DOI: 10.1016/j.jpsychires.2015.04.013

[65] Takahashi S, Glatt SJ, Uchiyama M, et al. Meta-analysis of data from the psychiatric genomics consortium and additional samples supports association of CACNA1C with risk for schizophrenia. Schizophrenia Research. Oct, 2015;**168**(1-2):429-433. DOI: 10.1016/j.schres.2015.07.033

[66] Perez-Becerril C, Morris AG, Mortimer A, et al. Common variants in the chromosome 2p23 region containing the SLC30A3 (ZnT3) gene are associated with schizophrenia in female but not male individuals in a large collection of European samples. Psychiatry Research. Dec 30, 2016;**246**:335-340. DOI: 10.1016/j.psychres.2016.09.052

[67] Chang H, Zhang C, Xiao X, et al. Further evidence of VRK2 rs2312147 associated with schizophrenia. The World Journal of Biological Psychiatry. Sep 2016;**17**(6):457-466. DOI: 10.1080/15622975.2016.1200746

[68] Xiao X, Li M. Replication of Han Chinese GWAS loci for schizophrenia via meta-analysis of four independent samples. Schizophrenia Research. Apr 2016;**172**(1-3):75-77. DOI: 10.1016/j.schres.2016.02.019

[69] DeLisi LE. Is schizophrenia a lifetime disorder of brain plasticity, growth and aging? Schizophrenia Research. Feb 7, 1997;**23**(2):119-129. DOI: 10.1016/S0920-9964(96)00079-5

[70] Sequeira PA, Martin MV, Vawter MP. The first decade and beyond of transcriptional profiling in schizophrenia. Neurobiology of Disease. Jan 2012;**45**(1):23-36. DOI: 10.1016/j.nbd.2011.03.001

[71] Palaniyappan L. Progressive cortical reorganisation: A framework for investigating structural changes in schizophrenia. Neuroscience and Biobehavioral Reviews. Aug 2017;**79**:1-13. DOI: 10.1016/j.neubiorev.2017.04.028

[72] Dietsche B, Kircher T, Falkenberg I. Structural brain changes in schizophrenia at different stages of the illness: A selective review of longitudinal magnetic resonance imaging studies. The Australian and New Zealand Journal of Psychiatry. May 2017;**51**(5):500-508. DOI: 10.1177/0004867417699473

[73] Heilbronner U, Samara M, Leucht S, et al. The longitudinal course of schizophrenia across the lifespan: Clinical, cognitive, and neurobiological aspects. Harvard Review of Psychiatry. Mar-Apr 2016;**24**(2):118-128. DOI: 10.1097/HRP.0000000000000092

[74] van Os J, Rutten BP, Poulton R. Gene-environment interactions in schizophrenia: Review of epidemiological findings and future directions. Schizophrenia Bulletin. Nov 2008;**34**(6):1066-1082. DOI: 10.1093/schbul/sbn117

[75] Popov NT, Stoyanova VK, Madzhirova NP, Vachev TI. Epigenetic aspects in schizophrenia etiology and pathogenesis. Folia Medica (Plovdiv). Apr-Jun 2012;**54**(2):12-16. DOI: 10.2478/v10153-011-0082-x

[76] Karim S, Kamal MA, Iqbal Z, et al. Global expression studies of schizophrenic brain: A meta-analysis study linking neurological immune system with psychological disorders. CNS & Neurological Disorders Drug Targets. 2016;**15**(4):477-488. DOI: 10.2174/1871527315666160321105216

[77] Gardiner EJ, Cairns MJ, Liu B, et al. Gene expression analysis reveals schizophrenia-associated dysregulation of immune pathways in peripheral blood mononuclear cells. Journal of Psychiatric Research. Apr 2013;**47**(4):425-437. DOI: 10.1016/j.jpsychires.2012.11.007

[78] van Beveren NJ, Buitendijk GH, Swagemakers S, et al. Marked reduction of AKT1 expression and deregulation of AKT1-associated pathways in peripheral blood mononuclear cells of schizophrenia patients. PLoS One. 2012;**7**:e32618. DOI: 10.1371/journal.pone.0032618

[79] van Kesteren CF, Gremmels H, de Witte LD, et al. Immune involvement in the pathogenesis of schizophrenia: A meta-analysis on postmortem brain studies. Translational Psychiatry. Mar 28, 2017;**7**(3):e1075. DOI: 10.1038/tp.2017.4

[80] Li C, Feng Y, Coukos G, Zhang L. Therapeutic MicroRNA strategies in human cancer. The AAPS Journal. Dec 2009;**11**(4):747. DOI: 10.1208/s12248-009-9145-9

[81] Wilfred BR, Wang WX, Nelson PT. Energizing miRNA research: A review of the role of miRNAs in lipid metabolism, with a prediction that miR-103/107 regulates human metabolic pathways. Molecular Genetics and Metabolism. Jul 2007;**91**(3):209-217. DOI: 10.1016/j.ymgme.2007.03.011

[82] Fasanaro P, Greco S, Ivan M, et al. microRNA: Emerging therapeutic targets in acute ischemic diseases. Pharmacology & Therapeutics. Jan 2010;**125**(1):92-104. DOI: 10.1016/j.pharmthera.2009.10.003

[83] Lagos-Quintana M, Rauhut R, Yalcin A, et al. Identification of tissue-specific microRNAs from mouse. Curr Biology. Apr 30, 2002;**12**(9):735-739. DOI: 10.1016/S0960-9822(02)00809-6

[84] Bartel DP. MicroRNAs: Genomics, biogenesis, mechanism, and function. Cell. Jan 23, 2004;**116**(2):281-297. DOI: 10.1016/S0092-8674(04)00045-5

[85] Wienholds E, Kloosterman WP, Miska E, et al. MicroRNA expression in zebrafish embryonic development. Science. Jul 8, 2005;**309**(5732):310-311. DOI: 10.1126/science.1114519

[86] Cuellar TL, McManus MT. MicroRNAs and endocrine biology. The Journal of Endocri nology. Dec 2005;**187**(3):327-332. DOI: 10.1677/joe.1.06426

[87] Chen CZ, Li L, Lodish HF, Bartel DP. MicroRNAs modulate hematopoietic lineage differentiation. Science. Jan 2, 2004;**303**(5654):83-86. DOI: 10.1126/science.1091903

[88] Trang P, Weidhaas JB, Slack FJ. MicroRNAs as potential cancer therapeutics. Oncogene. Dec 2008;**27**(Suppl 2):S52-S57. DOI: 10.1038/onc.2009.353

[89] Lai CY, Scarr E, Udawela M, et al. Biomarkers in schizophrenia: A focus on blood based diagnostics and theranostics. World Journal of Psychiatry. Mar 22, 2016;**6**(1):102-117. DOI: 10.5498/wjp.v6.i1.102

[90] Kuzman MR, Medved V, Terzic J, Krainc D. Genome-wide expression analysis of peripheral blood identifies candidate biomarkers for schizophrenia. Journal of Psychiatric Research. 2009;**43**:1073-1077. DOI: 10.1016/j.jpsychires.2009.03.005

[91] Dupont C, Armant DR, Brenner CA. Epigenetics: Definition, mechanisms and clinical perspective. Seminars in Reproductive Medicine. Sep 2009;**27**(5):351-357. DOI: 10.1055/s-0029-1237423

[92] Turner B. Defining an epigenetic code. Nature Cell Biology. 2007;**9**(1):2-6. DOI: 10.1038/ncb0107-2

[93] Sweatt JD, Tamminga CA. An epigenomics approach to individual differences and its translation to neuropsychiatric conditions. Dialogues in Clinical Neuroscience. Sep 2016;**18**(3):289-298

[94] Dempster E, Viana J, Pidsley R, Mill J. Epigenetic studies of schizophrenia: Progress, predicaments, and promises for the future. Schizophrenia Bulletin. Jan 2013;**39**(1):11-16. DOI: 10.1093/schbul/sbs139

[95] Karsli-Ceppioglu S. Epigenetic mechanisms in psychiatric diseases and epigenetic therapy. Drug Development Research. Nov 2016;**77**(7):407-413. DOI: 10.1002/ddr.21340

[96] Cariaga-Martinez A, Alelú-Paz R. Rethinking the epigenetic framework to unravel the molecular pathology of schizophrenia. International Journal of Molecular Sciences. Apr 7, 2017;**18**(4):pii:E790. DOI: 10.3390/ijms18040790

[97] Ibi D, González-Maeso J. Epigenetic signaling in schizophrenia. Cellular Signalling. Oct 2015;**27**(10):2131-2136. DOI: 10.1016/j.cellsig.2015.06.003

[98] Fullard JF, Halene TB, Giambartolomei C, et al. Understanding the genetic liability to schizophrenia through the neuroepigenome. Schizophrenia Research. Nov 2016;**177**(1-3): 115-124. DOI: 10.1016/j.schres.2016.01.039

[99] Javidfar B, Park R, Kassim BS, et al. The epigenomics of schizophrenia, in the mouse. American Journal of Medical Genetics. Part B, Neuropsychiatric Genetics. Sep 2017;**174**(6): 631-640. DOI: 10.1002/ajmg.b.32566

[100] Svrakic DM, Zorumski CF, Svrakic NM, et al. Risk architecture of schizophrenia: The role of epigenetics. Current Opinion in Psychiatry. Mar 2013;**26**(2):188-195. DOI: 10.1097/YCO.0b013e32835d8329

[101] Glatt SJ, Stone WS, Nossova N, et al. Similarities and differences in peripheral blood gene-expression signatures of individuals with schizophrenia and their first-degree biological relatives. American Journal of Medical Genetics. Part B, Neuropsychiatric Genetics. 2011;**156B**:869-887. DOI: 10.1002/ajmg.b.31239

[102] Akbarian S. Epigenetic mechanisms in schizophrenia. Dialogues in Clinical Neuro science. Sep 2014;**16**(3):405-417

[103] Rivollier F, Lotersztajn L, Chaumette B, et al. Epigenetics of schizophrenia: A review. Encephale. Oct 2014;**40**(5):380-386. DOI: 10.1016/j.encep.2014.06.005

[104] Negrón-Oyarzo I, Lara-Vásquez A, Palacios-García I, et al. Schizophrenia and reelin: A model based on prenatal stress to study epigenetics, brain development and behavior. Biological Research. Mar 11, 2016;**49**:16. DOI: 10.1186/s40659-016-0076-5

[105] Mitchell AC, Jiang Y, Peter C, Akbarian S. Transcriptional regulation of GAD1 GABA synthesis gene in the prefrontal cortex of subjects with schizophrenia. Schizophrenia Research. Sep 2015;**167**(1-3):28-34. DOI: 10.1016/j.schres.2014.10.020

[106] Huang HS, Akbarian S. GAD1 mRNA expression and DNA methylation in prefrontal cortex of subjects with schizophrenia. PLoS One. Aug 29, 2007;**2**(8):e809. DOI: 10.1371/journal.pone.0000809

[107] Murgatroyd C, Patchev AV, Wu Y, et al. Dynamic DNA methylation programs persistent adverse effects of early-life stress. Nature Neuroscience. Dec 2009;**12**(12):1559-1566. DOI: 10.1038/nn.2436

[108] Jin LV, Zuo ZY, Su WY, et al. Pathway-based analysis tools for complex diseases. Genomics, Proteomics & Bioinformatics. Oct 2014;**12**(5):210-220. DOI: 10.1016/j.gpb.2014.10.002

[109] Ramanan VK, Shen L, Moore JH, Saykin AJ. Pathway analysis of genomic data: Concepts, methods, and prospects for future development. Trends in Genetics. Jul 2012;**28**(7):323-332. DOI: 10.1016/j.tig.2012.03.004

[110] Khatri P, Sirota M, Butte AJ. Ten years of pathway analysis: Current approaches and outstanding challenges. PLoS Computational Biology. 2012;**8**(2):e1002375. DOI: 10.1371/journal.pcbi.1002375

[111] Hirschhorn JN. Genomewide association studies--illuminating biologic pathways. The New England Journal of Medicine. Apr 23, 2009;**360**(17):1699-1701. DOI: 10.1056/NEJMp0808934

[112] Mistry M, Gillis J, Pavlidis P. Meta-analysis of gene coexpression networks in the post-mortem prefrontal cortex of patients with schizophrenia and unaffected controls. BMC Neuroscience. Sep 26, 2013;**14**:105. DOI: 10.1186/1471-2202-14-105

[113] Xu K, Schadt EE, Pollard KS, et al. Genomic and network patterns of schizophrenia genetic variation in human evolutionary accelerated regions. Molecular Biology and Evolution. May 2015;**32**(5):1148-1160. DOI: 10.1093/molbev/msv031

[114] Green DR, Llambi F. Cell death signaling. Cold Spring Harbor Perspectives in Biology. Dec 1, 2015;**7**(12). DOI: 10.1101/cshperspect.a006080

[115] Lavrik IN. Systems biology of death receptor networks: Live and let die. Cell Death & Disease. May 29, 2014;**5**:e1259. DOI: 10.1038/cddis.2014.160

[116] Catts VS, Weickert CS. Gene expression analysis implicates a death receptor pathway in schizophrenia pathology. PLoS One. 2012;**7**(4):e35511. DOI: 10.1371/journal.pone.0035511

[117] Docherty AR, Bigdeli TB, Edwards AC, et al. Genome-wide gene pathway analysis of psychotic illness symptom dimensions based on a new schizophrenia-specific model of the OPCRIT. Schizophrenia Research. May 2015;**164**(1-3):181-186. DOI: 10.1016/j.schres.2015.02.013

[118] Luo X, Huang L, Han L, et al. Systematic prioritization and integrative analysis of copy number variations in schizophrenia reveal key schizophrenia susceptibility genes. Schizophrenia Bulletin. Nov 2014;**40**(6):1285-1299. DOI: 10.1093/schbul/sbu045

[119] Collier DA, Eastwood BJ, Malki K, Mokrab Y. Advances in the genetics of schizophrenia: Toward a network and pathway view for drug discovery. Annals of the New York Academy of Sciences. Feb 2016;**1366**(1):61-75. DOI: 10.1111/nyas.13066

[120] Matsumoto M, Walton NM, Yamada H, et al. The impact of genetics on future drug discovery in schizophrenia. Expert Opinion on Drug Discovery. Jul 2017;**12**(7):673-686. DOI: 10.1080/17460441.2017.1324419

# 10

# Repetitive Transcranial Magnetic Stimulation Treating Impulsivity in Borderline Personality Disorder and Attention Deficit/Hyperactivity Disorder

Tomas Sverak, Pavla Linhartova, Adam Fiala and Tomas Kasparek

**Abstract**

The need for novel treatment approaches that target impulsivity symptoms in neuropsychiatric disorders is clear. Repetitive transcranial magnetic stimulation (rTMS) allows selective neuromodulation of regions involved in the functional neuroanatomy of neuropsychiatric disorders. This chapter presents impulsivity in psychiatry, especially in borderline personality disorder (BPD) and attention-deficit hyperactivity disorder (ADHD), its neural underpinnings, and its possible treatment by rTMS. We reviewed available studies on rTMS in impulsivity in BPD and ADHD published before August 13, 2017, systematically searching in the PubMed, Web of Science, and Scopus databases. The results are discussed in the context of the latest neuropsychological models of impulsivity and their underlying functional neuroanatomy. rTMS treatment of impulsivity in BPD and ADHD seems to be a plausible approach. The functional neuroanatomy of processes related to impulsive behavior and decision making in these disorders is linked with abnormalities in the fronto-limbic structures that can be targeted and modulated by rTMS. Although limited evidence is available, rTMS seems to be a safe and potentially effective method of impulsivity treatment in patients with BPD and ADHD. However, more studies are needed to determine the most efficient cortical location and design for rTMS treatment of impulsivity.

**Keywords:** transcranial magnetic stimulation, rTMS, impulsivity, inhibition, decision making, reward processing, emotion regulation, borderline personality disorder, ADHD

# 1. Introduction

Impulsivity is a heterogeneous construct; problems with self-control can include impairment in different neural processes, such as behavioral inhibition, reward processing, and emotion regulation. This chapter shows that various frontal cortical regions have been found to underlie impulsivity. Therefore, repetitive transcranial magnetic stimulation (rTMS) is a potential treatment option since the key brain areas for impulsivity are easily accessed by TMS. So far, only a few studies have used rTMS for impulsivity reduction, or in other words for improving self-control, mainly in patients with BPD and ADHD. A proper theoretical justification based on impulsivity neuroimaging studies should precede the rTMS target selection and treatment design. However, the heterogeneous nature of impulsivity has led to find differences in the methodology of these studies. Several different tasks are used for measuring impulsivity and for neuroimaging, and these tasks also differ in their parameters across studies. We provide a review of impulsivity dimensions, measures, processes, and their neural substrates in the first part of this chapter. We then review the neural correlates of impulsivity and existing studies on rTMS of impulsivity in patients with BPD and ADHD. We conclude by suggesting future directions in rTMS treatment of impulsive behavior.

# 2. Impulsivity

Impulsivity can be broadly defined as a premature or unwanted behavior or act on the spur of the moment without considering consequences. Increased impulsivity can be frequently observed in patients with various neuropsychiatric diseases, especially borderline personality disorder (BPD) and attention-deficit/hyperactivity disorder (ADHD). Impulsivity is a diagnostic criterion for both BPD and ADHD according to DMS-V. Moreover, difficulties with self-control are commonly observed in a number of otherwise different neuropsychiatric disorders, including substance abuse disorders and addiction [1], eating disorders [2], bipolar disorder [3], antisocial personality disorder [4], schizophrenia [5], and Parkinson's disease [6]. Increased impulsivity significantly worsens the quality of everyday life, complicates treatment, and can have serious consequences. Impulsivity is manifested by a wide range of risky and (self) destructive behavior, such as drug abuse, dangerous sexual behavior, reckless driving, gambling, binge eating and buying, aggression, and self-harm, including suicidality. Both pharmacologic and psychotherapeutic approaches are used to treat impulsivity; however, psychiatry lacks effective impulsivity-focused treatment.

## 2.1. Dimensions of impulsivity

Theoretical conceptions of impulsivity are each closely related to different forms of measurement. In the personality approach, impulsivity is considered to be a personality trait, which is measured by self-report questionnaires. The most commonly used impulsivity questionnaires are the Barratt Impulsiveness Scale (BIS) [7] and the UPPS-P[1] Scale [8, 9]. Whereas the validity

[1] The name of the scale was derived from first letters of the scale dimensions: (Negative) **U**rgency, (Lack of) **P**remeditation, (Lack of) **P**erseverance, **S**ensation Seeking, **P**ositive Urgency.

of the BIS has been recently questioned [10–13], the UPPS-P Scale currently constitutes the most complex up-to-date self-report measure of impulsivity and can be recommended for impulsivity treatment evaluation. The behavioral approach to impulsivity is more relevant for rTMS treatment. Under this view, impulsive behavior follows from the impairment of a neurobiological function, namely behavioral inhibition, leading to Impulsive Action, with reward processing leading to Impulsive Choices. Different behavioral tasks are used for measuring and neuroimaging of these functions. In the current literature, authors use different labels for the same impulsivity dimensions, which can complicate understanding of the topic. Impulsivity facet specification should always stem from the task that has been used for its measurement.

#### 2.1.1. *Behavioral inhibition and Impulsive Action*

Behavioral models of impulsivity can be divided into two areas. The first area is based on behavioral inhibition impairment, and the second is based on reward processing impairment. Behavioral inhibition can be defined as the ability to control one's behavior, namely to inhibit, postpone, or interrupt one's undesired or premature actions. Impairment in behavioral inhibition leads to Impulsive Action [14] (or Rapid-Response Impulsivity [15], etc.). Impulsive Action can be further distinguished into Waiting Impulsivity and Stopping Impulsivity [16]. Waiting Impulsivity is the ability to withhold one's own unwanted actions, whereas Stopping Impulsivity is the ability to interrupt one's own already ongoing actions. The most commonly used tasks for measuring behavioral inhibition are the Go/No-Go Task (GNG) [17] for Waiting Impulsivity and the Stop Signal Task (SST) for Stopping Impulsivity [18, 19].

#### 2.1.2. *Reward processing and Impulsive Choice*

Reward processing is crucial for decision making, and its impairment leads to a decreased ability to postpone immediate rewards or gains even at the expense of negative future consequences. Immediate rewards preference can be associated with hypersensitivity to hedonic stimuli [20] or, on the other hand, general hyposensitivity to both positive and negative feedbacks [21, 22]. Impairment in reward processing leads to so-called Impulsive Choice [14] (or Choice Impulsivity [15], etc.). Manifestations of Impulsive Choice include decreased tolerance for waiting for a reward, preference of immediate rewards without considering future consequences, and even decreased ability to learn from negative consequences.

The most commonly used task for measuring Impulsive Choice is the Delay Discounting (DD) [23]. In DD, subjects make a series of choices between a higher, but delayed, reward (usually monetary), and a lower and immediate, reward, resulting in a discounting parameter that expresses how quickly the present value of a reward to the subject declines with a delay of its delivery. Other tasks related to Impulsive Choice focus on decision making using rewards and punishments (Iowa Gambling Task) or risk-taking (e.g. Balloon Analog Risk Task).

#### 2.1.3. *Emotion regulation and emotional impulsivity*

The influence of emotions on impulsivity was neglected in impulsivity models for a long time. However, some patients have a significant tendency to act impulsively under the influence of both negative and positive emotions, known as Negative and Positive Urgency [8, 9]. Other authors refer to cold and hot (i.e. emotional) impulsivity [24]. For example, patients with BPD show more pronounced behavioral inhibition impairment under the influence of stress [25], while in emotionally neutral situations, they might not show any difference in behavioral inhibition from healthy people [26, 27]. Moreover, emotional impulsivity in patients with BPD is often manifested by (self) destructive behaviors such as self-harm, suicidal behavior, aggression, substance abuse, and other dangerous impulsive behavior [28]. We hypothesize that impulsive behavior can occur as an attempt to handle the emotional tension that the person is unable to regulate by more adaptive means. In other words, behavioral inhibition impairment and impulsive decision making can occur as a result of insufficient emotion-regulation abilities. Impulsive, most often self-destructive behavior (getting hurt, taking drugs, etc.) can lead to momentary relief but almost always has negative consequences, including remorse, (self-)harm, and social condemnation. Thus, emotional impulsivity is a very dangerous phenomenon to which we should pay attention and which we should try to prevent in patients. In the treatment of patients with high emotional impulsivity, it is necessary to address not only behavioral inhibition or decision making, but also emotion-regulation skills.

Regarding the measurement of emotional impulsivity, the UPPS-P questionnaire includes dimensions of Negative Urgency and Positive Urgency. Previously mentioned, behavioral tests can be used in emotional variants, e.g. after stress induction or using emotional stimuli instead of neutral stimuli.

### 2.2. Neural correlates of behavioral inhibition

In neuroimaging studies of behavioral inhibition, a neuroimaging method is used while subjects perform a behavioral inhibition task. Studies using functional magnetic resonance imaging (fMRI) of behavioral inhibition are the most important for rTMS target selection. Swick et al. [29] performed a large meta-analysis of fMRI studies using Go/No-Go Tasks (GNG; 48 papers) and Stop Signal Tasks (SST; 21 papers) in healthy people. The authors found that the No-Go condition in GNG is associated with increased activity in the fronto-parietal network including the superior, middle, and inferior frontal cortical areas, including the dorsolateral prefrontal cortex (DLPFC), insula, dorsal medial frontal cortex including the (pre-) supplementary motor area (SMA/pre-SMA), and the inferior parietal lobule (IPL). All the largest clusters were bilateral but predominantly right-sided. Other activations included the right precuneus, left putamen/claustrum, posterior cingulate cortex, superior temporal cortex, and right inferior occipital cortex. In SST, the Stop condition was associated with a similar activation pattern, but compared to GNG, the activation was more pronounced in the left insula extending to the thalamus and putamen and the thalamus and posterior cingulate cortex. GNG activation was generally more right-sided and the maximal overlap between activations from the two tasks was found in the right insula and the SMA/pre-SMA. The important finding of this meta-analysis is that GNG and SST apparently do not measure the same processes, and thus the results from the two tasks cannot be combined. The authors further discuss that the SMA/pre-SMA could be the critical area for behavioral inhibition specifically, whereas the DLPFC could reflect more generally attentional executive control or top-down cognitive control, even though the previous literature on behavioral inhibition was mainly focused on the right DLPFC or inferior frontal gyrus (IFG).

Another two meta-analyses [30, 31] explored the hypothesis that the DLPFC and IFG are more related to attentional cognitive control than to behavioral inhibition itself. Simmonds et al. [30] reviewed 11 studies and compared activations between GNG tasks with stable No-Go stimulus and variable No-Go stimulus, with the variable stimulus putting higher demands on cognitive control components such as attention, stimulus recognition, and working memory. The authors found that the IFG and DLPFC, as well as the insula and IPL, were more activated in more cognitively demanding tasks. On the other hand, common activations in all tasks were found in the SMA and the left fusiform gyrus. A second meta-analysis [31] reviewed 30 studies and compared activations from simple and complex GNG tasks. Simple tasks should include only one invariable Go and No-Go stimulus and an even ratio of Go to No-Go stimuli; complex tasks are more complicated and cognitively demanding. Activations only in complex tasks were found in the right IFG, right DLPFC, right SMA/pre-SMA, insula, and right IPL. Common activations in both tasks were found in bilateral DLPFC, left IPL, and right superior temporal gyrus. The authors of the meta-analyses hypothesize that regions activated commonly in all tasks are related specifically to behavioral inhibition, but areas activated only in complex tasks are related to cognitive control. However, the results of the two meta-analyses differ substantially.

To summarize, the most commonly activated frontal regions during inhibition tasks are the right DLPFC and IFG and the SMA/pre-SMA. However, the specific role of the different regions remains unclear. Recent studies have importantly revealed that neural activity associated with behavioral inhibition is task related.

### 2.3. Neural correlates of reward processing

The most important network for performance in Delay Discounting according to the current literature is the cortico-striatal loop, including the prefrontal, cingulate, and posterior parietal cortex in the cortical part and the nucleus accumbens/ventral Striatum (NAcc/VS) and amygdala in the striatal part. Within this network, the NAcc/VS and amygdala are thought to be related to reward processing and reward learning; the prefrontal cortex (PFC) is associated with decision making and conflict resolution [32]. Amygdala activity was found to be associated with immediate (i.e. more impulsive) choices [33], while PFC region activity is associated with delayed (i.e. less impulsive) choices [34]. Another approach to studying the neural correlates of Delay Discounting distinguishes hard choices, in which two options have subjectively similar values for the subject, and easy choices, in which one option has a subjectively much higher value for the subject. The idea is that in hard choices, people should engage in decision making with greater effort because they should consider the pros and cons of each of the possibilities more precisely. Existing studies [35–39] show that regardless of population type, hard choices, in comparison to easy choices, are associated with higher activity in the fronto-parietal network, including the DLPFC and/or ventro-lateral prefrontal cortex (VLPFC), the anterior cingulate cortex (ACC), the IPL, and the intraparietal sulcus. Moreover, more impulsive individuals tend to show lower activity in these regions during DD, suggesting insufficient effort or decision-making ability engaged in more difficult choices.

### 2.4. Neural correlates of emotion regulation

Impaired emotion regulation can be found frequently among psychiatric patients with different diagnoses and is often associated with dangerous impulsive behavior. Studies on humans and animals have largely established the amygdala as a key region in emotion processing. The amygdala was found to be involved in emotional implicit learning, memory, social perception, emotion inhibition, and emotion regulation [40, 41]. The amygdala activity during emotion processing is regulated by a prefrontal-limbic negative coupling which represents top-down cognitive emotion control. Specifically, the decrease in amygdala activity has been shown to be associated with increases in various lateral and medial PFC areas [42–45]. Patients with emotion-regulation deficits show exaggerated amygdala response to emotional stimuli and disrupted amygdala-prefrontal connectivity [46–49]. Further, real-time fMRI neurofeedback studies showed that successful regulation of amygdala activity increases connectivity between the amygdala and DLPFC or VLPFC [50, 51], representing an increase in cognitive emotion-regulation abilities.

### 2.5. Possible targets for rTMS treatment of impulsivity

According to existing literature on neural correlates of impulsivity, the most suitable targets for rTMS impulsivity treatment seem to be the right lateral PFC areas, mainly the DLPFC or VLPFC. High frequency (HF) rTMS is used over these regions with the aim of the treatment should be to promote activity in the prefrontal areas. Lateral PFC activity, especially in the right hemisphere, has been consistently shown to be associated with successful behavioral inhibition, less impulsive decision making, and better emotion regulation. All of the areas mentioned could be improved through the application of HF rTMS treatment over the (right) DLPFC or VLPFC. Another promising candidate for rTMS application is SMA/pre-SMA that appears to be a crucial area for behavioral inhibition.

## 3. Transcranial magnetic stimulation in borderline personality disorder

According to DSM-V, BPD is characterized by a pervasive pattern of instability in interpersonal relationships, self-image, and affects, and marked impulsivity that begins by early adulthood and is present in a variety of contexts. BPD patients also have a high risk of mortality due to suicidal behavior. Up to 10% of BPD patients commit suicide; this rate is almost 50 times higher than in the general population [52]. BPD symptoms severely reduce patients' quality of life and impair their psychosocial functioning [49, 53]. The median prevalence of BPD is estimated from 1.6% up to 5.9% in the general population, up to 10% in psychiatric outpatients, and up to 20% in psychiatric inpatients [28, 54, 55]. BPD is about five times more common among first-degree biological relatives of those with the disorder than in the general population and it is also diagnosed predominantly (about 75%) in women [55]. One of the core elements of BDP is impaired emotion processing and impulsivity. BPD patients have impaired emotion-regulation abilities combined with emotional vulnerability characterized by marked sensitivity to emotional stimuli (low threshold) and unusually strong reactions (high amplitude) that abnormally slowly return to baseline (long duration) [56]. As mentioned earlier, impulsivity in BPD patients often appears under the emotional influence and usually manifests in various dangerous and (self-) destructive behavior.

### 3.1. Neurobiology and neurophysiology of impulsivity in BPD

BPD patients show impairment across various frontal regions and fronto-limbic connections crucial for behavioral inhibition, decision making, and emotion regulation. Functionally, patients with BPD show increased amygdala reactivity and altered PFC responses including in the DLPFC and ACC and sensorial processing areas, including the superior temporal gyrus in face processing and the visual cortex in response to emotional stimuli, as compared to healthy people [49, 56–58]. Anatomically, patients with BPD were found to have reduced gray matter volume in the amygdala, insula, DLPFC, and orbitofrontal cortex (OFC) compared with healthy controls [49, 59]. Positron Emission Tomography (PET) studies have revealed altered baseline metabolism in the prefrontal regions in BPD patients [60–62]. Disinhibited impulsive aggression in BPD patients has been associated with serotonergic neurotransmission, which is also affected by the PFC [62]. In conclusion, neuroimaging studies indicate that hyperactivity in the amygdala could be a consequence of weak inhibitory control of limbic emotion reactivity by PFC areas.

Some studies tried to use TMS for assessing cortical neurophysiology in BPD, including cortical excitability and inhibitory and excitatory mechanisms [63]. From this point of view, impulsivity could stem from increased or decreased excitability in some brain structures. BPD patients were found to have shorter cortical silent periods (CSP) in the right hemisphere than healthy controls [64, 65]. It is assumed that CSP measures $GABA_B$ inhibitory activity [66]. A similar reduction of CSP was also found in ADHD [67] and in patients with tic disorder [68]. Some authors hypothesized that the GABA neurotransmitter is the main inhibition neurotransmitter and the reduction of GABA activity could result in impulsive behavior and affective instability [64]. Another hypothesis is that intracortical inhibition is more linked with shifts in cortical glutamate and glutamine concentrations than with GABA neurotransmitter levels. But glutamate probably specifically interacts with $GABA_B$ receptors, so the higher glutamate and glutamine concentrations seem to be linked to the higher levels of receptor activity revealed by proton magnetic resonance spectroscopy [69]. Further studies to examine these neurophysiology markers in BPD and how they could be used for therapeutic rTMS would be appropriate.

### 3.2. Review of rTMS treatment studies in BPD

We searched for relevant studies through the PubMed (http://www.ncbi.nlm.nih.gov/pubmed/), Web of Science (https://apps.webofknowledge.com/), and Scopus (https://www.scopus.com/) databases published before August 13, 2017. The following terms were used to search for publication titles: (borderline OR BPD) AND (TMS OR rTMS OR "transcranial magnetic stimulation"). We found seven (PubMed), six (Web of Science), and seven (Scopus) publications. After excluding duplicates and nonrelevant contributions (e.g. theoretical articles), five studies were included in the review [70–74].

The first rTMS study in BPD [70] was a case report published in 2013. A 22-year-old female BPD patient received high frequency (HF) 10 Hz stimulation over her left DLPFC at 100% of her individual motor threshold (MT). The trains lasted 5 s and intertrain intervals were 55 s; the whole protocol had 10 sessions (1500 pulses per session, one session per day). The results revealed a decrease in depression levels (Beck Depression Inventory score from 20 to 7 to 2),[2] negative affect experiences (Positive and Negative Affect Schedule score from 38 to 36 to 22), impulsivity (Barratt Impulsiveness Scale score from 71 to 67 to 61), and BPD symptom score

[2]The effects are presented from before the stimulation, immediately after the stimulation, and 1 month after the stimulation.

(SCID-II score from 13 to 11 to 6) directly after the treatment and 1 month after the treatment, respectively. Reassessment after 3 months showed regression in the symptoms. According to the patient's reports, the rTMS therapy led to decreased sleep duration, increased emotional control and stability, behavioral self-awareness, increased motivation for change, sociability, self-esteem, happiness, attention to the behavior of others, and planning ability.

Cailhol et al. [71] performed a randomized controlled stimulation of 10 BPD patients by HF 10 Hz rTMS over the right DLPFC. Five patients received active stimulation, and five patients received sham stimulation. One patient was excluded. The right DLPFC was targeted as 6 cm anterior to M1, stimulation was done at 80% intensity of individual MT, trains lasted 5 s and intertrain intervals lasted 25 s (2000 per session, 10 sessions in total). The response rate was defined as a 30% reduction in the Borderline Personality Severity Index (BPDSI) after the stimulation; this was reached by two patients from the active group and one patient from the sham group. BPDSI scores were significantly lower for the active rTMS group than for the sham stimulation group after 3 months of affective instability and anger. Performance in the Tower of London test improved only in the rTMS active group. The stimulation was well tolerated without any adverse events. The authors hypothesized that PFC activity could be increased by rTMS neuromodulation and thereby downregulate the subcortical structures. The effect of rTMS on anger and affect instability in BPD patients could be explained by this hypothesis.

Another stimulation design was presented by De Vidovich et al. [72], who stimulated the left cerebellum in BPD patients. This cerebellar stimulation was used based on cerebellar projections to the PFC through the ventrolateral thalamic nucleus (VL), which was observed in animal studies [75, 76]. Further, one tractography study in humans found that about 40% of fiber tracts from the cerebellum through the superior cerebellar peduncle actually reach the PFC through the VL [77]. In the study itself, eight patients with BPD and eight healthy controls received 1 Hz stimulation on 80% of MT for 10 min over the left lateral cerebellum (1 cm inferior and 3 cm left to the union). The effect of the rTMS was measured by the Affective Go No-Go task (AGN), using two categories of words (positive/negative and fruits/insect). The first and second block of the task included only the first category; the third and fourth part included both categories. BPD patients generally scored worse than healthy controls in AGN, especially in the latter category before the stimulation. After rTMS, their performance became equivalent to the healthy control performance. The stimulation was well tolerated, with no adverse events. These data support previous findings that inhibition performance in BPD patients is impaired when cognitive demands are high, and the situation requires complex associative capacities [78, 79]. The results suggest that LF cerebellar rTMS could have a facilitating effect on the PFC.

Feffer et al. [73] stimulated three women (39, 32, and 42 years old) with BPD and depression comorbidity. The severity of depression symptoms was measured by Beck Depression Inventory II (BDI-II). Two patients received bilateral intermittent (iTBS) stimulation of the DMPFC targeted by neuronavigation; the stimulation had 20 sessions (1 session per day), 1200 pulses per session (600 pulses to each hemisphere). The BDI-II score of the first patient was reduced from 56 to 16 points; the score of the second patient was reduced from 20 to 12 points. The third patient received 20 sessions (1 session per day) of 20 Hz bilateral stimulation to the DMPFC localized by neuronavigation. The duration of the train was 2.5 s and the duration of the intertrain interval was 10 s. Stimulation of each hemisphere contained 1500 pulses in one session. The BDI-II score of the third patient was reduced from 29 to 10 points. The stimulation was well tolerated without any adverse events. Two of the patients described a mild headache at the point of stimulation. All three of them subjectively described better control of emotional and behavior impulses and better emotional regulation.

The last study is from Reyes-López et al. [74]. They stimulated 29 BPD patients divided into two groups with two stimulation designs. One stimulation group received 1 Hz stimulation to the right DLPFC (15 patients), 900 pulses per session. The second group received 5 Hz stimulation to the left DLPFC, trains lasted 10 s, intertrain intervals were also 10 s, 1500 pulses per session (14 patients). The whole stimulation had 15 sessions (1 session per day); the DLPFC was targeted as 5 cm above the maximum stimulation point in the motor area and patients were stimulated on 100% of their individual MT. There was a significant reduction in the Clinical Global Impression Scale for BPD (CGI-BPD) score from baseline after rTMS, with a 29.4% change for 1 Hz group and 28.7% for 5 Hz group. The Borderline Evaluation of Severity over Time (BEST) scores were also reduced for both groups (1 Hz group: 20.4% reduction from baseline; 5 Hz group: 36.9% reduction from baseline). Scores in BIS were also reduced significantly (1 Hz group: 18.96% reduction from baseline; 5 Hz group: 11.83% reduction from baseline). The reduction in BDI scores was 49% for 1 Hz group and 60% for 5 Hz group. Lastly, the Hamilton Anxiety Rating Scale (HAM-A) score was also reduced by 60.3% for 1 Hz group and by 58.7% for 5 Hz group. These results show that both stimulation protocols were effective in reducing BPD symptoms, such as fear of abandonment, impulsivity, emotional instability, and anger.

### 3.3. Conclusions and future directions of rTMS treatment paradigms in BPD

Most existing studies used rTMS targeted to the left or right DLPFC or DMPFC; one study targeted the cerebellum. Both high and low-frequency protocols were used. Many authors connected the BPD symptoms with hypometabolism in the prefrontal regions and hyperactivation of the amygdala. Current studies have reported various effects of rTMS treatment, mostly after HF treatment in BPD patients, including improved self-control, emotion regulation, mood, anxiety, and executive functions. Some studies also reported effects after sham stimulation. Consequently, it is difficult to make any recommendation regarding rTMS targeting and protocol parameters. We might also speculate that targeting any PFC region by rTMS could improve BPD symptoms thanks to the rich cortico-cortical and cortico-limbic projections from the prefrontal regions. The low-frequency stimulation of the cerebellum could be also used to reduce BPD symptoms based on the cerebellothalamocortical tracts. One question is the laterality of rTMS treatment in BPD patients. Neuroimaging studies of impulsivity usually find a greater association with action control with the right prefrontal regions. Differences in the CSP between patients with BPD and healthy controls were found, especially in the right hemisphere [64]. However, current studies show effects for both right and left prefrontal stimulation protocols.

Another question was raised by the study by Reyes-López et al. [74]. They used low-frequency rTMS in the right DLPFC and found similar effects as after high-frequency rTMS over the same area. These findings contradict previous findings and theoretical underpinnings about hypometabolism in PFC in BPD patients and about the effect of low-frequency rTMS. For example, low and high-frequency rTMS over the left DLPFC in depressed patients have been found to have opposite effects [80].

### 3.4. Summary of rTMS treatment in BPD

The existing studies suggest that rTMS is a well-tolerated treatment in patients with BPD and is a potentially highly useful tool for reducing BPD symptoms including impulsivity and emotion regulation. There is a lack of double-blind randomized controlled studies with sufficient sample sizes. Current studies differ substantially in both rTMS cortical targets and stimulation protocols. Most studies have found an effect of high-frequency rTMS over the right DLPFC, but there are also studies that found low-frequency DLPFC, left-sided DLPFC, and cerebellar rTMS effective. More double-blind placebo-controlled studies and studies directly comparing different stimulation protocols in BPD are needed, and the duration of the therapeutic effects should be assessed.

## 4. rTMS in attention-deficit/hyperactivity disorder treatment

ADHD, in the ICD-10 represented by hyperkinetic disorder, is one of the most common mental disorders among children, with a prevalence of 3–7% [81]. ADHD was long viewed as a childhood diagnosis; however, many studies in the last decades have demonstrated that symptoms persist to adulthood in up to 80% of patients [82]. The latest revision of the Diagnostic and Statistical Manual of Mental Disorders (DSM-V) reexamined the diagnostic criteria and allowed the classification of ADHD as a lifelong disorder with the condition of onset before the 12th year of life [55]. ADHD symptom heredity is considered to be as high as 75% [83]. Like many neuropsychiatric disorders, ADHD seems to be a result of the complex interplay of genetic and environmental factors and has been recently viewed as a neurodevelopmental disorder [81].

The three typical symptoms of childhood ADHD—attention deficit, hyperactivity, and impulsivity—are partially modified during the lifespan. In adulthood, feelings of internal restlessness, disorganization, and unrestrainability, and some behavioral difficulties, including impaired executive functions, prevail [84]. The treatment of ADHD in children as well as in adults is an ongoing topic in psychiatry. There are several possible treatment options in ADHD therapy. Treatment guidelines for both children and adult patients recommend using drugs such as methylphenidate and atomoxetine. However, about 20–50% of patients are considered nonresponders due to insufficient symptom reduction or severe side effects. Moreover, combining pharmacotherapy with psychotherapy (cognitive behavioral therapy, education, and focused complex programs) and other nonpharmacological methods is recommended in all cases [85].

### 4.1. Neurobiology and neurophysiology of impulsivity in ADHD

Neuroimaging studies indicate that ADHD might be a neurobiologically heterogeneous category of diseases. This would mean that there are several different disorder patterns which manifest by similar clinical symptoms or that dysfunctions in different functional systems could lead to similar symptoms. Data-mining techniques suggest three clusters of neuropsychological abnormities in ADHD: cognitive-behavioral management, time processing, and motivation. These clusters did not significantly overlap between individual subjects [86]. Similarly, a systematic review of the findings in executive function areas suggests that not all ADHD patients are impaired in the same region [87].

ADHD is characterized by a delay in cortical maturation, which is most substantial in the prefrontal regions [88]. Earlier neuroimaging studies described structural and functional abnormalities in patients with ADHD, suggesting a hypofunction of catecholamine projection from the basal ganglia into the PFC. This dysfunction manifests as a relative hypoactivity of the cortical dopamine system with a relative hyperactivity of striatal dopamine [89]. A meta-analysis of functional studies showed hypoactivity in the frontal regions (DLPFC, inferior PFC, OFC), anterior cingulum, superior parietal regions, caudate nucleus, and thalamus [90]. Duerden et al. [91] also observed that adolescents with ADHD had a significantly greater cortical thickness in the pre-supplementary motor area (SMA) than controls. Further, impaired functional connectivity between the frontal and parietal cortex and between the frontal and cerebellar cortex have been found in patients with ADHD during interference control tasks and time discrimination tasks [92] associated with interference control, activity timing, and time predictions. Striatal hypoactivation in ADHD can lead to the insufficient detection of behaviorally important stimuli, inability to orientate one's activities to long-term goals, and insufficient feedback effect from behavioral modification [93–95].

Several studies used TMS to investigate neurophysiological parameters in ADHD. A meta-analysis by Dutra et al. [96] identified no significant differences between ADHD and control groups in CSP, resting MT, and motor-evoked potential. However, there was a consistent finding in reduced short intracortical inhibition (SICI) in both children with ADHD [97–100] and adult ADHD patients [67]. SICI is a subthreshold conditioning stimulus followed by a suprathreshold test stimulus with an interstimulus interval of 1–6 ms. The motor-evoked potential which was evoked by the second suprathreshold stimulus should be reduced by 50–90% [101]. The SICI is described as probably measuring $GABA_A$-mediated cortical inhibition [66, 102]. A study by Hasan et al. [103] also reported increased intracortical facilitation (ICF) in adult ADHD patients compared to healthy controls when considering an interstimulus interval of 7 ms between paired pulses applied to the left hemisphere. ICF is measured by TMS when the magnetic evoked potential generated by the suprathreshold is usually facilitated at an interstimulus interval of 8–30 ms [101]. However, there are too few studies to make a more robust conclusion.

### 4.2. Review of rTMS treatment studies in ADHD

We searched for relevant studies through the PubMed (http://www.ncbi.nlm.nih.gov/pubmed/), Web of Science (https://apps.webofknowledge.com/), and Scopus (https://www.scopus.com/) databases published before August 13, 2017. The following terms were used to search in the publication titles: (ADHD OR "attention deficit hyperactivity disorder") AND (TMS OR rTMS OR "transcranial magnetic stimulation"). We found 20 (PubMed), 32 (Web of Science), and 25 (Scopus) articles. After excluding duplicates and nonrelevant contributions (e.g. theoretical articles), seven studies were included in the review.

Current studies examining the treatment of ADHD by rTMS use two main protocols. The first protocol is the low-frequency (LF) stimulation of the SMA, intended to suppress motor symptoms of hyperactivity. The other protocol uses HF rTMS over the DLPFC, intended to facilitate dopaminergic neurotransmission in the PFC and induce the release of endogenous dopamine in the nucleus caudate nucleus and NAcc [104]. This kind of stimulation could improve the symptoms of ADHD mostly in the cognitive domain (deficit of attention and impulsive cognitive style).

In his pilot study, Niederhofer [105] presented a case study of an adult ADHD patient. This study used LF 1 Hz rTMS protocol over the SMA in order to reduce the symptoms of hyperactivity. The results describe a significant improvement that lasted for at least 4 weeks. Three years later, Niederhofer repeated the same protocol with a 42-year-old female ADHD patient on a 20 mg daily dose of methylphenidate (MPH). After 21 days of 1 Hz rTMS (1200 pulses per session, each session lasting 1 h) over the SMA, the daily MPH dose was lowered to 10 mg; simultaneously, the 10 hyperactivity-associated items of the Conners scale improved from the initial 25 to 17 points (measured during the therapy and a week after the termination). The attention items did not show any difference [106].

The largest study was conducted by Bloch et al. [107]. They performed a randomized, cross-over, double-blind pilot study in 13 adult ADHD patients. They applied a single session of HF stimulation (42 × 2 s, 20 Hz stimuli at 100% of individual MT intensity, with a 30 s inter-stimulus interval) over the right DLPFC (located by measuring 5 cm anterior to the motor threshold). One patient dropped out of the study because the stimulation was painful, the other 12 completed the treatment and reported no side effects. The result of the study was a significant improvement in self-reported attention with no effects on mood or anxiety [positive and negative affect schedule (PANAS), visual analogue scales (VAS), and Cambridge neuropsychological test automated battery (CANTAB) were used]. No difference was found in the attention score when comparing the pre- and post-sham rTMS results. The limitation of that study was the fact that the symptoms were evaluated only before the treatment and 10 min after; therefore, no claims can be made about the long-term effects of this therapy.

Ustohal et al. [108] used a similar design in their own pilot study. They treated a 36-year-old male subject who was diagnosed with ADHD in childhood and experienced three major depression episodes in adulthood. The authors used HF 10 Hz frequency in 120% intensity of individual MT (10 s train, 30 s inter train interval, 1500 pulses per session). The study was divided into three sections, each lasting 1 week. In the first week, sham stimulation was applied; in the second week, the left DLPFC was stimulated; and in the third week, the right DLPFC was stimulated. In the first week, there was already a significant improvement in the d2 test of attention (from the initial 86.4 percentile to 98.2 percentile) and a small reduction on the depression scale (from MADRS 14 to 12). In the second week, there was a further reduction on the depression scale (MADRS score decreased to 7) and improvement in the d2 test of attention (98.9 percentile). On the first session of the third week, the patient described serious side effects—dysphoria, hypobulia, and increased tension. The MADRS score increased significantly (21 points). Therefore, the authors changed the target to the left DLPFC, which led to improved symptoms, reduced depression scale score (MADRS = 9), and improvement in the d2 test of attention (99.2 percentile). The authors discussed that these side effects may be related to the fact that LF rTMS of the right DLPFC is used in the treatment of depression [109] and, on the contrary, HF rTMS of this area has been used in patients with mania [110].

In another study, Weaver et al. [111] stimulated nine adolescents and young adults diagnosed with ADHD. They targeted the right DLPFC (located by measuring 5 cm anterior to the motor threshold) and used HF stimulation (10 Hz, 4 s trains, 26 s inter train interval, 2000 pulses per session) with 100% intensity of individual MT. This study had a double-blind design and each of the patients was stimulated for 2 weeks (10 sessions). Results showed an overall significant improvement in the clinical global impression-improvement (CGI-I) and the ADHD-IV scales in both groups combined ($P < 0.01$); no significant differences between active and sham stimulation were described. The study also described no negative side effects of the stimulation.

In another study [112], 25 children with ADHD underwent rTMS treatment. The primary motor cortex (M1) was stimulated using LF 1 Hz rTMS at low intensity—80% of the individual MT. This study did not evaluate the clinical effect of the stimulation, it only measured the effect of rTMS on electrophysiological parameters of the cortical excitability by EEG. The result of this study was a significant decrease of the N100 which was evoked by rTMS and lasted for at least 10 min after the stimulation. EEG source analysis indicated that the TMS-evoked N100 change reflected rTMS effects in the stimulated motor cortex and therefore the TMS-evoked N100 could represent a promising candidate marker to monitor rTMS effects on cortical excitability in children with ADHD. No serious side effects of the stimulation were described; three patients reported a mild headache.

Another study with child ADHD patients was conducted by Gómez et al. [113]. The aim of the study was to evaluate the tolerability and safety of LF rTMS in children with ADHD. The study group included 10 children aged from 7 to 12 years. These patients received 1 Hz stimulation (a total of 1500 stimuli in each session) over the left DLPFC (the site for stimulation was defined by the F3 electrode position (10/20 International System)) for 5 consecutive days, the intensity was set to 90% of the individual MT. The assumption was that 1 Hz stimulation over the left DLPFC could be as effective as 10 Hz stimulation to the homologous right area. Seventy percent of the patients reported a mild headache or a local discomfort lasting for few minutes as the most frequent side effect, 20% reported also a mild neck pain. Their parents and teachers were asked to fill out the symptoms checklist (SCL) for ADHD from DSM-IV, before and 1 week after completing the rTMS sessions. There was improvement in inattentiveness symptoms at school (score dropped from 16.7 to 8.6) and in hyperactivity/impulsivity at home (score dropped from 30.8 to 11.4).

None of these studies reported any severe side effects of rTMS; the only common side effect was a temporary and mild headache. Theoretically, there is a higher risk of paroxysmal reaction on rTMS in child patients due to their lower seizure threshold, but so far no study has reported such a side effect. If the personal history, entry EEG exam, and safety limits are performed properly, the risk of provoking a paroxysmal reaction is very low [114].

### 4.3. Conclusions and future directions of rTMS treatment paradigms in ADHD

Using rTMS in treating ADHD symptoms is still a relatively unexplored area. However, current studies suggest it might be a promising nonpharmacological approach or it could be used in combination with pharmacotherapy. The benefit of using rTMS in ADHD treatment is the minimal occurrence of side effects among current studies, none of which is a serious side effect. Studies have explored the effect of rTMS in only small numbers of patients using different methodology, including different stimulation parameters and application targets. Current studies focus mostly on reducing inattention and impulsivity by stimulating the DLPFC. The most widely used stimulation is high frequency rTMS over the right DLPFC. However, a study by Ustohal et al. [108] showed that this protocol can have a negative effect on patient's depression symptoms and suggests another stimulation site, such as left DLPFC, at least for patients with a personal history of depression. However, this side effect has only been observed in a single patient. Another treatment protocol to consider is low frequency rTMS over the left DLPFC, which could possibly have a similar effect. Hyperactivity symptoms of ADHD could also be reduced by using low frequency rTMS over the SMA; however, only two patients have been stimulated by this protocol, and further research is needed. There is a lack of reliable data on the duration of the therapeutic effect. Further understanding of the neurophysiological mechanisms of the effect and assessment of adequate stimulation parameters are required.

### 4.4. Summary of rTMS treatment in ADHD

Studies suggest that rTMS is a well-tolerated treatment in patients with ADHD and potentially a highly useful tool for reducing ADHD symptoms including impulsivity, motor hyperactivity, and reduced attention. There are not yet double-blind randomized controlled studies with sufficient sample sizes. The current studies differ substantially in both rTMS cortical targets and stimulation protocols. Most studies suggest stimulation over the right DLPFC by high frequency rTMS; another potentially promising protocol in ADHD is low frequency rTMS over the SMA. More double-blind placebo-controlled studies and evidence about the therapeutic effect of rTMS in ADHD patients are needed.

## 5. Conclusion

The most important application of rTMS for impulsivity reduction in BDP and ADHD seems to be stimulation over the left or right DLPFC, the SMA, or the cerebellum. However, it should be stressed that the neural activity associated with impulsivity differs according to the task parameters used during neuroimaging. This applies for studies of behavioral inhibition, Delay Discounting, and emotion regulation. This problem might be overcome by navigating rTMS individually according to functional fMRI from a specific task administered to the patients before stimulation. rTMS seems to be well tolerated without any adverse events in BPD and ADHD patients. The results of rTMS impulsivity treatment studies are promising, but double-blind studies with larger active and sham group sizes are needed to optimize the treatment results.

## Acknowledgements

This contribution was supported by the Ministry of Health of the Czech Republic, grant no. 15-30062A. The authors like to thank Ms. Anne Johnson for proof-reading.

## Author details

Tomas Sverak[1,2]*, Pavla Linhartova[1], Adam Fiala[1] and Tomas Kasparek[1]

*Address all correspondence to: tomas.sverak@mail.muni.cz

1 Department of Psychiatry, Masaryk University and University Hospital Brno, Czech Republic

2 Central European Institute of Technology (CEITEC MU), Masaryk University, Brno, Czech Republic

## References

[1] Smith JL, Mattick RP, Jamadar SD, Iredale JM. Deficits in behavioural inhibition in substance abuse and addiction: A meta-analysis. Drug and Alcohol Dependence. 2014;**145**:1-33

[2] Schag K, Schönleber J, Teufel M, Zipfel S, Giel KE. Food-related impulsivity in obesity and binge eating disorder—A systematic review. Obesity Reviews: An Official Journal of the International Association for the Study of Obesity. 2013;**14**(6):477-495

[3] Najt P, Perez J, Sanches M, Peluso MAM, Glahn D, Soares JC. Impulsivity and bipolar disorder. European Neuropsychopharmacology. 2007;**17**(5):313-320

[4] Turner D, Sebastian A, Tüscher O. Impulsivity and cluster B personality disorders. Current Psychiatry Reports. 2017;**19**(3):15

[5] Ouzir M. Impulsivity in schizophrenia: A comprehensive update. Aggression and Violent Behavior. 2013;**18**(2):247-254

[6] Maloney EM, Djamshidian A, Sullivan SSO. Phenomenology and epidemiology of impulsive-compulsive behaviours in Parkinsons disease, atypical Parkinsonian disorders and non-Parkinsonian populations. Journal of the Neurological Sciences. 2017;**374**:47-52

[7] Patton JH, Stanford MS, Barratt ES. Factor structure of the Barratt Impulsiveness Scale. Journal of Clinical Psychology. 1995;**51**(6):768-774

[8] Whiteside SP, Lynam DR. The five factor model and impulsivity: Using a structural model of personality to understand impulsivity. Personality and Individual Differences. 2001;**30**(4):669-689

[9] Cyders MA, Smith GT. Mood-based rash action and its components: Positive and negative urgency. Personality and Individual Differences. 2007;**43**(4):839-850

[10] Haden SC, Shiva A. Trait impulsivity in a forensic inpatient sample: An evaluation of the Barratt impulsiveness scale. Behavioral Sciences & the Law. 2008;**26**:675-690

[11] Ireland JL, Archer J. Impulsivity among adult prisoners: A confirmatory factor analysis study of the Barratt Impulsivity Scale. Personality and Individual Differences. 2008; **45**(4):286-292

[12] Reise SP, Moore TM, Sabb FW, Brown AK, London ED. The Barratt Impulsiveness Scale—11: Reassessment of its structure in a community sample. Psychological Assessment. 2013; **25**(2):631-642

[13] Vasconcelos AG, Malloy-Diniz L, Correa H. Systematic review of psychometric proprieties of barrattimpulsiveness scale version 11 (BIS-11). Clinical Neuropsychiatry. 2012; **9**(2):61-74

[14] Winstanley CA, Eagle DM, Robbins TW. Behavioral models of impulsivity in relation to ADHD: Translation between clinical and preclinical studies. Clinical Psychology Review. 2006;**26**(4):379-395

[15] Hamilton KR, Littlefield AK, Anastasio NC, Cunningham KA, Fink LHL, Wing VC, et al. Rapid-response impulsivity: Definitions, measurement issues, and clinical implications. Personality Disorders: Theory, Research, and Treatment. 2015;**6**(2):168-181

[16] Robinson ESJ, Eagle DM, Economidou D, Theobald DEH, Mar AC, Murphy ER, et al. Behavioural characterisation of high impulsivity on the 5-choice serial reaction time task: Specific deficits in "waiting" versus "stopping". Behavioural Brain Research. 2009; **196**(2):310-316

[17] Wright L, Lipszyc J, Dupuis A, Thayapararajah SW, Schachar R. Response inhibition and psychopathology: A meta-analysis of go/no-go task performance. Journal of Abnormal Psychology. 2014;**123**(2):429-439

[18] Verbruggen F, Logan GD. Models of response inhibition in the stop-signal and stop-change paradigms. Neuroscience and Biobehavioral Reviews. 2009;**33**(5):647-661

[19] Logan GD. On the ability to inhibit thought and action: A users' guide to the stop signal paradigm. In: Dagenbach D, Carr TH, editors. Inhibitory Processes in Attention, Memory, and Laguage. San Diego: Academic; 1994

[20] Weafer J, Burkhardt A, de Wit H. Sweet taste liking is associated with impulsive behaviors in humans. Frontiers in Behavioral Neuroscience. 2014;**8**(June):228

[21] Lole L, Gonsalvez CJ, Barry RJ. Reward and punishment hyposensitivity in problem gamblers: A study of event-related potentials using a principal components analysis. Clinical Neurophysiology. 2015;**126**(7):1295-1309

[22] Völlm B, Richardson P, McKie S, Elliott R, Dolan M, Deakin B. Neuronal correlates of reward and loss in Cluster B personality disorders: A functional magnetic resonance imaging study. Psychiatry Research: Neuroimaging. 2007;**156**(2):151-167

[23] Ainslie G. Specious reward: A behavioral theory of impulsiveness and impulse control. Psychological Bulletin. 1975;**82**(4):463-496

[24] Sebastian A, Jacob G, Lieb K, Tüscher O. Impulsivity in borderline personality disorder: A matter of disturbed impulse control or a facet of emotional dysregulation? Current Psychiatry Reports. 2013;**15**(2):339

[25] Krause-Utz A, Cackowski S, Daffner S, Sobanski E, Plichta MM, Bohus M, et al. Delay discounting and response disinhibition under acute experimental stress in women with borderline personality disorder and adult attention deficit hyperactivity disorder. Psychological Medicine. 2016;**46**:3137-3149

[26] Cackowski S, Reitz AC, Ende G, Kleindienst N, Bohus M, Schmahl C, et al. Impact of stress on different components of impulsivity in borderline personality disorder. Psychological Medicine. 2014;**44**(August):3329-3340

[27] Barker V, Romaniuk L, Cardinal RN, Pope M, Nicol K, Hall J. Impulsivity in borderline personality disorder. Psychological Medicine. 2015;**45**:1955-1964

[28] Lieb K, Zanarini MC, Schmahl C, Linehan MM, Bohus M. Borderline personality disorder. Lancet. 2004;**364**(364):453-461

[29] Swick D, Ashley V, Turken U. Are the neural correlates of stopping and not going identical? Quantitative meta-analysis of two response inhibition tasks. NeuroImage. 2011; **56**(3):1655-1665

[30] Simmonds DJ, Pekar JJ, Mostofsky SH. Meta-analysis of Go/No-go tasks demonstrating that fMRI activation associated with response inhibition is task-dependent. Neuropsychologia. 2008;**46**(1):224-232

[31] Criaud M, Boulinguez P. Have we been asking the right questions when assessing response inhibition in go/no-go tasks with fMRI? A meta-analysis and critical review. Neuroscience and Biobehavioral Reviews. 2013;**37**(1):11-23

[32] Winstanley CA. The neural and neurochemical basis of delay discounting. In: Madden GJ, Bickel WK, editors. Impulsivity: The Behavioral and Neurological Science of Discounting. Washington: American Psychological Association. 2002. pp. 95-122

[33] Ludwig VU, Nüsser C, Goschke T, Wittfoth-Schardt D, Wiers CE, Erk S, et al. Delay discounting without decision-making: Medial prefrontal cortex and amygdala activations reflect immediacy processing and correlate with impulsivity and anxious-depressive traits. Frontiers in Behavioral Neuroscience. 2015;**9**(280):1-15

[34] McClure SM, York MK, Montague PR. The neural substrates of reward processing in humans: The modern role of fMRI. Neuroscience. 2004;**10**(3):260-268

[35] Kishinevsky FI, Cox JE, Murdaugh DL, Stoeckel LE, Cook EW, Weller REFMRI. Reactivity on a delay discounting task predicts weight gain in obese women. Appetite. 2012; **58**(2):582-592

[36] Stoeckel LE, Murdaugh DL, Cox JE, Cook EW, Weller RE. Greater impulsivity is associated with decreased brain activation in obese women during a delay discounting task. Brain Imaging and Behavior. 2013;**7**(2):116-128

[37] Monterosso JR, Ainslle G, Xu J, Cordova X, Domier CP, London ED. Frontoparietal cortical activity of methamphetamine-dependent and comparison subjects performing a delay discounting task. Human Brain Mapping. 2007;**28**(5):383-393

[38] Meade CS, Lowen SB, MacLean RR, Key MD, Lukas SE. fMRI brain activation during a delay discounting task in HIV-positive adults with and without cocaine dependence. Psychiatry Research. 2011;**192**(3):167-175

[39] Clewett D, Luo S, Hsu E, Ainslie G, Mather M, Monterosso J. Increased functional coupling between the left fronto-parietal network and anterior insula predicts steeper delay discounting in smokers. Human Brain Mapping. 2014;**35**(8):3774-3787

[40] Armony JL. Current emotion research in behavioral neuroscience: The role(s) of the amygdala. Emotion Review. 2013;**5**(1):104-115

[41] Phelps EA, LeDoux JE. Contributions of the amygdala to emotion processing: From animal models to human behavior. Neuron. 2005;**48**(2):175-187

[42] Nimrod J, Sarkheil P, Zilverstand A, Kilian-hütten N, Schneider F, Goebel R, et al. NeuroImage self-regulation of human brain activity using simultaneous real-time fMRI and EEG neurofeedback. NeuroImage. 2016;**125**(6):1-18

[43] Paret C, Ruf M, Fungisai M, Kluetsch R, Demirakca T, Jungkunz M, et al. NeuroImage fMRI neurofeedback of amygdala response to aversive stimuli enhances prefrontal—Limbic brain connectivity. NeuroImage. 2016;**125**:182-188

[44] Kober H, Barrett LF, Joseph J, Bliss-Moreau E, Lindquist K, Wager TD. Functional grouping and cortical-subcortical interactions in emotion: A meta-analysis of neuroimaging studies. NeuroImage. 2008;**42**(2):998-1031

[45] Zotev V, Phillips R, Young KD, Drevets WC, Bodurka J. Prefrontal control of the amygdala during real-time fMRI neurofeedback training of emotion regulation. PLoS One. 2013;**8**(11):e79184

[46] Wei S, Geng H, Jiang X, Zhou Q, Chang M. Amygdala-prefrontal cortex resting-state functional connectivity varies with first depressive or manic episode in bipolar disorder. Neuroscience Letters. 2017;**641**:51-55

[47] Cisler JM. Childhood trauma and functional connectivity between amygdala and medial prefrontal cortex: A dynamic functional connectivity and large-scale network. Perspective. 2017;**11**(May):1-11

[48] Vargas C, López-Jaramillo C, Vieta E. A systematic literature review of resting state network-functional MRI in bipolar disorder. Journal of Affective Disorders. 2013;**150**(3): 727-735

[49] Schulze L, Schmahl C, Niedtfeld I. Neural correlates of disturbed emotion processing in borderline personality disorder: A multimodal meta-analysis. Biological Psychiatry. 2016;**79**(2):97-106

[50] Paret C, Kluetsch R, Zaehringer J, Ruf M, Demirakca T, Bohus M, et al. Alterations of amygdala-prefrontal connectivity with real-time fMRI neurofeedback in BPD patients. Social Cognitive and Affective Neuroscience. 2016;**11**(6):952-960

[51] Nicholson AA, Rabellino D, Densmore M, Frewen PA, Paret C, Kluetsch R, et al. The neurobiology of emotion regulation in posttraumatic stress disorder: Amygdala downregulation via real-time fMRI neurofeedback. Human Brain Mapping. 2017;**38**(1):541-560

[52] Oldham JM, Gabbard GO, Soloff P, Spiegel D, Stone M, Phillips KA. Practice guideline for the treatment of patients with borderline personality disorder. American Psychiatric Association. 2001;**3**(October):1-82

[53] Ansell EB, Sanislow CA, McGlashan TH, Grilo CM. Psychosocial impairment and treatment utilization by patients with borderline personality disorder, other personality disorders, mood and anxiety disorders, and a healthy comparison group. Comprehensive Psychiatry. 2007;**48**(4):329-336

[54] Torgersen S, Kringlen E. The prevalence of personality disorders in a community sample. Archives of General Psychiatry. 2001;**58**(6):590-596

[55] American Psychiatric Association. Diagnostic and Statistical Manual of Mental Disorders. Arlington: American Psychiatric Association; 2013. 991 p

[56] Donegan NH, Sanislow CA, Blumberg HP, Fulbright RK, Lacadie C, Skudlarski P, et al. Amygdala hyperreactivity in borderline personality disorder: Implications for emotional dysregulation. Biological Psychiatry. 2003;**54**(11):1284-1293

[57] Koenigsberg HW, Siever LJ, Lee H, Pizzarello S, New AS, Goodman M, et al. Neural correlates of emotion processing in borderline personality disorder. Psychiatry Research: Neuroimaging. 2009;**172**(3):192-199

[58] Mitchell AE, Dickens GL, Picchioni MM. Facial emotion processing in borderline personality disorder: A systematic review and meta-analysis. Neuropsychology Review. 2014;**24**(2):166-184

[59] Brunner R, Henze R, Parzer P, Kramer J, Feigl N, Lutz K, et al. Reduced prefrontal and orbitofrontal gray matter in female adolescents with borderline personality disorder: Is it disorder specific? NeuroImage. 2010;**49**(1):114-120

[60] De La Fuente JM, Goldman S, Stanus E, Vizuete C, Morlán I, Bobes J, et al. Brain glucose metabolism in borderline personality disorder. Journal of Psychiatric Research. 1997; **31**(5):531-541

[61] Soloff PH, Meltzer CC, Becker C, Greer PJ, Kelly TM, Constantine D. Impulsivity and prefrontal hypometabolism in borderline personality disorder. Psychiatry Research: Neuroimaging. 2003;**123**(3):153-163

[62] Soloff PH, Meltzer CC, Greer PJ, Constantine D, Kelly TM. A fenfluramine-activated FDGPET study of borderline personality disorder. Biological Psychiatry. 2000 Mar;**47**(6): 540-547

[63] Camprodon JA, Pascual-Leone A. Multimodal applications of transcranial magnetic stimulation for circuit-based psychiatry. JAMA Psychiatry. 2016 Apr 1;**73**(4):407

[64] Barnow S, Völker KA, Möller B, Freyberger HJ, Spitzer C, Grabe HJ, et al. Neurophysiological correlates of borderline personality disorder: A transcranial magnetic stimulation study. Biological Psychiatry. 2009;**65**(4):313-318

[65] Lang S, Stopsack M, Kotchoubey B, Frick C, Grabe HJ, Spitzer C, et al. Cortical inhibition in alexithymic patients with borderline personality disorder. Biological Psychology. 2011;**88**(2-3):227-232

[66] Radhu N, de Jesus DR, Ravindran LN, Zanjani A, Fitzgerald PB, Daskalakis ZJ. A meta-analysis of cortical inhibition and excitability using transcranial magnetic stimulation in psychiatric disorders. Clinical Neurophysiology. 2013;**124**(7):1309-1320

[67] Richter MM, Ehlis A-C, Jacob CP, Fallgatter AJ. Cortical excitability in adult patients with attention-deficit/hyperactivity disorder (ADHD). Neuroscience Letters. 2007;**419**(2):137-141

[68] Moll GH, Heinrich H, Gevensleben H, Rothenberger A. Tic distribution and inhibitory processes in the sensorimotor circuit during adolescence: A cross-sectional TMS study. Neuroscience Letters. 2006;**403**(1-2):96-99

[69] Tremblay S, Beaule V, Proulx S, de Beaumont L, Marjanska M, Doyon J, et al. Relationship between transcranial magnetic stimulation measures of intracortical inhibition and spectroscopy measures of GABA and glutamate+glutamine. Journal of Neurophysiology. 2013;**109**(5):1343-1349

[70] Arbabi M, Hafizi S, Ansari S, Oghabian MA, Hasani N. High frequency TMS for the management of borderline personality disorder: A case report. Asian Journal of Psychiatry. 2013;**6**(6):614-617

[71] Cailhol L, Roussignol B, Klein R, Bousquet B, Simonetta-Moreau M, Schmitt L, et al. Borderline personality disorder and rTMS: A pilot trial. Psychiatry Research. 2014;**216**(1):155-157

[72] De Vidovich GZ, Muffatti R, Monaco J, Caramia N, Broglia D, Caverzasi E, et al. Repetitive TMS on left cerebellum affects impulsivity in borderline personality disorder: A pilot study. Frontiers in Human Neuroscience. 2016;**10**(December):1-11

[73] Feffer K, Peters SK, Bhui K, Giacobbe P, Downar J. Successful dorsomedial prefrontal rTMS for major depression in borderline personality disorder: Three cases. Brain Stimulation. 2017;(February):2-3

[74] Reyes-López J, Ricardo-Garcell J, Armas-Castañeda G, García-Anaya M, Arango-De Montis I, González-Olvera JJ, et al. Clinical improvement in patients with borderline personality disorder after treatment with repetitive transcranial magnetic stimulation: Preliminary results. Revista Brasileira de Psiquiatria. 2017

[75] Çavdar S, lýz Onat FY, Yananli HR, Şehirli ÜS, Tulay C, Saka E, et al. Cerebellar connections to the rostral reticular nucleus of the thalamus in the rat. Journal of Anatomy. 2002;**201**(6):485-491

[76] Yamamoto T, Yoshida K, Yoshikawa H, Kishimoto Y, Oka H. The medial dorsal nucleus is one of the thalamic relays of the cerebellocerebral responses to the frontal association cortex in the monkey: Horseradish peroxidase and fluorescent dye double staining study. Brain Research. 1992;**579**(2):315-320

[77] Palesi F, Tournier JD, Calamante F, Muhlert N, Castellazzi G, Chard D, et al. Contralateral cerebello-thalamo-cortical pathways with prominent involvement of associative areas in humans in vivo. Brain Structure & Function. 2015;**220**(6):3369-3384

[78] Finn PR, Justus A, Mazas C, Steinmetz JE. Working memory, executive processes and the effects of alcohol on Go/No-Go learning: Testing a model of behavioral regulation and impulsivity. Psychopharmacology. 1999;**146**(4):465-472

[79] Hinson JM, Jameson TL, Whitney P. Impulsive decision making and working memory. Journal of Experimental Psychology. Learning, Memory, and Cognition. 2003;**29**(2):298-306

[80] Speer AM, Benson BE, Kimbrell TK, Wassermann EM, Willis MW, Herscovitch P, et al. Opposite effects of high and low frequency rTMS on mood in depressed patients: Relationship to baseline cerebral activity on PET. Journal of Affective Disorders. 2009;**115**(3):386-394

[81] Barkley RA. Attention-Deficit Hyperactivity Disorder. A Handbook for Diagnosis and Treatment. 3rd ed. New York, NY, US: Guilford Press; 2006

[82] Ramsay JR, Rostain A. Cognitive-Behavioral Therapy for Adult ADHD: An Integrative Psychosocial and Medical Approach. New York, NY, US: Routledge/Taylor & Francis Group; 2008 (Practical clinical guidebooks series)

[83] Faraone SV, Perlis RH, Doyle AE, Smoller JW, Goralnick JJ, Holmgren MA, et al. Molecular genetics of attention-deficit/hyperactivity disorder. Biological Psychiatry. 2005 Jun;**57**(11):1313-1323

[84] Barkley RA. Deficient emotional self-regulation: A core component of attention-deficit/hyperactivity disorder. Journal of ADHD & Related Disorders. 2010;**1**(2):5-37

[85] Torgersen T, Gjervan B, Rasmussen K. Treatment of adult ADHD: Is current knowledge useful to clinicians? Neuropsychiatric Disease and Treatment. 2008 Feb;**4**(1):177-186

[86] Sonuga-Barke EJS. Disambiguating inhibitory dysfunction in attention-deficit/hyperactivity disorder: Toward the decomposition of developmental brain phenotypes. Biological Psychiatry. 2010;**67**(7):599-601

[87] Nigg JT, Willcutt EG, Doyle AE, Sonuga-Barke EJS. Causal heterogeneity in attention-deficit/hyperactivity disorder: Do we need neuropsychologically impaired subtypes? Biological Psychiatry. 2005;**57**(11):1224-1230

[88] Shaw P, Eckstrand K, Sharp W, Blumenthal J, Lerch JP, Greenstein D, et al. Attention-deficit/hyperactivity disorder is characterized by a delay in cortical maturation. Proceedings of the National Academy of Sciences. 2007;**104**(49):19649-19654

[89] Todd RD, Neuman RJ, Lobos EA, Jong Y-JI, Reich W, Heath AC. Lack of association of dopamine D4 receptor gene polymorphisms with ADHD subtypes in a population sample of twins. American Journal of Medical Genetics. 2001 Jul;**105**(5):432-438

[90] Dickstein SG, Bannon K, Xavier Castellanos F, Milham MP. The neural correlates of attention deficit hyperactivity disorder: An ALE meta-analysis. Journal of Child Psychology and Psychiatry and Allied Disciplines. 2006;**47**(10):1051-1062

[91] Duerden EG, Tannock R, Dockstader C. Altered cortical morphology in sensorimotor processing regions in adolescents and adults with attention-deficit/hyperactivity disorder. Brain Research. 2012;**1445**:82-91

[92] Vloet TD, Gilsbach S, Neufang S, Fink GR, Herpertz-Dahlmann B, Konrad K. Neural mechanisms of interference control and time discrimination in attention-deficit/hyperactivity disorder. Journal of the American Academy of Child and Adolescent Psychiatry. 2010;**49**(4):356-367

[93] Bush G. Cingulate, frontal, and parietal cortical dysfunction in attention-deficit/hyperactivity disorder. Biological Psychiatry. 2011;**69**(12):1160-1167

[94] Kašpárek T, Theiner P, Filová A. Neurobiologie hyperkinetické poruchy pohledem zobrazovacích metod. Česká a slovenská psychiatrie. 2013 Apr;**109**(2):73-80

[95] Scheres A, Milham MP, Knutson B, Castellanos FX. Ventral striatal hyporesponsiveness during reward anticipation in attention-deficit/hyperactivity disorder. Biological Psychiatry. 2007;**61**(5):720-724

[96] Dutra TG, Baltar A, Monte-Silva KK. Motor cortex excitability in attention-deficit hyperactivity disorder (ADHD): A systematic review and meta-analysis. Research in Developmental Disabilities. 2016;**56**:1-9

[97] Gilbert DL, Isaacs KM, Augusta M, Macneil LK, Mostofsky SH. Motor cortex inhibition A marker of ADHD behavior and motor development in children. Neurology. 2011;**76**(7):615-621

[98] Moll GH, Heinrich H, Trott G-E, Wirth S, Rothenberger A. Deficient intracortical inhibition in drug-naive children with attention-deficit hyperactivity disorder is enhanced by methylphenidate. Neuroscience Letters. 2000;**284**(1):121-125

[99] Moll GH, Heinrich H, Trott G-E, Wirth S, Bock N, Rothenberger A. Children with comorbid attention-deficit-hyperactivity disorder and tic disorder: Evidence for additive inhibitory deficits within the motor system. Annals of Neurology. 2001 Mar 1;**49**(3):393-396

[100] Wu SW, Gilbert DL, Shahana N, Huddleston DA, Mostofsky SH. Transcranial magnetic stimulation measures in attention-deficit/hyperactivity disorder. Pediatric Neurology. 2012;**47**(3):177-185

[101] Wagle-Shukla A, Ni Z, Gunraj CA, Bahl N, Chen R. Effects of short interval intracortical inhibition and intracortical facilitation on short interval intracortical facilitation in human primary motor cortex. The Journal of Physiology. 2009;**587**(23):5665-5678

[102] Kaster TS, de Jesus D, Radhu N, Farzan F, Blumberger DM, Rajji TK, et al. Clozapine potentiation of GABA mediated cortical inhibition in treatment resistant schizophrenia. Schizophrenia Research. 2015;**165**(2-3):157-162

[103] Hasan A, Schneider M, Schneider-Axmann T, Ruge D, Retz W, Rösler M, et al. A similar but distinctive pattern of impaired cortical excitability in first-episode schizophrenia and ADHD. Neuropsychobiology. 2013;**67**(2):74-83

[104] Strafella AP, Paus T, Barrett J, Dagher A. Repetitive transcranial magnetic stimulation of the human prefrontal cortex induces dopamine release in the caudate nucleus. Journal of Neuroscience. 2001;**21**(15):RC157

[105] Niederhofer H. Effectiveness of the repetitive transcranical magnetic stimulation (rTMS) of 1 Hz for attention-deficit hyperactivity disorder (ADHD). Psychiatria Danubina. 2008 Mar;**20**(1):91-92

[106] Niederhofer H. Additional biological therapies for attention-deficit hyperactivity disorder: Repetitive transcranical magnetic stimulation of 1 Hz helps to reduce methylphenidate. Clinical Practice. 2011 Dec;**2**(1):e8

[107] Bloch Y, Harel EV, Aviram S, Govezensky J, Ratzoni G, Levkovitz Y. Positive effects of repetitive transcranial magnetic stimulation on attention in ADHD Subjects: A randomized controlled pilot study. The World Journal of Biological Psychiatry. The official Journal of the World Federation of Societies of Biological Psychiatry. 2010 Aug;**11**(5):755-758

[108] Ustohal L, Prikryl R, Kucerova HP, Sisrova M, Stehnova I, Venclikova S, et al. Emotional side effects after high-frequency RTMS of the right dorsolateral prefrontal cortex in an adult patient with ADHD and comorbid depression. Psychiatria Danubina. 2012;**24**(1):102-103

[109] Lefaucheur J, André-obadia N, Antal A, Ayache SS, Baeken C, Benninger DH, et al. Evidence-based guidelines on the therapeutic use of repetitive transcranial magnetic stimulation ( rTMS). Clinical Neurophysiology. 2014;**125**(11):2150-2206

[110] Saba G, Rocamora JF, Kalalou K, Benadhira R, Plaze M, Lipski H, et al. Repetitive transcranial magnetic stimulation as an add-on therapy in the treatment of mania: A case series of eight patients. Psychiatry Research. 2004;**128**(2):199-202

[111] Weaver L, Rostain AL, Mace W, Akhtar U, Moss E, O'Reardon JP. Transcranial magnetic stimulation (TMS) in the treatment of attention-deficit/hyperactivity disorder in adolescents and young adults: A pilot study. The Journal of ECT. 2012 Jun;**28**(2):98-103

[112] Helfrich C, Pierau SS, Freitag CM, Roeper J, Ziemann U, Bender S. Monitoring cortical excitability during repetitive Transcranial magnetic stimulation in children with ADHD: A single-blind, sham-controlled TMS-EEG study. PLoS One. 2012;**7**(11):e50073

[113] Gómez L, Vidal B, Morales L, Báez M, Maragoto C, Galvizu R, et al. Low frequency repetitive transcranial magnetic stimulation in children with attention deficit/hyperactivity disorder. Preliminary results. Brain Stimulation. 2014;**7**(5):760-762

[114] D'Agati D, Bloch Y, Levkovitz Y, Reti I. rTMS for adolescents: Safety and efficacy considerations. Psychiatry Research. 2010 May;**177**(3):280-285

# 11

# Immune System Dysregulation and Autoimmunity in Schizophrenia: IgGs from Sera of Patients with Several Catalytic Activities

Valentina N. Buneva, Evgeny A. Ermakov and Georgy A. Nevinsky

**Abstract**

Schizophrenia is usually a progressive mental illness with very different polymorphic symptoms. Several different theories of schizophrenia were discussed; the causes of this disease are not yet clear. Destruction of DNA, RNA, and myelin basic protein (MBP) by inflammation caused by autoimmune reactions has been revealed. Healthy humans usually do not develop abzymes. It was shown that DNase, RNase, and MBP-hydrolyzing abzymes are easily detectable at the beginning of different autoimmune diseases (AIDs). During the development of spontaneous and induced AIDs in mice, a specific reorganization of their immune system associated with the generation of abzymes hydrolyzing different autoantigens was revealed. SCZ is currently not assigned to classical autoimmune diseases. However, the sera of approximately 30% of SCZ patients demonstrated a high level of anti-DNA Abs (comparing to 37% of SLE patients); abzymes hydrolyzing DNA, RNA, and MBP were revealed in 80–100% of SCZ patients. The site-specific hydrolysis of four known SCZ-specific microRNA playing an important role in the regulation of several genes functioning was revealed. Anti-MBP IgGs hydrolyze specifically only MBP but not other proteins. The data indicate that SCZ patients may to a certain extent show similar to SLE and MS patients' typical signs of autoimmune processes.

**Keywords:** schizophrenia, autoimmunity, catalytic antibodies, hydrolysis of autoantigens

# 1. Introduction

Schizophrenia (SCZ) is a highly heritable brain disorder, and it is one of the most relevant problems of psychiatry [1]. The prevalence of SCZ in the human population is approximately 1%, and this disease is the most severe mental diseases [2]. Schizophrenia is a progressive mental illness demonstrating polymorphic symptomatology and resulting in the persistent violation of social adaptation and ability to work. In SCZ, a violation of synaptic transmission resulting in neuronal damage and severe dysfunction was observed [3–5]. These changes often may begin to arise in utero or early childhood [6, 7].

Several different theories of SCZ were discussed, but all of them cannot be definitively concluded for or against the degenerative or neurodevelopmental hypothesis and did not provide clarity concerning the mechanism of schizophrenia development [8].

The dopamine hypothesis of schizophrenia is a model, attributing symptoms of SCZ to a disturbed and hyperactive dopaminergic signal transduction. Since dysfunction of the glutamatergic system is a widely known fact in SCZ [9–12], it is possible that misbalance of dopamine-glutamate homeostasis can lead to the patient's development of generalized oxidative stress [13, 14]. The known theory, however, does not posit dopamine overabundance as a complete explanation of SCZ. Rather, the overactivation of D2 receptors, specifically, is one effect of the global chemical synaptic dysregulation observed in this disorder.

Detection of neurotropic effect which was postulated is associated with the damages of cell membranes [15, 16]. It is believed that the brain cell membranes damage causes the formation of autoantigens and as the consequence autoantibodies (Abs) [17–19]. Interestingly, Abs to glutamate receptors were revealed in SCZ and many other diseases including typical autoimmune ones [20]. Anti-NMDA-NR1, anti-AMPA-GluR3, anti-NMDA-NR2A/B, and anti-mGluR1 or anti-mGluR5 antibodies were found in subpopulations of patients not only with SCZ but also with encephalitis, epilepsy, SLE, neuropsychiatric SLE, cerebellar ataxia, Sjogren's syndrome, and mania or stroke [20]. These autoimmune Abs against anti-glutamate receptors can bind neurons in few brain regions, activate receptors of glutamate, decrease glutamate receptor's expression, activate blood-brain barrier endothelial cells, damage the brain, impair glutamate-induced signaling and function, kill neurons, and induce psychiatric/behavioral/cognitive abnormalities [20]. The association between SCZ and various inflammatory-autoimmune diseases was reported in several epidemiological surveys. Several studies demonstrated that individuals with SCZ are somehow less likely to have rheumatoid arthritis [21]. Some other autoimmune (AI) disorders have also been linked to schizophrenia, particularly Hashimoto's thyroiditis and celiac disease [22, 23].

During the last decade, new data about increasing recognition of central nervous system (CNS) syndromes associated with autoimmune processes leading to the production of autoantibodies to CNS cell surface antigens were obtained [24]. Most of these syndromes present outstanding mental and cognitive symptoms, among the variety of neurological manifestations such as seizures, movement disorders, and autonomic dysfunction, and is best described as "autoimmune encephalopathy."

The causes of schizophrenia include environmental and genetic factors [25]. Recently, a genome-wide microarray study in postmortem brains of SCZ patients has explored expression profiling of immune-modulatory genes [26]. Genetic factors in SCZ include a variety of common and rare genetic variants [27]. It was shown that SCZ is a multifactorial disease, the pathogenesis of which can contribute to numerous genes and the products of their transcription [28]. Therefore, in research of schizophrenia pathogenesis, understanding a possible role of microRNAs may be important. Short non-coding microRNAs (18–25 nucleotides) can individually regulate up to several hundred genes. Disturbances in microRNA (microRNA-regulated gene network) lead to alteration in the expression of many genes. The expression of different microRNAs in plasma [29, 30], mononuclear cells of peripheral blood [31] as well as in various brain regions [32, 33] in patients with SCZ was detected. In addition, genome-wide association study shows, in SCZ, a close association of a single-nucleotide polymorphism of miR-137 and miR-9-5p [34–36]. MicroRNA miR-137 plays an important role in the differentiation of embryonic stem cells, proliferation, and differentiation of neurons, the maturation of the synapses [37]. The miR-137 inhibits AMPA receptor-mediated synaptic transmission by decreasing the expression of the GluA1 subunit of this receptor [38]; influences the release of neurotransmitters from synaptic vesicles and disrupts synaptic plasticity [39]. Interestingly, one of the genes regulating the expression of miR-137, is a protein zinc finger 804A (zinc finger protein 804 A-ZNF804A), which in turn inhibits the expression of catechol-O-methyltransferase (catechol-O-methyltransferase), and D2 receptor of dopamine [37], which leads to a disruption in dopamine neurotransmission. In the regulation of expression of the D2 receptor of dopamine is also involved in the miR-9-5p [36]. It is shown that miR-9-5p is involved in neuronal migration and that the expression of miR-9-5p in patients with schizophrenia is reduced in neuronal cells precursors (neural progenitor cells) [40]. It was also found that miR-219 plays an important role in the differentiation of oligodendrocytes and myelination of axons of neuronal cells [41].

It is known that enzymes can play important role in the pathogenesis of different diseases: dysfunction of enzymes systems involved in the metabolism of biogenic amines (indolamine, catecholamines) during mental disorders including SCZ [23, 42].

The above data testify to the fact that some patients with SCZ are clearly showing signs of typical autoimmune pathologies. However, the importance of immunological changes resulting in the loss of the tolerance to self-antigens in the pathogenesis of SCZ is currently not accepted. Summarizing all existing hypotheses, one can say that SCZ is a very multifactorial disease including some variations in the functioning of neurotransmitter systems associated with the changes in the rate of synthesis or breakdown of the neurotransmitter, possible modifications of the structure of the relevant receptors, genetic predisposition and a dysregulation between the immune and nervous systems, important role of genetic factors and microRNAs, as well as enzymatic systems.

Despite the fact that SCZ is not currently attributed to typical autoimmune diseases, the immune system and dysregulation of immune cells, including autoimmune processes in this disease, are not to be excluded [17–20, 24]. Schizophrenia, autoimmunity and immune system dysregulation are reviewed in [43, 44]. Thus, the search of the importance of different mechanisms of SCZ development including possible autoimmune factors is undoubtedly actual. In this connection, some literature data should be mentioned. Catalytically active artificial antibodies or abzymes (Abzs) against transition chemical reaction states were well studied (reviewed in [45–47]). In the last three decades, it was shown that auto-antibodies from the blood of patients with different AIDs can possess enzymatic activities and that their occurrence is a specific feature of these pathologies (reviewed in [47–53]). Similarly to artificial Abzs to transition states of chemical reactions [45–47], natural abzymes are Abs raised directly against enzyme substrates acting as haptens of proteins mimicking transition states of catalytic reactions. In addition, anti-idiotypic Abs against catalytic centers of enzymes can be induced in AIDs, and they also possess catalytic activities [47–56].

Even in the sera of healthy mammals, auto-antibodies to different peptides, proteins, DNA, and RNA are detectable, and their titers vary significantly [47–57]. The sera of SLE patients usually contain DNA and anti-DNA Abs in increased concentrations, and SLE is usually considered to be associated with the autoimmunization of patients with DNA. However, the sera of patients with several different autoimmune diseases contain DNA and anti-DNA Abs [57], as well as RNA and anti-RNA Abs in high concentrations [58–61]. Many anti-DNA Abs are directed against histone-DNA nucleosomal complexes appearing from internucleosomal cleavage during apoptosis [62].

Despite the fact that the blood of healthy donors usually contains autoantibodies to DNA, RNA, and many different proteins, these Abs usually do not possess catalytic activities [47–56]. It was shown, that in the case of different autoimmune patients, experimental mice abzymes with DNase, protease, and amylase activities are the earliest and statistically significant markers of autoimmune pathology onset and following development [63–69]. Enzymatic activities of Abs are detectable even at the stage of pre-disease when there is no visible markers of autoimmune diseases and changes in proteinuria, and the anti-antigen titers including DNA and proteins are within the typical ranges of these indicators for healthy humans and experimental mice [63–69]. Therefore, a detectable level of Ab activities can be considered as valuable index even at the beginning of the pathology (pre-disease) and obvious pathology conditions of spontaneous or induced autoimmune diseases [63–69].

Natural polyclonal IgGs and/or IgAs and IgMs hydrolyzing mononucleotides, DNA, RNA, oligopeptides, proteins, and polysaccharides, from the sera of patients with several AIDs and several viral diseases with significant autoimmune reactions were revealed (reviewed in [47–56]). Bence-Jones proteins of multiple myeloma patients [70], DNase abzymes from SLE [71] and MS [51] are cytotoxic, induce nuclear DNA fragmentation and cause cell death by apoptosis, leading to increase in the concentration of many different cell components including DNA, RNA, and proteins in patients with various AIDS. Abzymes with RNase activity in autoimmune diseases are of particular interest. The same polyclonal preparations of Abzs hydrolyzed RNA approximately 10-fold to 300-fold faster than DNA [72–74].

It has been recently shown that myelin basic protein (MBP)-hydrolyzing activity is an intrinsic property of IgGs of SLE patients [75–78] as well as IgGs, IgMs, and IgAs from the sera of MS patients [79–82]. In MS and SLE, anti-MBP abzymes with protease activity can attack MBP of the myelin-proteolipid sheath of axons and can play an important harmful role in MS and SLE pathogenesis [75–82].

In this review, an analysis of the catalytic activities of currently described abzymes in the blood of patients with SCZ was carried out. These abzymes of SCZ with different catalytic activities are compared with other Abzs in AIDs. In addition, a possible role of defects of immune systems leading to the production of abzymes is discussed.

Taking into accoIn this review, an analysis of the catalytic activities of currently described abzymes in the blood of patients with SCZ. These abzymes of SCZ with different catalytic activities are compared with other Abzs in AIDs. In addition, a possible role of defects of immune systems leading to the production of abzymes is discussed.unt the ability of autoimmune patient's abzymes to hydrolyze RNA together with the important role of microRNAs in proliferation, differentiation, and maturation of neuronal cells and the relationship of microRNAs with the development of SCZ, the aim of present chapter was to analyze the RNA-hydrolyzing activity of Abs of schizophrenia patients. In addition, we have described substrate specificity antibodies in the hydrolysis of specific for schizophrenia microRNA.

As mentioned above, schizophrenia is not attributed to the classic autoimmune diseases. At the same time, it was recently shown that the sera of ~30% of SCZ patients showed a higher content of anti-DNA Abs (comparing to 37% of SLE patients), while DNase abzymes were revealed in 80% of SCZ patients [83]. In addition, it was shown that abzymes hydrolyzing MBP were revealed in 82% of the SC patients. These data can indicate for at least a pronounced autoimmune component in patients with SCZ. Interestingly, the researchers of the London medical Institute Oliver House advanced theory, according to which schizophrenia is the result of a lesion of immune system of the brain (http://the-newspapers.com/2017/11/08/schizophrenia-has-announced-a-disease-of-the-immune-system).

## 2. Abzymes with DNase activity

The generation of auto-Abs to DNA usually occurs not only in patients with AI, viral, and bacterial diseases but also in healthy humans [23, 24, 32–35, 55]. We have compared the relative levels of Abs interacting with DNA in sera of 20 SCZ patients and 20 healthy donors. The levels of Abs interacting with single-stranded (ss) DNA ($A_{450}$/ml) for 20 healthy donors were detectable; they varied from 0.07 to 0.14 specific units (average value—0.13 ± 0.02) and, on average, they were 1.3-fold higher ($P = 6.3 \times 10^{-4}$) than those interacting with double-stranded (ds) DNA varying from 0.1 to 0.18 (0.1 ± 0.02) [83, 84]. The average level of Abs ($A_{450}$/ml) for the total group of patients with SCZ interacting with ssDNA (range from 0.1 to 1.4; average value 0.23 ± 0.13) was only 1.1-fold lower ($P = 6.9 \times 10^{-4}$) than that for interacting with dsDNA (range from 0.15 to 0.44; average value 0.25 ± 0.07). The average level of Abs interacting with dsDNA for healthy donors is 2.5-fold lower ($P = 1.0 \times 10^{-6}$) than that for SCZ patients, while for antibodies interacting with ssDNA, it is lower only 1.8-fold ($P = 0.05$). Several SCZ patients are characterized by very high levels of Abs interacting with ssDNA and dsDNA (0.31–1.4 $A_{450}$/ml) characterizing patients with SLE (0.51 ± 0.50 and 0.66 ± 0.48 $A_{450}$/ml, respectively) and with MS (0.22 ± 0.18 and 0.39 ± 0.26 $A_{450}$/ml, respectively) [53–56].

The average relative level of Abs interacting with dsDNA (0.23 ± 0.05 $A_{450}$/ml) for SCZ patients with positive symptoms was 1.2-fold lower than that for patients with negative symptoms

(0.28 ± 0.07 $A_{450}$/ml) (**Table 2**). At the same time, the average level of Abs interacting with ssDNA (0.3 ± 0.22 $A_{450}$/ml) for patients with positive symptoms was 1.9-fold higher than that for SCZ patients demonstrating negative symptoms (0.16 ± 0.07 $A_{450}$/ml). It was accepted that increased concentration of anti-DNA Abs is a characteristic of patients with SLE. However, concentration of anti-DNA Abs compared with healthy donors is higher in patients with SLE (37% of patients), MS (17–18%), Sjogren's syndrome (18%), Hashimoto thyroiditis (23%), rheumatoid arthritis (7% of patients), and myasthenia gravis (6%) [57]. Overall, ~30% of SCZ patients (comparable with SLE patients 37% [57]) displayed higher content of Abs interacting with ss- and dsDNA when compared to healthy donors.

As mentioned above, polyclonal natural DNA-hydrolyzing IgGs and/or IgAs and IgMs were revealed in blood sera of patients with several AI and viral diseases (reviewed in [47–57]). Electrophoretically and immunologically homogeneous IgGs were obtained from the sera of 20 SCZ patients and 20 healthy volunteers by sequential chromatography of the serum proteins on Protein A-Sepharose using conditions providing removing non-specifically bound proteins, followed by FPLC gel filtration in an acidic buffer destroying immune complexes as in [75–81]. For some experiments, equimolar mixtures of 20 IgG preparations of SCZ patients (scz-$IgG_{mix}$) and 20 preparations of healthy donors (healthy-$IgG_{mix}$) were used [83]. To show that IgGs of SCZ patients possess DNase activity, we have checked several known strict criteria [52–56, 85]. The following main criteria were used [83]: (a) Abs should be electrophoretically homogeneous (**Figure 1A**); (b) Abs after gel filtration in an acidic buffer (pH 2.6) dissociating strong noncovalent complexes IgGs must possess DNase activity and the peak of the activity should tracked exactly with the intact Abs (**Figure 1B**); (c) immobilized polyclonal antibodies against the human Abs should completely absorb the DNase activity; (d) among criteria, there is an hardest one; if it is carried out, all other criteria are also met. To exclude any possible artifacts due to hypothetical traces of contaminating canonical DNases, scz-$IgG_{mix}$ preparation was subjected to SDS-PAGE in a gel containing polymeric DNA, and its DNase activity was analyzed after gel incubation in the standard reaction buffer (**Figure 1C**). Ethidium bromide staining of the gels revealed sharp dark bands against a fluorescent DNA background only in the position of intact $IgG_{mix}$ before (lane 3) and only in the position of light chains after Abs reduction with DTT (lane 4). There was no revealed DNase activity of healthy-$IgG_{mix}$ before (lane 5) and after Abs reduction with DTT (lane 6).

The intact IgGs have molecular masses (~150 kDa) significantly higher than for all canonical human DNases (35–36 kDa), while DNases have higher molecular masses than light chains of IgGs (22–25 kDa). SDS usually dissociates all protein complexes. The detection of DNase activity only in the gel zones of intact IgGs and their light chains as well as the absence of any other activity and protein bands (**Figure 1C**) ensure direct evidence that SCZ IgGs hydrolyze DNA and are not contaminated with canonical DNases. Several other strict criteria were also fulfilled (see below).

We have shown that the DNase activity of IgGs purified by chromatography on Protein G-Sepharose followed by FPLC gel filtration can be used for the evaluation of their relative activity (RA) without additional purification. The RAs of SCZ patients IgGs were significantly varied from patient to patient. However, 16 of 20 samples (80%) had high or detectable DNase activity. The distributions of the RAs for IgGs of different SCZ patients with positive and

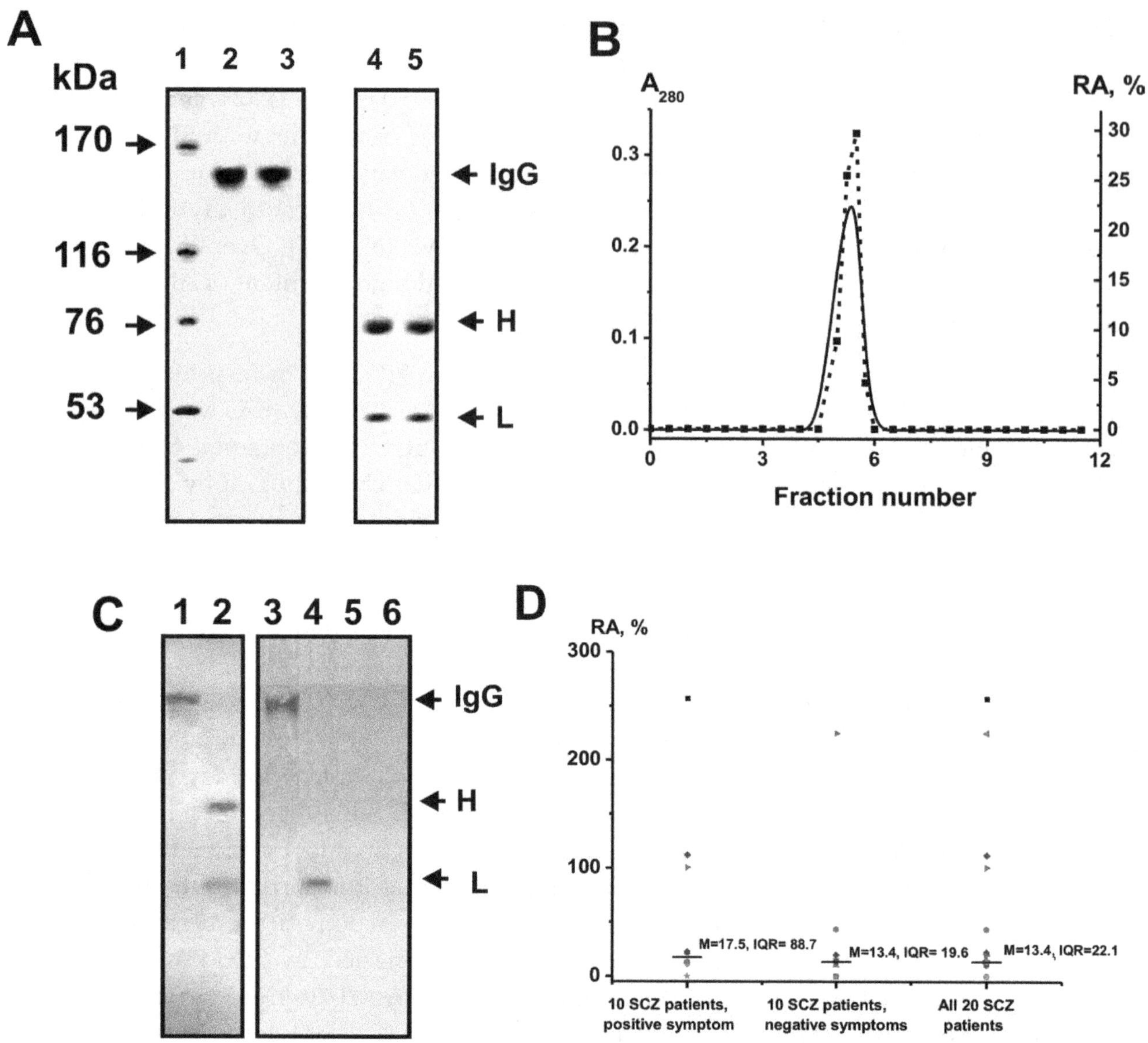


**Figure 1.** SDS-PAGE analysis of $IgG_{mix}$ (7 μg) corresponding to the mixtures of scz-$IgG_{mix}$ (lane 2) from the sera of 20 patients with SCZ and healthy-$IgG_{mix}$ (lane 3) corresponding to 20 healthy donors in a nonreducing 3–16% gradient gel or in a reducing 12% gel (lanes 4 and 5, respectively) followed by silver staining (A); the lane 1 arrows indicate the positions of molecular mass markers. The application of the strict criteria is to prove that the DNase activity of Abs is the intrinsic property of scz-$IgG_{mix}$. FPLC gel filtration of scz-$IgG_{mix}$ on a Superdex 200 column using an acidic buffer (pH 2.6) after IgGs pre-incubation in the same buffer (B): (■), relative activity (RA, %) of IgGs in the hydrolysis of supercoiled DNA; (—), absorbance at 280 nm (A280). A complete hydrolysis of 18 μg/ml scDNA for 2 h was taken for 100%. The initial rate determination error from three experiments in each case did not exceed 7–10%. Assay of DNase activity of scz-$IgG_{mix}$ from schizophrenia patients in-gel containing thymus DNA before (lane 3) and after IgGs reduction with DTT (lane 4); lane 5 corresponds to healthy-IgGmix before treatment with DTT (C). DNase activity was revealed after gel staining with ethidium bromide as a dark band on the fluorescent background. There was no revealed catalytic activity of healthy-$IgG_{mix}$ before its reduction (lane 5). A part of the used gel was stained with Coomassie R250 to find the position of intact scz-$IgG_{mix}$ before (lane 1) as well as its free heavy and light chains after Ab reduction (lane 2). The distribution of the RAs (in the hydrolysis of scDNA) corresponding to SCZ patients with positive and negative symptoms within different ranges (D). The median (M; solid lines) and interquartile ranges (IQR) were estimated using the Mann-Whitney test.

negative symptoms are shown in **Figure 1D**. Finally, to compare RAs of DNase IgGs of SCZ patients with those for patients with other diseases, the values of apparent $k_{cat}$ in the hydrolysis of DNA for every IgG preparation ($k_{cat}$ = V (M/min)/ [IgGs] (M) and average values of parameters were calculated (**Table 1**) [83].

One of the criteria of Abs' activity is their higher affinity for substrates comparing with canonical DNases. The $K_m$ and $k_{cat}$ values for scDNA hydrolysis were estimated. First, IgG-19 corresponds to the patient with negative symptoms (NS) of SCZ, while IgG-1 and IgG-6 to patients with positive symptoms (**Table 1**). The $K_m$ value for IgG-19 ($K_m$ = 95 ± 18 nM) was comparable with that for IgG-1 ($K_m$ = 85.0 ± 12.0 nM) and IgG-6 ($K_m$ = 80.0 ± 12.0 nM), while $k_{cat}$ for IgG-19 ((2.7 ± 0.3) × $10^{-3}$ $min^{-1}$) and IgG-6 ((3.0 ± 0.3) × $10^{-3}$ $min^{-1}$) were comparable, but lower than that for IgG-1 ((7.9 ± 0.5) × $10^{-3}$ $min^{-1}$). Thus, the affinity of scDNA for SCZ IgGs was in the range 80–95 nM, which corresponds to typical $K_d$ (and $K_m$) values for interactions of antibodies with antigens; it is approximately 3–4 orders of magnitude higher than affinity of DNase I for scDNA ($K_m$ = 46–58 μM) [86].

| Number of patients (sex) | Abs to dsDNA, $A_{450}$/ml | Abs to ssDNA, $A_{450}$/ml | Relative hydrolysis of DNA, % | $k_{cat}$ ×$10^5$,$min^{-1}$ |
|---|---|---|---|---|
| | 1 | 2 | 3 | 4 |
| | **Positive symptoms (PS)** | | | |
| 1 (M) | 0.35 | 1.4 | 257$^{\mu}$ | 39.6$^{***}$ |
| 2 (M) | 0.19 | 0.11 | 11.7 | 1.8 |
| 3 (M) | 0.2 | 0.31 | 22.2 | 3.4 |
| 4 (M) | 0.19 | 0.16 | 11 | 1.7 |
| 5 (M) | 0.24 | 0.19 | 12 | 1.9 |
| 6 (M) | 0.15 | 0.11 | 100.4 | 15.5 |
| 7 (M) | 0.21 | 0.14 | 112 | 17.3 |
| 8 (F) | 0.2 | 0.23 | 22 | 3.4 |
| 9 (F) | 0.34 | 0.25 | 13 | 2.0 |
| 10 (F) | 0.18 | 0.11 | 0 | 0 |
| Average (PS) | 0.23±0.05 | 0.30±0.22 | 56.1±60.2 | 8.7±9.3 |
| M (IQR) (PS)ϒ | 0.20 (0.05) | 0.18 (0.14) | 17.5 (88.7) | 2.7 (13.7) |
| Correl. coeff. (PS) | Groups 1–2 (0.71) | | 1–3 (0.46) | 2–3 (0.84) |
| Negative symptoms (NS) | | | | |
| 11 (M) | 0.48 | 0.23 | 0$^{\mu}$ | 0 |
| 12 (M) | 0.28 | 0.2 | 0 | 0 |
| 13 (M) | 0.21 | 0.13 | 10.4 | 1.6 |
| 14 (M) | 0.22 | 0.16 | 15.0 | 2.3 |
| 15 (M) | 0.23 | 0.1 | 13.3 | 2.1 |
| 16 (F) | 0.44 | 0.12 | 225 | 34.7 |
| 17 (F) | 0.24 | 0.11 | 19.6 | 3.0 |
| 18 (F) | 0.17 | 0.19 | 13.6 | 2.1 |
| 19 (F) | 0.25 | 0.16 | 43.4 | 6.7 |

| Number of patients (sex) | Abs to dsDNA, $A_{450}$/ml | Abs to ssDNA, $A_{450}$/ml | Relative hydrolysis of DNA, % | $k_{cat}$ ×10[5],min[-1] |
|---|---|---|---|---|
| | 1 | 2 | 3 | 4 |
| | Positive symptoms (PS) | | | |
| 20 (F) | 0.24 | 0.15 | 0 | 0 |
| Average (NS)[**] | 0.28±0.07 | 0.16±0.03 | 34.0±40.1 | 5.3±6.2 |
| M (IQR) (NS) | 0.24 (0.06) | 0.16 (0.07) | 13.4 (19.6) | 2.1 (3.0) |
| Average, total group | 0.25±0.07 | 0.23±0.13 | 45.1±50.4 | 7.0 (7.9) |
| M (IQR), total group[ϒ] | 0.23 (0.07) | 0.16±0.1 | 13.4 (22.1) | 2.1 (3.4) |
| Correl. coeff. (NS) | 1–2 (0.3) | 1–3 (0.5) | 2–3 (0.35) | |
| Correl. coeff., complete group | 1–2 (0.3) | 1–3 (0.4) | 2–3 (0.62) | |

[*]For each value, a mean of three measurements is reported; the error of the determination of values did not exceed 7–10%.

[**]Average values are reported as mean ± S.E; they were recalculated to standard conditions and complete hydrolysis of 18 μg/ml scDNA after 1 h of incubation in the presence of 0.1 mg/ml IgG was taken for 100%.

[***]The average apparent $k_{cat}$ values of the reaction of DNA hydrolysis were calculated using average RA values: $k_{cat}$ = V (M/min)/ [IgGs] (M), 18 μg/ml scDNA was used.

[μ]Statistical significance of differences in DNase activity between schizophrenia patients with positive and negative symptoms ($P = 0.026$).

[ϒ]The median (M) and interquartile ranges (IQR) were calculated using the Mann-Whitney test.

**Table 1.** The relative concentration of fnti-DNA Abs, RAs (%), and the apparent $k_{cat}$ values characterizing hydrolysis of scDNA by IgGs from the sera of SCZ patients.[*]

## 3. Abzymes with RNase activity

It was shown in several articles that IgGs from the sera of healthy humans cannot hydrolyze RNA [87–90]. At the same time, IgGs from the sera of patients with SLE, MS, Hashimoto's thyroiditis and some other autoimmune pathologies effectively hydrolyze different ribopolynucleotides and tRNAs [87–90].

Electrophoretically and immunologically homogeneous IgGs purified from the sera of 35 SCZ patients according to [75–83] as described above were used [91]. On the first step, we used a mixture of equal amounts of 35 polyclonal IgGs (scz-$IgG_{mix}$) and 15 healthy donors. Then, we checked the fulfillment of the strict criteria described above. The homogeneity of the typical 150-kDa $IgG_{mix}$ was confirmed by SDS-PAGE with silver staining similar to **Figure 1**. The activity peak of the $IgG_{mix}$ treated with acidic buffer (pH 2.6) coincided under gel filtration exactly with the peak of intact Abs (**Figure 2A**) Immobilized polyclonal mouse IgGs against the light chains of human IgGs completely bind the RNase activity. Scz-$IgG_{mix}$ was subjected to SDS-PAGE in a gel co-polymerized with polymeric yeast RNA, and its RNase activity was revealed after the gel incubation in the standard reaction buffer only in the position of intact scz-$IgG_{mix}$. (**Figure 2B**). Canonical human RNases have significantly lower molecular masses (13–15 kDa) than the intact IgGs (150 kDa). Therefore, the activity detection in the gel zones

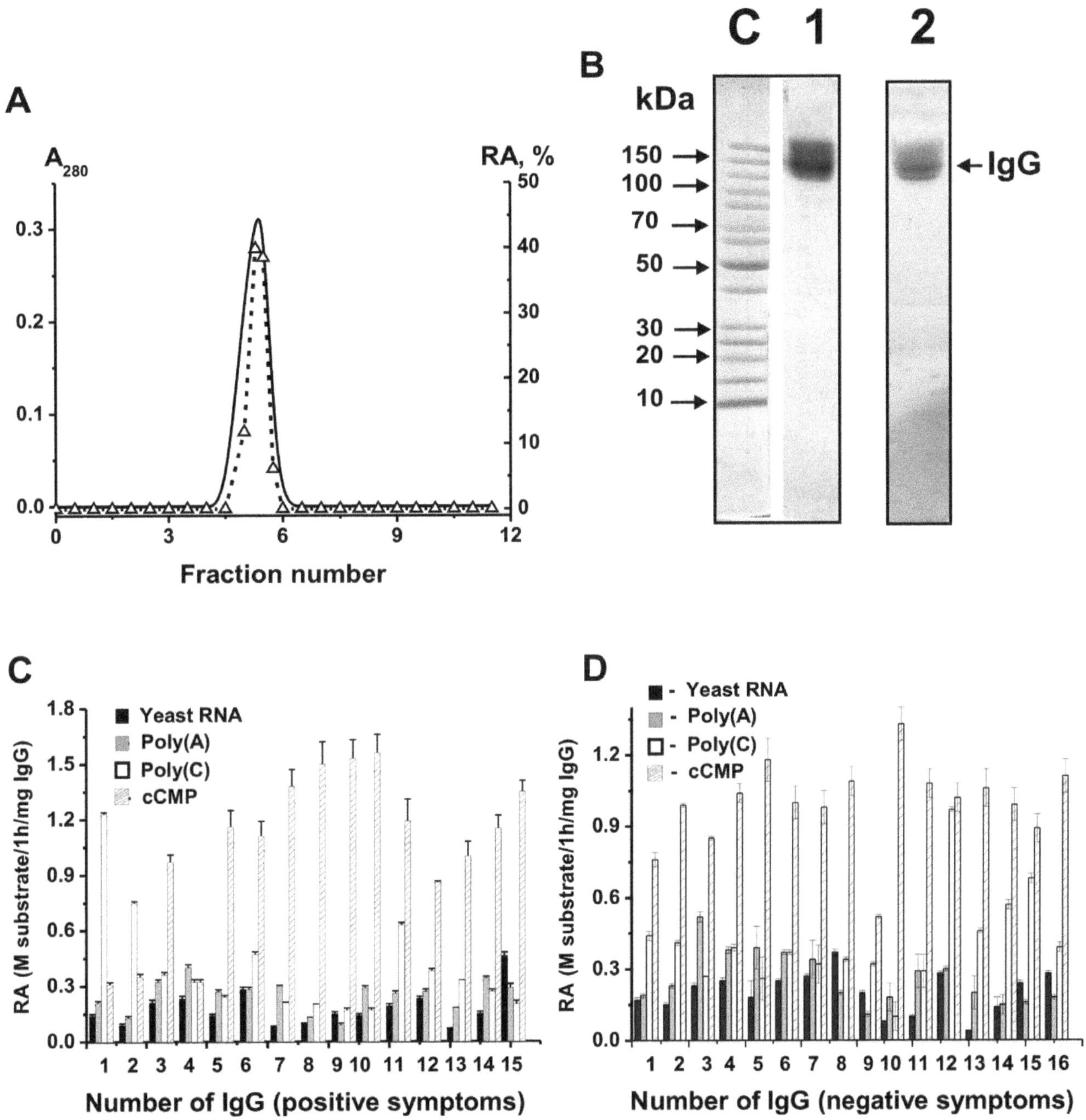


**Figure 2.** Verification of the strict criteria to prove that the RNase activity of IgGs is an intrinsic property of $IgG_{mix}$. FPLC gel filtration of scz-$IgG_{mix}$ on a Superdex 200 column equilibrated with an acidic buffer (pH 2.6) after its pre-incubation in the same buffer (A): (—), absorbance at 280 nm ($A_{280}$); (Δ), relative activity (RA, %) of $IgG_{mix}$ in the cleavage of RNA. A complete hydrolysis of poly(C) for 7 h was taken for 100%. The error in the initial rate estimation from two experiments in each case did not exceed 7–10%. Assay of RNase activity of scz-$IgG_{mix}$ in-gel containing polymeric yeast RNA (lane 2). RNase activity was detected after gel staining with ethidium bromide as a dark band on the fluorescent background. A gel part was stained with Coomassie R250 to show the position of intact scz-$IgG_{mix}$ (lane 1). Lane C corresponds to molecular mass markers. Relative activity of individual IgGs of patients with positive (C) and negative (D) symptoms of SCZ in the hydrolysis of yeast RNA, poly(A), poly(C), and cCMP.

of only intact scz-$IgG_{mix}$ together with the absence of any other activity and protein bands (**Figure 2B**) guarantee direct evidence that schizophrenia IgGs cleave RNA and IgGs are not contaminated by canonical RNases. Several other strict criteria were also fulfilled (see below).

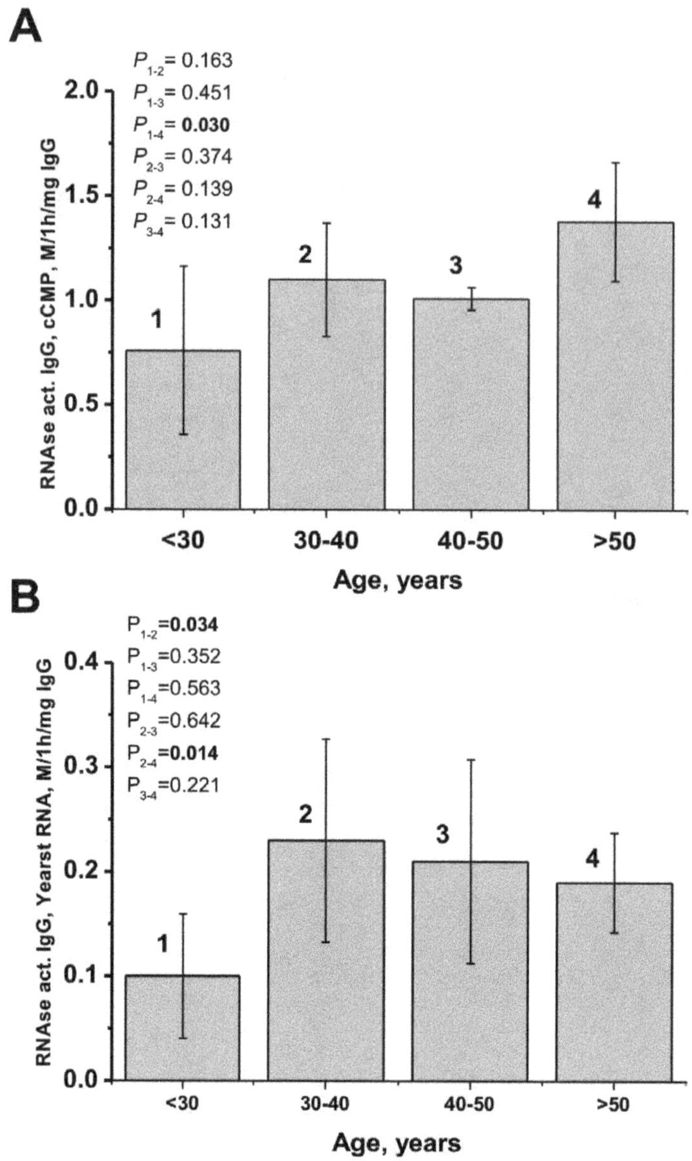


**Figure 3.** Dependencies of average activities of IgGs of four groups of SCZ patients with different age in the hydrolysis of cCMP (A) and poly(C) (B).

The relative activities of IgGs significantly varied from patient to patient. However, all 15 samples of patients with positive and 16 ones with negative symptoms of SCZ demonstrated detectable or high RNase activity (**Figure 2C** and **D**). The relative average activity for patients with SCZ positive symptoms varied essentially (M/1 h/mg IgG): cCMP (0.31–1.56; average value (AV) = 1.05 ± 0.43), poly(C) (0.17–1.23 AV = 0.4 ± 0.29), poly(A) (0.09–0.4; AV = 0.25 ± 0.09), and yeast total RNA (0.08–0.46 AV = 0.18 ± 0.1) (**Figure 2C**). Similar situation was observed for patients with negative symptoms (M/1 h/mg IgG): cCMP (0.52–1.18; AV = 0.99 ± 0.18), poly(C) (0.1–0.68, AV = 0.41 ± 0.2), poly(A) (0.11–0.52; AV = 0.20 ± 0.11), and yeast total RNA (0.4–3.1 AV = 1.68 ± 0.71) (**Figure 2D**). The difference in average activities of IgGs from patients with positive and negative symptoms was very small: cCMP (1.1-fold), poly(C) (1.03-fold), poly(A) (1.3-fold), and yeast total RNA (1.1-fold). According to non-parametric Kruskal-Wallis analysis, in none of these cases, there was a statistically significant difference ($P > 0.2$). Interestingly, a clear correlation of the RNase RAs with the duration of SCZ was not observed ($P = -0.015 \pm 0.14$) except with activity of IgGs in poly(C) hydrolysis (+ 0.47). The tendency of increase in activity of IgGs in the hydrolysis of cCMP and poly(C) with age of SCZ patients was revealed (**Figure 3**). A statistically significant difference in the mean values of the relative activity in the case of cCMP hydrolysis was observed for a group of patients younger than 30 and over 50 years old ($P = 0.03$) (**Figure 3A**). For activity in poly(C) hydrolysis, statistically significant difference was revealed between the groups younger 30 and 30–40 ($P = 0.034$) as well as group of patients over 50 years old ($P = 0.014$) (**Figure 3B**). In addition, a good statistically significant correlation was observed between the activity in hydrolysis of cCMP (CC = + 0.896) and composite index of SCZ, demonstrating a difference between parameters of positive symptoms and negative symptoms and showing the prevailing symptoms. Interestingly, a moderate but statistically significant negative correlation was observed between the efficiency of poly(C) hydrolysis and PANSS + (or PANSS Positive scale) evaluating signs that are redundant in relation to normal mental status (−0.43).

## 4. Hydrolysis of microRNAs

As mentioned above, some microRNAs regulate up to several hundred genes in the pathogenesis of SCZ [34–41]. We have analyzed the hydrolysis by SCZ abzymes' four known microRNAs playing an important role in SCZ [91]. **Figures 4–7** demonstrate typical patterns of miR-137, miR-9-5p, miR-219-2-3p, and miR-219a-5p hydrolysis; specific % of the hydrolysis for each IgG and the average percent of microRNAs hydrolysis by 21 different Abs were estimated. Percentage of the microRNA hydrolysis by different IgGs in the same conditions varied and average values decreased in the following order: miR-219a-5p (the range: 7.4–99.7%, AV = 71.0 ± 32.7%) ≥ miR-137 (14.9–99.9%, AV = 66.2 ± 29.2%) ≥ miR-9-5p (3.1–99.9%, AV = 56.7 ± 32.9%) ≥ miR-219a-2-3p (7.4–99.7%, AV = 52.4 ± 34.5%) (**Figures 2–5**). The correlation coefficients between sets of RAs in the hydrolysis of all 4 microRNAs are quite high, 0.84–0.93.

Spatial structures of microRNAs having minimal energy were calculated; **Figure 8A–D** show position of major, moderate, and minor sites of four microRNA hydrolysis by different IgGs (average % of the RNAs hydrolysis by 21 IgG preparations) [91]. One can see that three major sites of microRNAs hydrolysis are located in their loops or duplex parts directly articulated with the loops. The major sites of the hydrolysis of four microRNAs are different, but more often the cleavages occur after or before G-base: miR-219a-5p—6G-7U; 13C-14G, and 8C-9C; miR-137—5 U-6G, 8 U–9 U, and 10A-11A; miR-9-5p—6G-7G, 8 U–9 U, and 13 U-14A; miR-219a-2-3p—5 U-6 U, 8 U-9G, and 13G–14G (**Figure 8**).

We have estimated the $K_m$ and $V_{max}$ ($k_{cat}$) values for microRNA hydrolysis using different preparations [91]. The dependencies of the initial rate on the microRNA concentration in the reaction catalyzed by IgGs were consistent with Michaelis-Menten kinetics. The $K_m$ and $k_{cat}$ values were to some extent comparable for all microRNAs: miR-137, $K_m = 3.5 \pm 0.2$ μM,

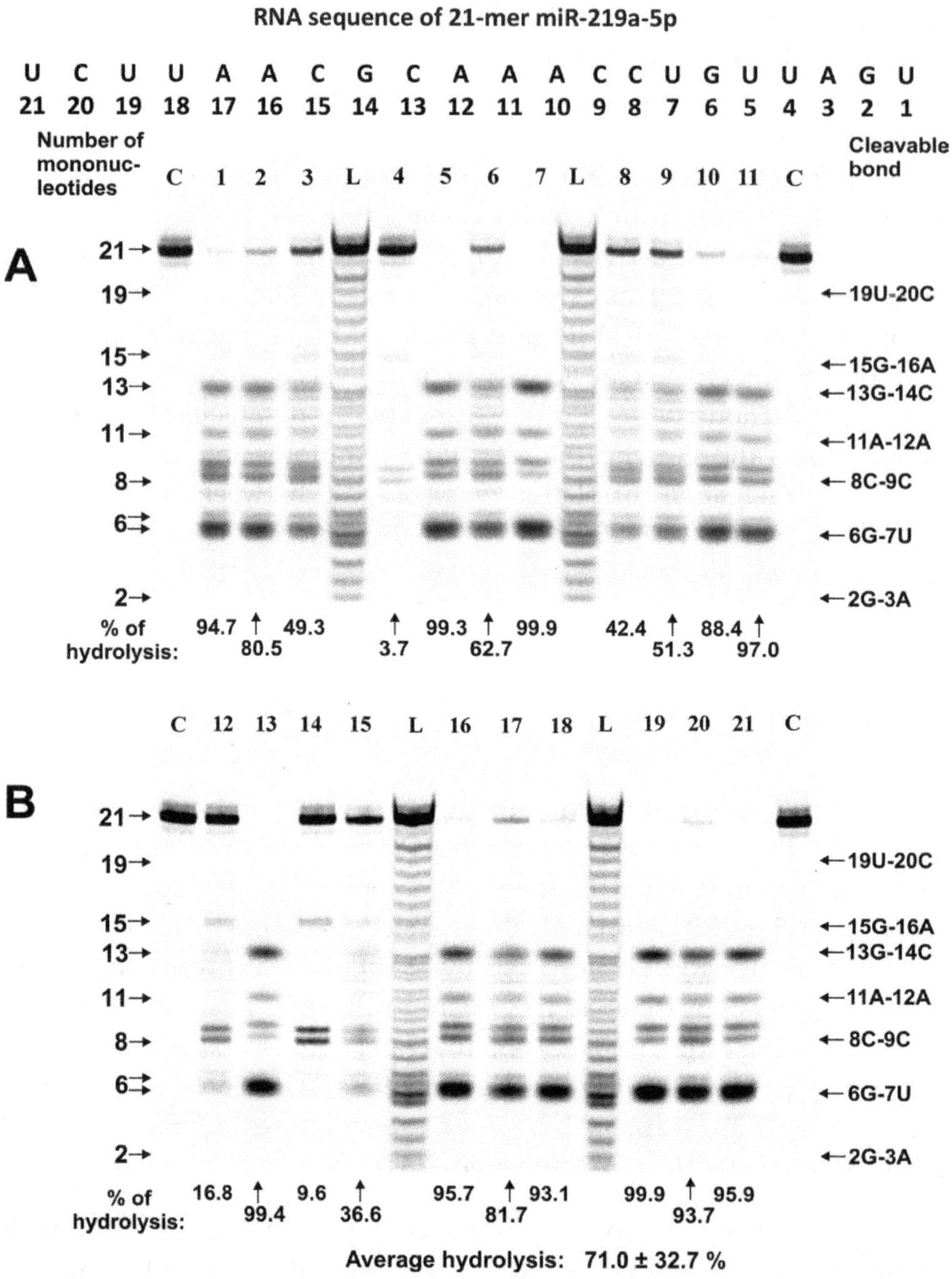


**Figure 4.** The patterns of flu- miR-219a-5p (0.01 mg/ml) hydrolysis by IgGs (0.1 mg/ml) from sera of 21 SCZ patients. The hydrolysis products were detected by their fluorescence due to the fluorescent residue (flu) on their 5′-ends. The numbers of antibodies, lengths of the products, and the percentage of microRNA hydrolysis by each preparation are indicated in panels A and B.

$k_{cat} = 0.14 \pm 0.009$ min$^{-1}$; miR-9-5p, $K_m = 2.4 \pm 0.13$ μM, $k_{cat} = 0.083 \pm 0.003$ min$^{-1}$; miR-219-2-3p. $K_m = 1.7 \pm 0.12$ μM, $k_{cat} = 0.10 \pm 0.008$ min$^{-1}$; miR-219a-5p $K_m = 4.5 \pm 0.2$ μM, $k_{cat} = 0.17 \pm 0.02$ min$^{-1}$.

Many anti-DNA Abs are directed against histone-DNA nucleosomal complexes appearing from internucleosomal cleavage during apoptosis [62]. In addition, cell apoptosis leads to the increase in blood the concentration of different nucleases, RNA and its complexes with various

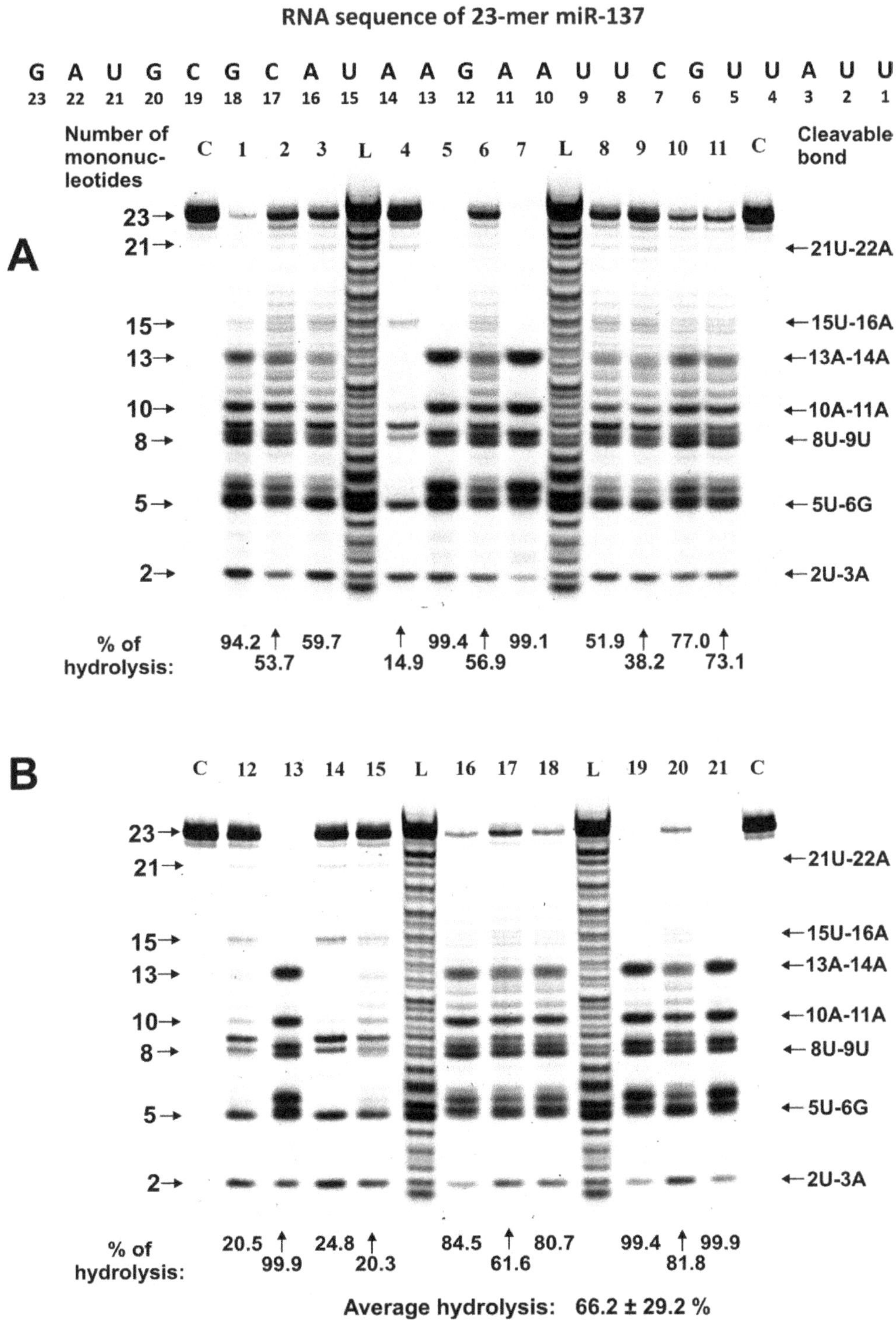


**Figure 5.** The patterns of Flu-miR-9-5p (0.01 mg/ml) hydrolysis by IgGs (0.1 mg/ml) from sera of 21 different SCZ patients. The hydrolysis products were detected by their fluorescence due to the fluorescent residue (Flu) on their 5′-ends. The numbers of antibodies, lengths of the products, and the percentage of microRNA hydrolysis by each preparation are indicated in panels A and B.

proteins. It was shown that the formation of DNA- and RNA-hydrolyzing Abs occurs after immunization of rabbits with RNA, DNA, DNase I, DNase II, and pancreatic RNase [92–96]. In addition, several monoclonal IgGs against B-DNA of different sequences (from SLE mice) efficiently hydrolyze ss- and dsRNA and DNA in a sequence-independent manner and the

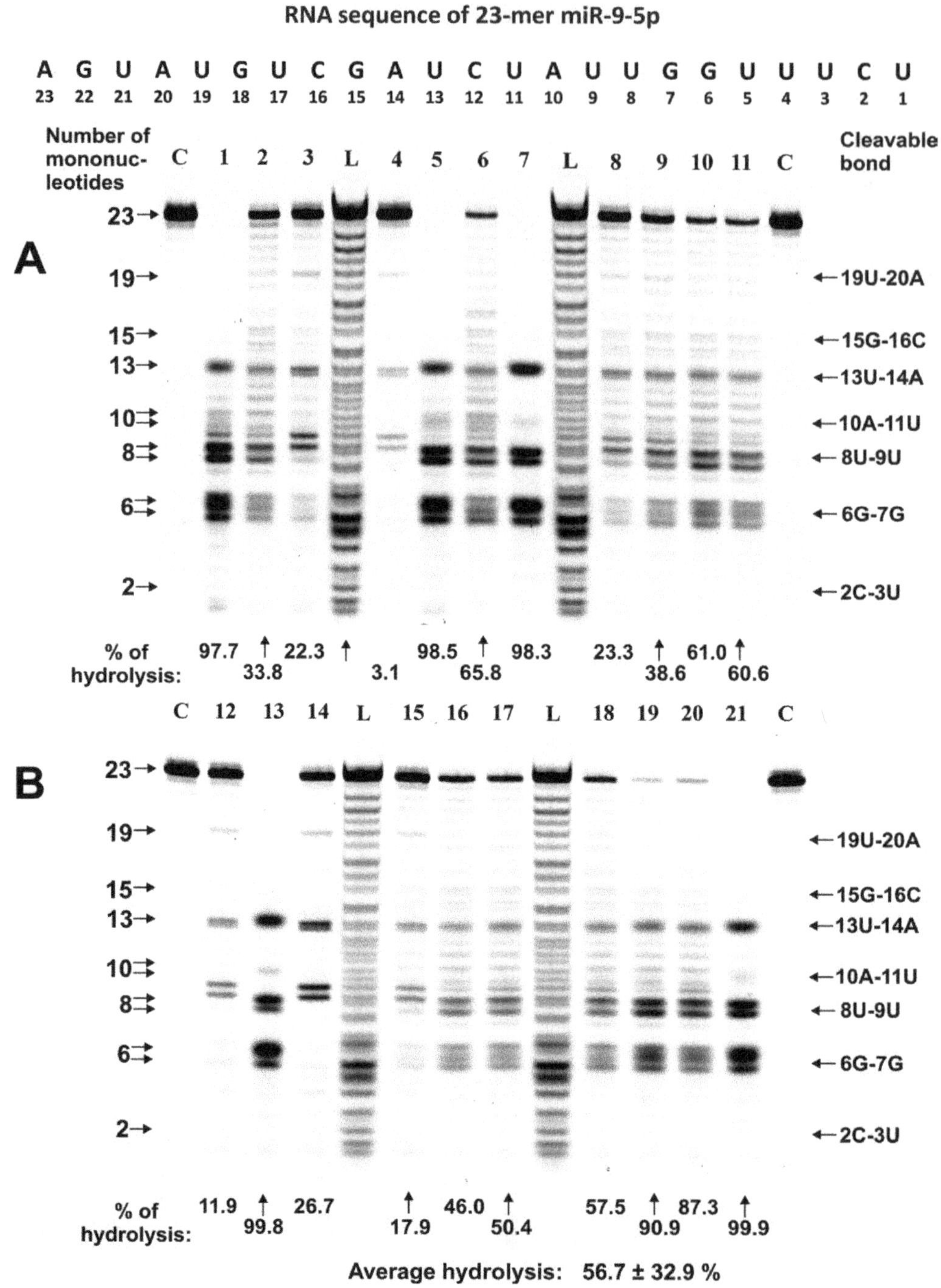


**Figure 6.** The patterns of Flu-miR-137 (0.01 mg/ml) hydrolysis by IgGs (0.1 mg/ml) from sera of 21 different SCZ patients. The hydrolysis products were detected by their fluorescence due to the fluorescent residue (Flu) on their 5′-ends. The numbers of antibodies, lengths of the products, and the percentage of microRNA hydrolysis by each preparation are indicated in panels A and B.

RNase activity was by a factor of 30–100 higher than that of DNA [97]. Thus, DNase and RNase abzymes can appear in the blood of autoimmune patients due to several very different ways. Since IgGs hydrolyze different homo-polynucleotides and cleavage of four microRNA is site-specific (**Figures 4–8**), one can assume that some sets of RNase abzymes may be specific for some RNAs, while others are not.

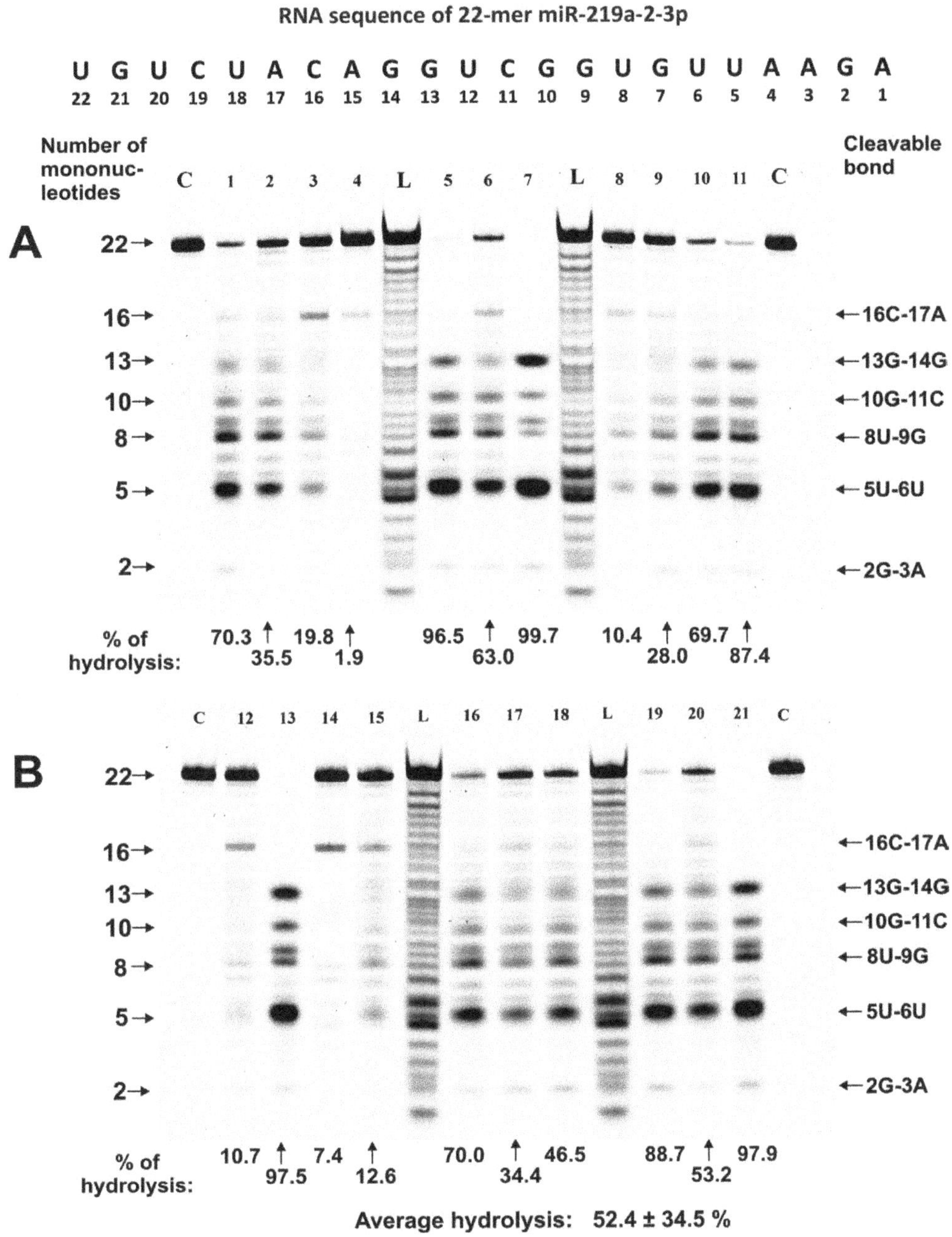


**Figure 7.** The patterns of Flu-miR-219a-2-3p (0.01 mg/ml) hydrolysis by IgGs (0.1 mg/ml) from sera of 21 different SCZ patients. The hydrolysis products were detected by their fluorescence due to the fluorescent residue (Flu) on their 5′-ends. The numbers of antibodies, lengths of the products, and the percentage of microRNA hydrolysis by each preparation are indicated in panels A and B.

It was shown that 90–95% of Abs SLE and MS patients effectively hydrolyze DNA [47–56]. It was shown that a very high percent IgGs of SCZ patients (80–82%) are active the hydrolysis of DNA [83]. At the same time, similar to SLE and MS [47–56], all 100% schizophrenia IgGs effectively hydrolyze different RNAs [91]. It was shown previously that the appearance of abzymes hydrolyzing DNA and RNA is among the clear and earliest signs of autoimmune reactions [47–56]. In addition, light chains of IgGs from schizophrenia patients are similar to

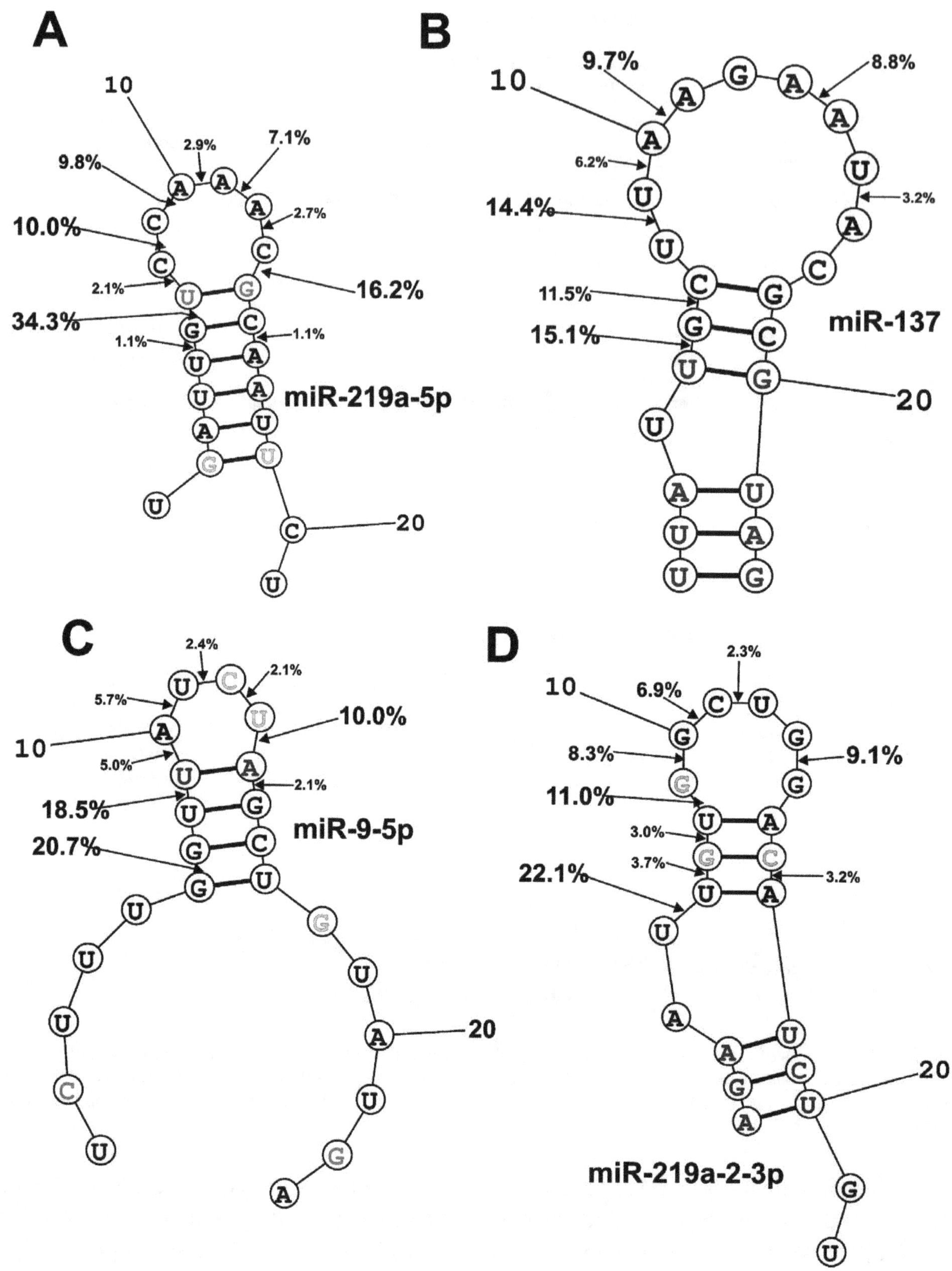


**Figure 8.** The average efficiency of four micro-RNAs hydrolysis by 21 IgG preparations in all sites of their cleavage (A–D). The position of major and moderate sites of different RNAs hydrolysis is shown.

those of SLE patients, but not to these chains of healthy donors [83]. These data indicate that in patients with SCZ similar to SLE, MS, and other AIDS, there is a trespassing of the immune system leading to the production of abzymes with DNase and RNase activities.

## 5. Hydrolysis of myelin basic protein

Serum anti-MBP Abs in MS and SLE patients were reported in several articles [75, 76, 79–81, 98, 99]. The relative levels of antibodies against MBP in the sera of 28 patients with SCZ and 15 healthy donors were compared by ELISA (**Table 2**). The concentrations of auto-Abs against MBP for healthy donors were not zero and changed from 0.02 to 0.16 $A_{450}$ units, in average 0.09 ± 0.04 $A_{450}$ units [75, 76, 79–81, 100, 101]. Relative indexes of anti-MBP Abs for 28 SCZ patients varied from 0.04 to 0.26 $A_{450}$ units, in average 0.16 ± 0.068 $A_{450}$ units. For patients with positive symptoms of SCZ, average value (0.18 ± 0.066 $A_{450}$ units) was 1.3-fold higher than that for patients with negative symptoms (0.14 ± 0.067 $A_{450}$ units), but this difference was statistically

| Number of patients (Sex) | Abs to MBP, $A_{450}$/ml | Relative % of hydrolysis | $k_{cat} \times 10^3$, min$^{-1}$ |
|---|---|---|---|
| | Positive symptoms of SCZ | | |
| | Parameters 1 | Parameters 2 | |
| 1 (M) | 0.32* | 10.5** | 9.8*** |
| 2 (M) | 0.24 | 50.0 | 46.8 |
| 3 (M) | 0.13 | 20.5 | 19.2 |
| 4 (M) | 0.07 | 0.5 | 0.5 |
| 5 (F) | 0.13 | 1.0 | 1.0 |
| 6 (F) | 0.18 | 18.5 | 17.3 |
| 7 (F) | 0.15 | 15.0 | 14.0 |
| 8 (F) | 0.09 | 0.5 | 0.5 |
| 9 (F) | 0.17 | 17.5 | 16.4 |
| 10 (F) | 0.20 | 4.5 | 4.2 |
| 11 (F) | 0.18 | 15.0 | 14.0 |
| 12 (M) | 0.14 | 0 | 0 |
| 13 (F) | 0.20 | 0 | 0 |
| 14 (M) | 0.26 | 0 | 0 |
| Average value | 0.18 ± 0.066 | 11.0 ± 13.7 | 10.3 ± 12.9 |
| | Negative symptoms of SCZ | | |
| | Parameters 3 | Parameters 4 | |
| 15 (M) | 0.17* | 50.0** | 46.8*** |

| Number of patients (Sex) | Abs to MBP, $A_{450}$/ml | Relative % of hydrolysis | $k_{cat} \times 10^3$, min$^{-1}$ |
|---|---|---|---|
| | Positive symptoms of SCZ | | |
| | Parameters 1 | Parameters 2 | |
| 16 (M) | 0.19 | 49.5 | 46.3 |
| 17 (F) | 0.22 | 13.5 | 12.6 |
| 18 (M) | 0.17 | 47.0 | 44.0 |
| 19 (M) | 0.08 | 50.0 | 46.8 |
| 20 (F) | 0.04 | 25.0 | 23.4 |
| 21 (F) | 0.17 | 10.5 | 9.8 |
| 22 (M) | 0.26 | 14.0 | 13.1 |
| 23 (F) | 0.03 | 26.5 | 24.8 |
| 24 (M) | 0.11 | 6.5 | 6.1 |
| 25 (F) | 0.18 | 43.5 | 40.7 |
| 26(F) | 0.16 | 43.5 | 40.7 |
| 27 (F) | 0.08 | 0.0 | 0.0 |
| 28 (M) | 0.12 | 0.0 | 0.0 |
| Average value | 0.14 ± 0.067 | 27.1 ± 19.6 | 25.4 ± 18.4 |
| Correl. coefficient | Parameters 1 and 2 (0.28), Parameters 3 and 4 (0.10); Parameters 1 + 3 and 2 + 4 (0.04) | | |

*For each value, a mean of three measurements is reported; the error of the determination of values did not exceed 7–10%.

**Average values are reported as mean ± S.E; they were recalculated to standard conditions and complete hydrolysis of 0.33 mg/ml MBP after 5 h of incubation in the presence of 0.1 mg/ml IgG was taken for 100%.

***The average apparent $k_{cat}$ values in the reaction of MBP hydrolysis were calculated using average RA values (% of the hydrolysis at fixed concentration of MBP**): $k_{cat}$ = V (M/min)/ [IgGs] (M).

**Table 2.** Numbers of SCZ patients, their sex, and relative characteristics of patients antibodies.

insignificant ($P = 0.27$). Using the same approach and test system, it was previously shown that average index of anti-MBP antibodies for 25 MS patients is 0.8 ± 0.1 $A_{450}$ units [79] and, for SLE patients, it is 0.38 ± 0.08 $A_{450}$ units [75]. Thus, all SCZ patients analyzed by us demonstrated ~1.8-fold higher level of serum anti-MBP Abs than healthy individuals, but ~2.4-fold and 5.0-fold lower level than SLE and MS patients, respectively.

Electrophoretically and immunologically homogeneous polyclonal IgGs were separated from the sera of 28 SCZ patients and 15 healthy donors as described above. The homogeneity of the 150 kDa scz-$IgG_{mix}$ and healthy-IgGmix (mixtures of equal amounts IgGs from the sera of 28 SCZ patients and 15 healthy volunteers, respectively) was confirmed by SDS-PAGE similar to [83] **Figure 1A**.

We have applied several of known rigid criteria described above. The most important of these criteria are given below: (1) electrophoretic homogeneity of scz-$IgG_{mix}$ (**Figure 1A**); (2) complete

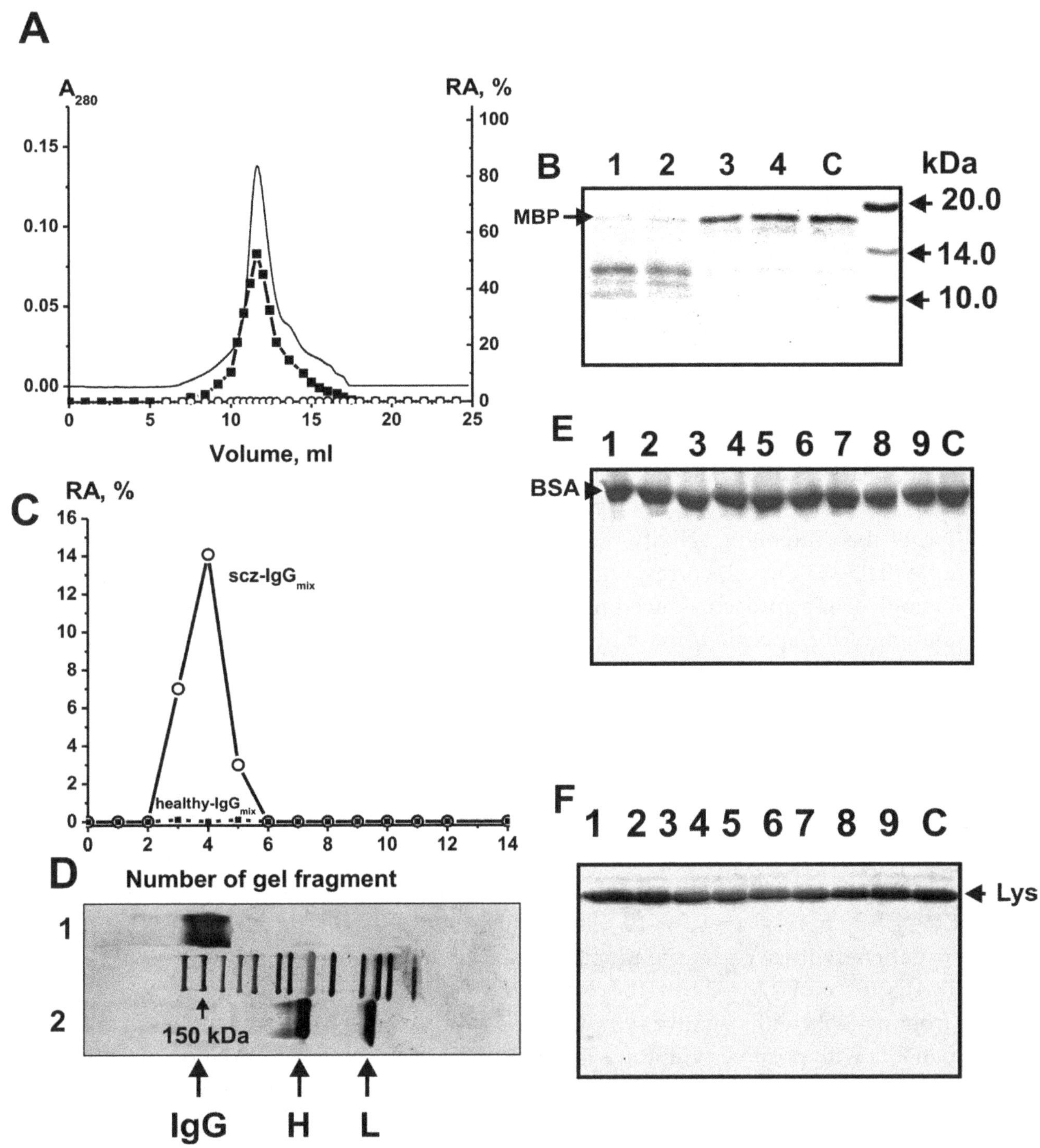


**Figure 9.** FPLC gel filtration of scz-$IgG_{mix}$ on a Superdex 200 column in an acidic buffer (pH 2.6) after IgGs pre-incubation in the same buffer (A): (—), absorbance at 280 nm ($A_{280}$); (■), relative activity (RA, %) of IgGs in the hydrolysis MBP. A complete hydrolysis of MBP for 5 h was taken for 100%. Assay of MBP-hydrolyzing activity of purified scz-$IgG_{mix}$ after SDS-PAGE in gradient 4-15 % gel, the gel was incubated under special conditions for renaturation of Abs (B). MBP (0.4 mg/ml) was incubated with 0.1 mg/ml scz-$IgG_{mix}$ for 24 h (lane 1) or scz-IgG-1 (lane 2) and with healthy-$IgG_{mix}$ (lane 3) or individual healthy-IgG-1 (lane 4), as well as in the absence of Abs (lane C). The RA (%) was revealed using the extracts of 2-3-mm many fragments of one longitudinal slice of the gel (C). The second control longitudinal slices of the same gels corresponding to $IgG_{mix}$ before (lane 1) and after (lane 2) treatment with DTT were stained with Coomassie R250 (D). Analysis of possible hydrolysis of bovine serum albumin (BSA) (E) and hen egg lysozyme (Lys) (F) by scz-$IgG_{mix}$ purified on MBP-Sepharose (lanes 1). Lanes 2-9 correspond to nine individual scz-IgGs, while lanes C to the proteins incubated in the absence of Abs (E and F).

adsorption of $IgG_{mix}$ hydrolyzing MBP by anti-IgG Sepharose leading to a disappearance of the catalytic activity of the solution; (3) FPLC gel-filtration of scz-$IgG_{mix}$ under conditions of "acidic shock" (pH 2.6) lead to revealing of the activity only in the peak corresponding exactly to 150 kDa IgGs (**Figure 9A**); (4) in contrast to scz-$IgG_{mix}$, healthy-$IgG_{mix}$ did not hydrolyze MBP (**Figure 9B**); (5) Scz-$IgG_{mix}$ purified on MBP-Sepharose hydrolyzed only MBP and was inactive in the hydrolysis of control proteins, bovine serum albumin (**Figure 9C**), and lactoferrin (**Figure 9D**); (6) scz-$IgG_{mix}$ was separated by SDS-PAGE, and their MBP-hydrolyzing activity was estimated after the extraction of proteins from the separated gel slices (**Figure 9E** and **F**). The electrophoretic mobility of low molecular mass canonical proteases (24–25 kDa) cannot coincide with that of intact IgGs (150 kDa). Therefore, the detection of protease activity in the gel fragments corresponding only to intact IgGs together with the absence of any other proteins and activity bands (**Figure 9E** and **F**) provides direct evidence that SCZ IgGs possess MBP-hydrolyzing activity.

The RAs of SCZ IgGs in the cleavage MBP was estimated from the decrease in the intensity of Coomassie-stained MBP band after electrophoresis according to [76–81]. For quantitative estimation of the proteolytic activity, we have found a relatively low concentration of each IgG sample (0.05–0.3 mg/ml) corresponding to the reaction of the first order (1–24 h; 15–45% of conversion). This approach allowed us to normalize the relative activity, like in the case of determination of the specific activity of enzymes [102], to standard condition; relative % of MBP hydrolysis after incubation for 5 h in the presence of 0.1 mg/ml (0.66 μM) IgGs.

Among 28 individual SCZ patients, the RAs of IgGs at a fixed concentration of MBP (0.33 mg/ml) were absent for five patients (17.9%): 3 of 14 patients (21.4%) with positive symptoms and 2 of 14 patients (14.3%) with negative symptoms (**Table 1**). The average relative activity (RA, %) and apparent $k_{cat}$ values ($k_{cat}$ = V/[IgG]) at fixed concentration of MBP (0.33 mg/ml; 18.3 μM) were calculated (**Table 2**). The apparent $k_{cat}$ values characterizing hydrolysis of MBP by 14 IgGs of patients with positive symptoms varied in the range 0–46.8 × $10^{-3}$ $min^{-1}$ (average 10.3 ± 12.9) × $10^{-3}$ $min^{-1}$; M = 0.7 × $10^{-3}$, IQR = (0.5–16.4) × $10^{-3}$). The apparent $k_{cat}$ values for 14 IgGs of patients with negative symptoms also varied in the range 0–46.8.0 × $10^{-3}$ $min^{-1}$ (average (25.4 ± 18.4) × $10^{-3}$ $min^{-1}$; M = 24.1 × $10^{-3}$, IQR = (9.8–44.0) × $10^{-3}$). Overall, the average $k_{cat}$ value of IgGs from patients with negative symptoms was approximately 2.5-fold higher than that for Abs of patients with positive symptoms (**Table 2**). The coefficient of correlation (CC) between the anti-MBP Abs titers ($A_{450}$) and RAs of 28 Abs was very low, 0.04. At the same time, CC for these values in the case of patients with positive symptoms (0.28) was 2.8-fold higher than that for patients with negative symptoms (0.10) (**Table 2**). According to Wald-Wolfowitz test, there is a statistically significant difference between $k_{cat}$ value of IgGs from patients with negative and positive symptoms ($P$ = 0.034). Interestingly, the CC (0.7–0.79) between the anti-MBP Abs titers ($A_{450}$) and RAs of Abs from SLE patients [8] was significantly higher than for SCZ patients.

It has been recently shown that abzymes against MBP from the sera of MS patients hydrolyze MBP at several clustered sites localized within four known antigenic determinants of human MBP and that four oligopeptides corresponding to these determinants of MBP are encephalytogenic and can play a negative role in the MS pathogenesis [79–82]. It is important that anti-MBP abzymes from the sera of SLE, MS, and SCZ patients hydrolyze MBP at the same four sites of antigenic determinants and effectively cleavage all four 17–25-mer OPs corresponding to these four determinants [75–80]. It was shown, that anti-MBP abzymes of SCZ patients can also cleavage these four OPs: OP21 and OP25 were the best substrates of SCZ abzymes.

We have estimated the $K_m$ and $k_{cat}$ values for the hydrolysis of MBP, OP21 (YLASASTM-DHARHGFLPRRHR) and OP25 (AQGTLSKIFKLGGRDSRSGSPMARR) in the case of two individual preparations of SCZ patients. The initial rate data obtained at increasing MBP, OP21, and OP25 concentrations were consistent with the Michaelis-Menten kinetics. Different abzymes usually demonstrate a significantly higher affinity to substrates in comparison with canonical proteases [45–56]. The affinity of intact MBP for SCZ IgGs was (in terms of $K_m$ values) in the range of 4.3–12.4 μM (**Table 2**), which corresponds to typical $K_d$ (and $K_m$) values for Ab-antigen interactions. These $K_m$ values for MBP of SCZ abzymes are to some extent comparable with the $K_m$ for MBP (~0.6–2.7 μM) reported previously for IgGs from SLE [75–78] and MS (0.9–5.0 μM) [81] patients. Interestingly, the $K_m$ values for scz-IgGs in the case OP21 and OP25 (49–770 μM) are to some extent lower compared with those for four OPs in the case of SLE. As it mentioned above, a detectable level of MBP-hydrolyzing abzymes was shown to be as an indicator of pre-disease, while increase in the activity of obvious pathology conditions of typical spontaneous or induced autoimmune diseases [63–68].

It was shown that DNase and RNase abzymes of autoimmune patients present a "cocktail" of Abs directly to DNA and RNA or their complexes with proteins and anti-idiotypic Abs against active centers of DNase I, DNase II, RNase and other enzymes hydrolyzing nucleic acids [92–96]. MBP-hydrolyzing Abs are produced from animals immunization with MBP and its encephalytogenic peptides [66–68]. In addition, immunization of experimental autoimmune encephalomyelitis (EAE) mice, a model of human MS, with myelin oligodendrocyte glycoprotein ($MOG_{35–55}$) leads to the production of both MBP- and DNA-hydrolyzing abzymes [66–68].

## 6. Abzymes with oxidation-reduction activities

Several publications show that some abzymes may form not only in patients with autoimmune pathologies but also in healthy humans. However, it is not currently clear which antigens can stimulate the formation of these abzymes in autoimmune patients and healthy donors.

Human organisms are constantly exposed to oxidative stress and various toxic components. The partially reduced oxygen species ($O^{2-}$, $H_2O_2$, and $OH^{\bullet}$) produced in all higher organisms and appeared in bodies through exposure to different compounds to ionizing radiation. They act as dangerous oxidants attacking lipids, proteins, DNA, and other different cellular components [103–107]. Oxidative damage of many cells has been considered as a very important pathophysiological factor in the development of many different diseases such as carcinogenesis, aging, multiple sclerosis (MS), and SCZ. It is believed that MS and SCZ have different pathogenetic mechanisms. MS is a neurodegenerative chronic disease of AI nature, associated with structural damage to the nerve fibers myelin sheath, while SCZ has neurotransmitter nature. It was, however, demonstrated that the oxidative stress activation is a major factor in the MS and SCZ [108–114]. In the case of SCZ, the cellular metabolism changes associated with alteration in the activity of enzymes including antioxidant enzymes were revealed [109, 112].

Several enzymes protecting various organisms from oxidative stress are known. Mammalian, plant, and bacterial peroxidases, glutathione peroxidases, oxidoreductases, oxidases, and dismutases are mostly metal ions-dependent enzymes [107, 115–118]. Metal ions having the variable valence (more often: $Fe_{2+}$, $Cu^{2+}$, and $Mn^{2+}$) participate in a transfer of electrons in the reactions of oxidation-reduction, catalyzed by enzymes [118].

A comparison of catalase, superoxide dismutase, $H_2O_2$-dependent peroxidase, and $H_2O_2$-independent oxidoreductase activities of polyclonal IgGs obtained from the sera of healthy Wistar rats have been carried out [119]. Approximately, 83% of IgGs possess superoxide dismutase activity, but all IgGs oxidized 3,3′-diaminobenzidine in the presence (peroxidase activity) and the absence of hydrogen peroxide (oxidoreductase activity). Only 17% of rat IgGs were shown to possess catalase activity. It was shown that small fractions of IgGs and their $F(ab)_2$ and Fab fragments of IgGs from sera healthy humans oxidize 3,3′-diaminobenzidine in the presence of $H_2O_2$ through a peroxidase and in the absence of $H_2O_2$ through an oxidoreductase activity [120, 121].

It was shown that some electrophoretically homogeneous IgGs (and their F(ab) and $F(ab)_2$ fragments) from the sera of patients with SCZ (36.4%) and from healthy donors (33.3%) possess catalase activity [122]. As in the case of the abzymes described above, it was shown that the catalase activity of all IgGs is their intrinsic property (**Figure 10**). The catalase RA of IgGs from the sera of individual of SCZ patients on average was 15.8-fold higher than that of healthy volunteers. After extensive dialysis against EDTA chelating metal ions of IgGs, the catalase RA of IgGs, on average decreases approximately 2.5–3.7-fold; all IgGs possess metal-independent and dependent catalase activity.

External $Me^{2+}$ ions added to non-dialyzed and dialyzed IgGs significantly increase their activity (**Figure 11**). $Co^{2+}$is the best activator of non-dialyzed and dialyzed IgGs, the activation of IgGs by $Mn^{2+}$, $Cu^{2+}$, and $Ni^{2+}$ ions is substantially lower than by $Co^{2+}$. All IgGs demonstrate several individual different expressed pH optima in the pH range from 4.0 to 9.5. These data speak for the individual repertoire of catalase IgGs in every person and an extreme diversity of abzymes in their pH optima and activation by different metal ions.

In this connection, it should be marked that polyclonal IgGs against different antigens from the blood sera of patients with AI diseases and with different activities are usually very heterogeneous in their affinity for specific antigens and can be separated into many subfractions by chromatography on antigens-Sepharoses [75, 76, 79, 123]. Pools of polyclonal abzymes can contain different proportions of light chains of κ- and λ-types, Abs demonstrating different pH optima, having different net charges, metal-independent or activated by different metal ions, and characterized by different substrate affinities and specificities [17, 39–43, 124]. It was shown that small fractions of IgGs of all four subclasses (IgG1–IgG4) from autoimmune patients are catalytically active in the hydrolysis of different substrates [47–56]. For analysis of myelin basic protein- and DNA-hydrolyzing activities of monoclonal light chains (MLChs) corresponding to SLE phagemid library of kappa MLChs were used [125–129]. It was shown that some hundreds of different monoclonal light chains hydrolyze DNA and other ones cleavage myelin basic protein; all MLChs demonstrated very different physicochemical and enzymatic properties [125–129]. It should be assumed that the extraordinary diversity of these

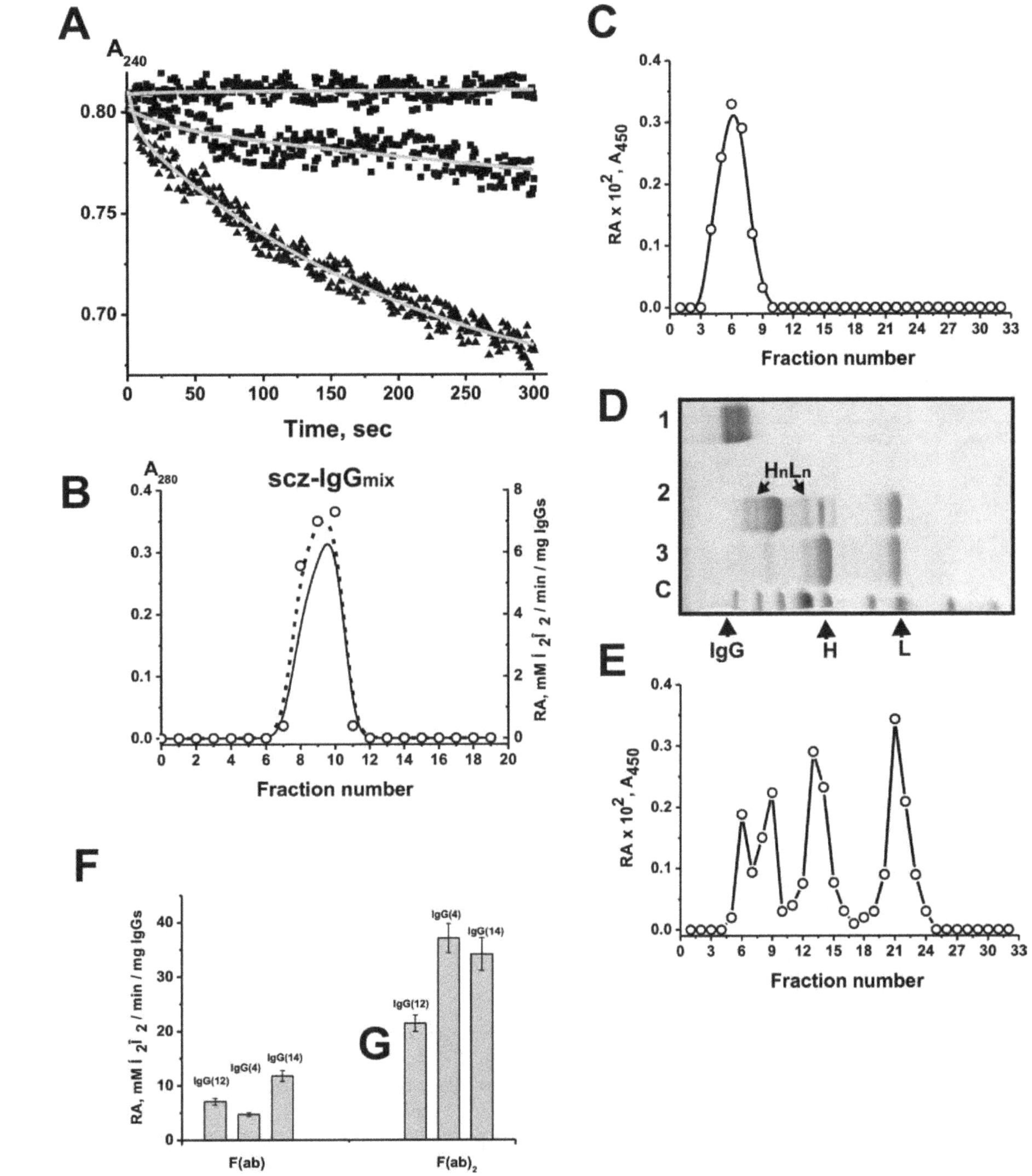


**Figure 10.** Typical time-dependencies of the decrease in 30 mM $H_2O_2$ absorbance at 240 nm ($A_{240}$) in the presence of 200 nM IgG-1 and IgG-11 as well as 2 nM IgG-8 corresponding to different individual patients (A). Checking of strict criteria proving that the catalase activity is intrinsic properties of scz-$IgG_{mix}$. Preparations of scz-$IgG_{mix}$ (equimolar mixture of 22 samples) were separated by FPLC gel filtration on a Superdex 200 column in an acidic buffer Gly-HCl pH 2.6 after Abs pre-incubation using the same buffer (B): (o), relative activity (RA) of the $IgG_{mix}$ in the degradation of $H_2O_2$; (—), absorbance at 280 nm ($A_{280}$); SDS-PAGE analysis of catalase activity of intact scz-$IgG_{mix}$ (C) as well as separated H, L chains and their $L_nH_n$ oligomers (E) in non-reducing SDS-PAGE using gradient 4–15%: Scz-IgGmix before (C) and after treatment of $IgG_{mix}$ with DTT (E); lane 1 of panel D corresponds to panel C and lane 2 to panel E. The RAs ($A_{240}$/min) were revealed using the extracts of 2–3-mm fragments of one gel longitudinal slice of corresponding $IgG_{mix}$ before (C) and after treatment with DTT (E). The control longitudinal slices of the same gels were stained with Coomassie R250 (D): lane 1 corresponds to intact $IgG_{mix}$, lane 2 to $IgG_{mix}$ incubated with 40 mM DTT for 10 min at 30° C, lane 3 to $IgG_{mix}$ boiled with DTT. Lane C (D) shows the positions of molecular mass standard markers. The relative activity of F(ab) and $F(ab)_2$ fragments of individual IgG-4, IgG-12, and IgG-14 (F). The average error of the initial rate determination from two experiments did not exceed 10–15%.

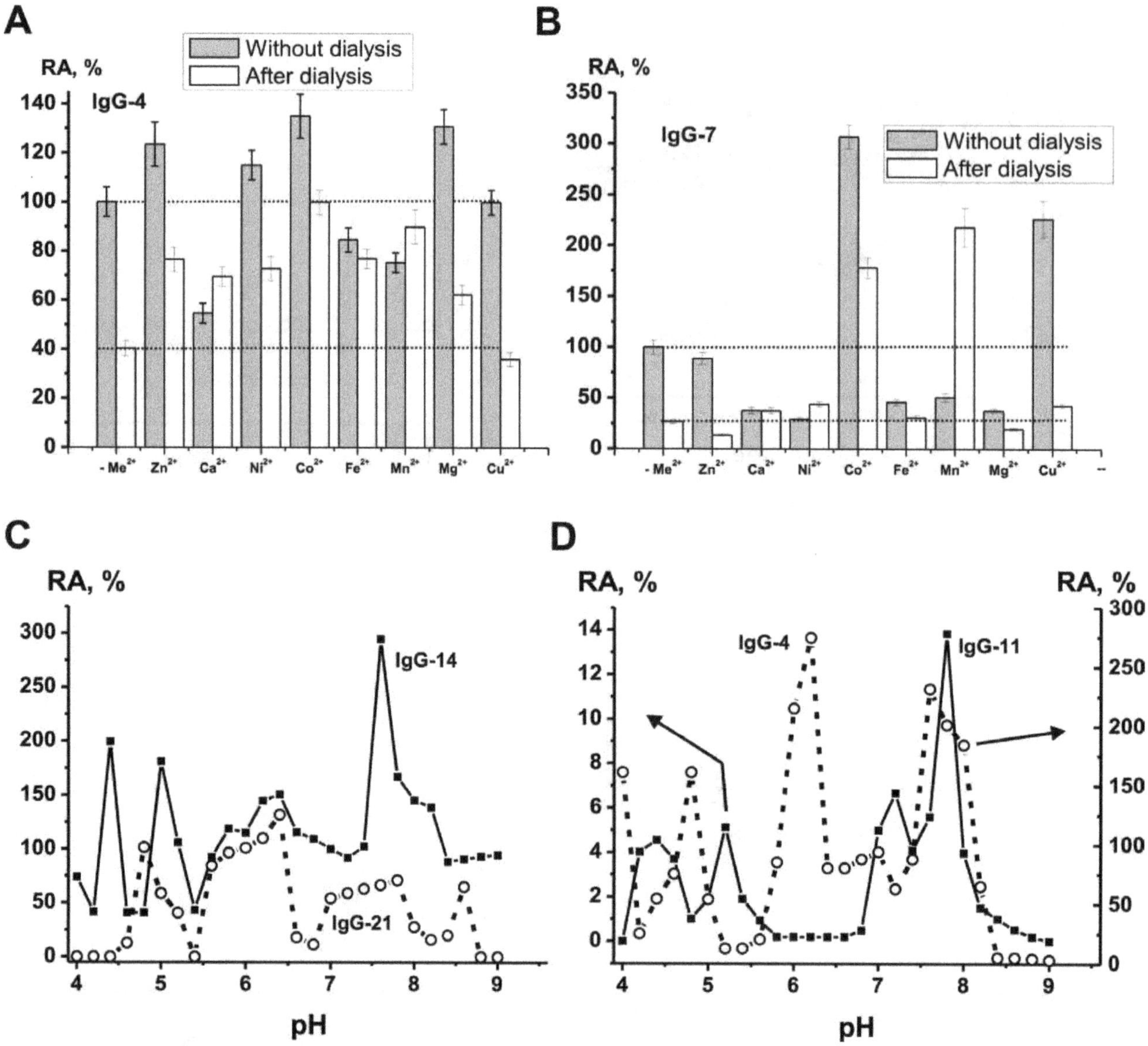


**Figure 11.** Effect of the dialysis of IgGs against EDTA for two individual scz-IgGs and different metal ions on the relative activity (RA, %) of dialyzed and non-dialyzed preparations (A and B). The RA of every non-dialyzed preparation was taken for 100%. Dependencies of the relative catalase activity of scz-IgGs on pH of the reaction mixture (C and D). All RAs of Abs before its preincubation were taken for 100%. The relative activity of IgG-14 at pH 7.0 was taken for 100%. All IgG preparations, metal ions, and conditions used marked on panels A–D. The errors in the determination of initial rate from three experiments in each case did not exceed 7–10%.

monoclonal light chains is mainly due to the significant differences in their variable regions responsible for substrate specificity and catalysis [125–129]. Heterogeneity is also observed in intact catalytic IgGs with kappa light chains, and it was shown that structural diversity (heterogeneity) might exist due to the constant region domain and specific role of metal ions of the catalytic light chains [130, 131]. A similar result of extreme catalytic heterogeneity is observed for abzymes with catalase activity.

It has been shown that immunoglobulins from humans and various animals have superoxide dismutase activity; they convert singlet oxygen $^1O^2$ into its reduced form $O^{2\bullet}$ [132, 133]. These abzymes use $H_2O$ as an electron source and attach it to $^1O^{2*}$ to form $H_2O_3$ as the first intermediate of several consecutive stages leading to the formation of $H_2O_2$. These data are believed to

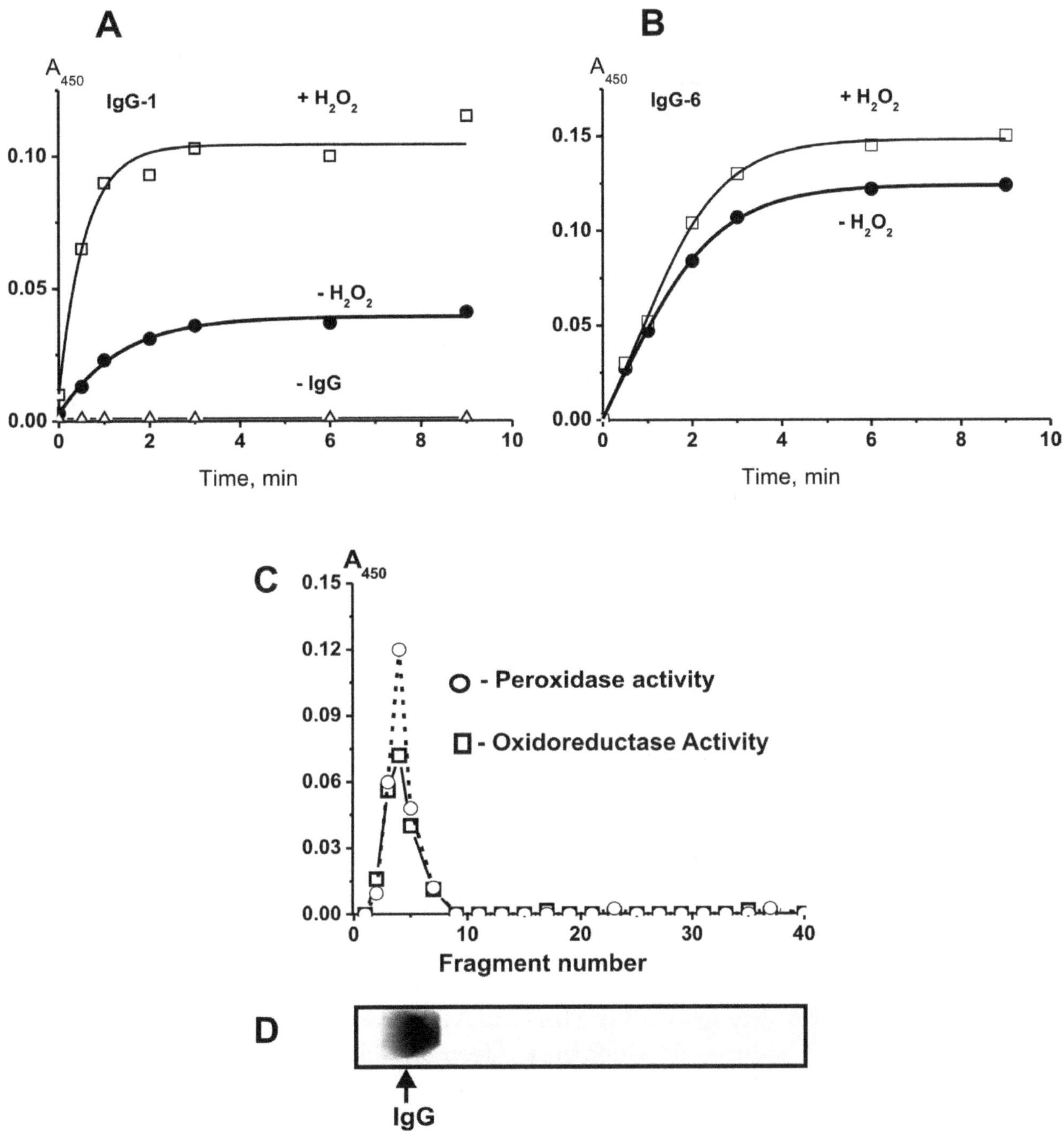


**Figure 12.** Typical kinetic curves of accumulation of a colored product ($A_{450}$) after DAB substrate oxidation by IgGs with peroxidase (in the presence of $H_2O_2$) (A) and with oxidoreductase (in the absence of $H_2O_2$) (B); activities in the oxidation of 3,3′-diaminobenzidine (0.2 mg/ml) in the case of 670 nM IgG-1 and IgG-6. Curve - IgG corresponds to the oxidation of the substrate in the absence of IgGs. SDS-PAGE analysis of peroxidase (o) and oxidoreductase (□) activities of $IgG_{mix}$ (20 μg) (C and D). After electrophoresis, the 4–15% gradient gel was treated using special conditions for renaturation of $IgG_{mix}$. The RAs were evaluated using extracts of 40 gel fragments (2–3 mm); 20 μl of extracts were added to the standard mixtures and incubated for 24 h. The second band of the same gel was used to determine the position of intact $IgG_{mix}$ (D); the gel was stained with Coomassie R250.

indicate the possibility of protecting mammalian organisms from $^1O^{2*}$ with Abs and raise the question of the possibility of a special evolution of immunoglobulins as a specific antioxidants of blood [132, 133]. For immunoglobulins, a mechanism has been discovered by which oxygen can be recovered and reused in phagocytosis, which indicates the possibility of the involvement of the immune system in microbial regulation. Even more surprising is the discovery of abzymes of higher eukaryotes that catalyze the formation of ozone used by cells in phagocytosis [134]. Taking this into account, one can put that Abs with superoxide dismutase activity can catalyze the conversion of the superoxide radical into hydrogen peroxide, and the abzymes with catalase activity neutralize the harmful effect of $H_2O_2$.

It was shown that IgGs from the blood of healthy Wistar rats possess high $H_2O_2$-dependent peroxidase (hereinafter peroxidase) and $H_2O_2$-independent oxidoreductase (hereinafter oxidoreductase) activities in the oxidation of horseradish peroxidase substrate—3,3′-diaminobenzidine and some other aromatic amines, phenols, and quinones [135–138]. Interestingly, the same activities were detected in IgG from the blood of healthy people [120, 121]. The relative peroxidase activity of IgG of healthy people in the absence of external metal ions varies very much from donor to donor, but on average, it is about five times lower than in rat IgGs [120, 121].

Electrophoretically and immunologically homogeneous preparations of IgG antibodies were isolated from blood sera of 18 patients with SCZ and 14 healthy donors by affinity chromatography on Protein G-Sepharose followed by high-efficiency gel filtration as described above. Using rigid criteria, it was shown that the oxidation of substrates is an intrinsic property of these polyclonal antibodies (**Figure 12**). The comparison of $H_2O_2$-dependent peroxidase and $H_2O_2$-independent oxidoreductase activities of IgGs of SCZ patients and healthy donors in the oxidation of 3,3′-diaminobenzidine was carried. All IgG preparations of SCZ patients and healthy donors had these activities, but the apparent $k_{cat}$ values varied in a very wide range (16.2–355.8 $min^{-1}$).

On average, the rate of oxidation of the substrate in the presence of $H_2O_2$ from the sera of SCZ patients and healthy donors was 1.3–1.5 times higher than in the absence of $H_2O_2$. The difference between the average peroxidase (1.8-fold) and oxidoreductase (1.5-fold) IgG activity from the sera of SCZ patients and healthy donors was statistically significant ($P = 0.008$). At the same time, the correlation coefficient of peroxidase and oxidoreductase activity of abzymes of SCZ patients was significantly higher (0.66) than for healthy donors (0.27).

The blood of healthy donors and patients with various autoimmune diseases including SLE and MS usually contains abzymes with amylase and ATPase activities [47–56]. In addition, the spontaneous and DNA-induced development of deep SLE-like pathology associated with a specific reorganization of the immune system in the case of autoimmune-prone MRL-lpr/lpr mice, leads to a production of IgGs hydrolyzing DNA, ATP, and polysaccharides [64, 65]. It was surprising that in the case of 18 patients with SCZ, amylase activity was detected only in IgG antibodies from one patient, but all 18 preparations were inactive in ATP hydrolysis. This indicates the possibility of the production of abzymes to various antigens in the case different autoimmune diseases.

## 7. Comparison of abzymes of patients with SCZ and other pathologies

It has been shown that antibodies hydrolyzing DNA, proteins, ATP, and polysaccharides can be considered the earliest and statistically significant markers of autoimmune pathologies in human patients and experimental mice with autoimmune diseases [47–56, 64–69]. Abzymes are found already in the early stages of different diseases when there are no visible markers of specific AIDs, and changes in proteinuria, auto-antibodies titers correspond to typical ranges of these indicators for healthy individuals. The detection of abzymes is significantly more sensitive than the detectable ELISA markers since catalysis is characterized by the development of the reaction product due to a large number of enzyme turns and the possibility of increasing the catalyst turnover due to the increase in the reaction time. It makes possible to detect even small amounts of abzymes in preparations of polyclonal Abs with a relatively low but reliably tested activity.

Antibodies against DNA were detected in an increased concentration, compared with that in healthy donors, in only 17–18% of patients with MS and 37% of patients with SLE [57], while DNA-hydrolyzing Abs in 90–95% of patients with MS [74] and SLE [72, 73]. This is because the increase in auto-Abs titers in patients with AIDs occurs only in the late stages or with exacerbations of these diseases. Thus, reliable detection of abzymes, from our point of view, can be considered as an indicator of even a painful condition (the onset of pathology), and even more development of spontaneous or induced AIDS [47–56, 64–69].

To diagnose MS, a number of medical Poseur criteria are usually used [139, 140], but the final reliable diagnosis is made after the tomography showing "plaques" in the brain that appear in the late stages of the disease. The presence of anti-DNA Abs in patients with MS traditionally was considered only as one of the additional evidences of a system imbalance in immunoregulation, which has no independent pathogenetic significance. However, only anti-DNA Abs as the main component of the intracerebral IgG response was found directly in the brain plaques and the cerebrospinal fluid, and they bind to the surface of neuronal cells and oligodendrocytes [141]. These data were interpreted as evidence of the leading role of anti-DNA Abs in the pathogenesis of MS [141].

Despite the absence of signs that meet the criteria of Poseur, we assumed a preliminary diagnosis of the "initial stage of MS" in the case of three patients [69], since they demonstrated Abs with high DNase activity in their blood. Approximately 1.5 years later, the indicators of these patients began to meet the criteria of Poseur and after 2–3 years, the patients had "plaques" in the brain.

In this connection, it should be mentioned that the sera of healthy donors do not contain Abs with DNase, RNase, and MBP-hydrolyzing activities [47–56]. In addition, there were no detected abzymes with such activities in patients with weak autoimmune reactions. Currently, IgGs and/or IgAs and IgMs hydrolyzing DNA/RNA have been revealed in the sera of patients with SLE [72, 73, 142, 143], Hashimoto thyroiditis [144], diabetes mellitus [53], MS [74, 145, 146], tick-borne encephalitis [147], and HIV infection [148] demonstrating strong autoimmune reactions. As it was shown on the example of Hashimoto thyroiditis, the typical therapy of patients with thyroxine resulted only in a temporary change of the hormone concentration in the blood but did not affect the level of DNase abzymes. However, treatment of patients with an immunosuppressive drug Plaquenil leads to a significant decrease in DNase antibodies associated with an increase in concentrations of thyroid hormone, elevation of the thyroid gland functional activity, and improvement of the patient's clinical state [144].

It should be mentioned that the average concentration of Abs interacting with dsDNA for SCZ patients (0.25 ± 0.07 $A_{450}$/ml) is 2.5-fold higher than that for healthy donors (0.1 ± 0.02 $A_{450}$/ml), but lower than for MS (0.39 ± 0.26 $A_{450}$/ml) and SLE (0.66 ± 0.48 $A_{450}$/ml) patients [53–56]. At the same time, concentrations of anti-DNA antibodies in comparison with healthy donors are higher in 30% patients with SCZ, which is comparable with that for SLE patients (37%) [83]. In addition, 80% IgGs of SCZ patients possess detectable or high DNase activity. Moreover, all 100% of IgGs of SCZ patients have RNase activity, and they can hydrolyze not only different polynucleotides and cCMP, but also specific for this pathology microRNAs [83]. Thus, these data point to the development of autoimmune processes in patients with schizophrenia similar to those of classical AIDS: SLE and MS [83].

Interestingly, SCZ patients demonstrated ~1.8-fold higher level of serum anti-MBP Abs than healthy individuals, but ~2.4- and 5..50-fold lower than those for SLE and MS patients, respectively [75]. A feature people with MS and SLE is the development of abzymes hydrolyzing not only DNA, but also MBP and polysaccharides [75–82]. It was shown that IgGs from the sera and cerebrospinal fluid (CSF) of MS patients are active in the hydrolysis of MBP, DNA, and polysaccharides [149–151]. In contrast to healthy donors, Abs from the sera of 82% of patients with SCZ showed a reliably tested or high activity in the hydrolysis of MBP [100, 101]. As mentioned above, the researchers of the London medical Institute Oliver House advanced theory, according to which schizophrenia is the result of a lesion of immune system of the brain. The set forth above data reveals a number of similarities between SCZ and MS.

In this connection, it should be mentioned that development of SLE in autoimmune-prone MRL-lpr/lpr mice and changes in EAE-like (experimental autoimmune encephalomyelitis) parameters in C57BL/6 mice can occur spontaneously and may be accelerated by immunization of mice with DNA [63–65] or with MOG [66–68], respectively. It was shown that IgGs from the sera of control C57BL/6 mice are catalytically inactive. During spontaneous development of EAE, a specific reorganization of the immune system of mice occurred leading to a condition which was associated with the generation of catalytically active IgGs hydrolyzing MBP, MOG (myelin oligodendrocyte glycoprotein) and DNA. These processes are associated with increased proteinuria, changes in the differentiation of mice bone marrow hematopoietic stem cells and an increase in proliferation of lymphocytes in bone marrow, spleen, and thymus as well as a significant suppression of cell apoptosis in these organs. The strongest alterations were found after mice immunization with MOG. Thus, a significant increase in DNase and protease activities of abzymes were shown to be the earliest statistically significant marker of EAE development. In connection with these, it is important to note that abzymes hydrolyzing DNA, MBP, and oligosaccharides were found in cerebrospinal fluid of MS patients and their activity on average approximately from 30 to 60-fold higher than those from the sera of the same patients [149–151]. This may indicate that the development of autoimmune processes can begin already in the human brain.

In MS, SLE, and SCZ, anti-MBP abzymes can attack MBP of the myelin-proteolipid sheath of axons leading to a disturbance of conduction of nerve impulses [53–56]. Overall, the destruction of the myelin sheath and the production of MBP-hydrolyzing Abs can be a common phenomenon for some different diseases including SCZ. Interestingly, neuropsychiatric involvement to some extent similar to MS and SCZ patients occurs in approximately 50%

patients with SLE and carries a poor forecast [152]. SLE mostly affects the central neural system, and within its cerebral complications, it has a particular propensity—perhaps more than any other systemic inflammatory disease—to cause psychiatric disorders. Some similar neuropsychiatric indicators of disease common to SLE, MS, and SCZ were observed [152]. The production of abzymes hydrolyzing MBP as well as DNA and RNA even more powerful indicate the development of significant autoimmune reactions in patients with SCZ. Thus, in different patients with SCZ, SLE, and MS, there are, in some extent, similarities in the violation of the immune system, production of abzymes, and neuropsychiatric disorders.

As it indicated above, the sera of healthy donors contain abzymes with different oxidation-reduction activities. Therefore, at first glance, the detection of abzymes with such activities in patients with SCZ may not have a pathophysiological significance. However, in SCZ patients, a dysfunction of the glutamatergic system is shown [9–12], while misbalance of dopamine-glutamate homeostasis can result in the patient's development of generalized oxidative stress [13, 14]. In SCZ patients, the cellular metabolism changes are associated with alteration in the activity of enzymes, including antioxidant enzymes [109, 112].

The difference between the average peroxidase (1.8-fold) and oxidoreductase (1.5-fold) IgG activity in the oxidation of 3,3′-diaminobenzidine from the sera of SCZ patients and healthy donors was moderate but statistically significant ($P = 0.008$). At the same time, the average relative catalase activity of IgGs from the sera of SCZ patients was 15.8-fold higher than from healthy donors. These data on the oxidation-reduction enzymatic activities of antibodies seem to be important for understanding the possibility of protecting a person from oxidative stress with the help of blood immunoglobulins.

## 8. Conclusion

It was shown that similar to patients with typical autoimmune pathologies, SLE and MS, sera of SCZ patients contain IgGs hydrolyzing DNA, RNA, MBP, and abzymes with catalase, peroxidase, and oxidoreductase activities. As mentioned above, an appearance of abzymes with nuclease and protease activities, which are absent in the blood of healthy donors, may be used as the earliest markers of autoimmune reactions in patients with different autoimmune diseases. Therefore, one cannot exclude that abzymes with these activities may in addition to other different important factors cooperatively promote activation of neuropathologic and psychiatric mechanisms in SCZ pathogenesis.

SCZ patients show some similarity with MS and SLE patients in the development of the same medical, biochemical, and immunological indexes appearing especially in late stages of these diseases. Thus, it is obvious that early diagnostics of SCZ requires the use of all known independent methods to exclude SLE, MS, and probably other possible diseases leading to a formation of MBP-, DNA-, and RNA-hydrolyzing abzymes. However, even revealing of these abzymes on early stages of SCZ may be very useful for detecting of autoimmune reactions in such patients. It is known that SLE, MS, and SCZ patients are usually treated with different drugs. SCZ is known as the progressive mental illness with very different polymorphic symptoms, which are similar to typical autoimmune diseases associated in addition with autoimmune reactions. Taking this into account, one cannot exclude that for a more effective treatment of schizophrenia, patients may be necessary to use some kind of medications suppressing the autoimmune reactions in this pathology. For example, it should be emphasized that the activity of MBP-hydrolyzing Abs attacking myelin-proteolipid shell of axons may be inhibited by MS therapeutic Copaxone [82].

DNase abzymes form SLE and MS patients are cytotoxic and induce apoptotic cell death. The decrease in activity of Abs with nuclease activities was achieved after treatment of patients with Hashimoto thyroiditis with Plaquenil [144]. It cannot be ruled out that any other drugs that are used to treat patients with other different autoimmune diseases can be effective in suppressing the autoimmune component in patients with schizophrenia.

In summary, as mentioned above, schizophrenia is not currently attributed to the typical autoimmune diseases. However, we have shown for the first time in several articles that poly-clonal IgGs from the sera of schizophrenia patients possess DNase, RNase, MBP-hydrolyzing, catalase, peroxidase, and oxidoreductase catalytic activities, which are the earliest markers of autoimmune reactions. It means that immune system dysregulation including autoimmunity together with other factors can be important for the development of schizophrenia.

## Acknowledgements

This research was made possible by grant from the Russian Science Foundation (No 16-15-10103) to G. A. Nevinsky).

## Author details

Valentina N. Buneva, Evgeny A. Ermakov and Georgy A. Nevinsky*

*Address all correspondence to: nevinsky@niboch.nsc.ru

Institute of Chemical Biology and Fundamental Medicine of Siberian Division of Russian Academy of Sciences, Novosibirsk, Russia

## References

[1] Meyer-Lindenberg A. Neuroimaging and the question of neurodegeneration in schizophrenia. Progress in Neurobiology. 2011;**95**:514-516. DOI: 10.1016/j.pneurobio.2011.07.007

[2] Goldner EM, Hsu L, Waraich P, Somers JM. Prevalence and incidence studies of schizophrenic disorders: A systematic review of the literature. Canadian Journal of Psychiatry. 2002;**47**:833-843. DOI: 10.1177/070674370204700904

[3] Beasley CL, Pennington K, Behan A, Wait R, Dunn MJ, Cotter D. Proteomic analysis of the anterior cingulate cortex in the major psychiatric disorders: Evidence for disease-associated changes. Proteomics. 2006;**6**:3414-3425. DOI: 10.1002/pmic.200500069

[4] Lewis DA, Hashimoto T, Volk DW. Cortical inhibitory neurons and schizophrenia. Nature Reviews. Neuroscience. 2005;**6**:312. DOI: 10.1038/nrn1648

[5] Reynolds LM, Reynolds GP. Differential regional N-acetylaspartate deficits in postmortem brain in schizophrenia, bipolar disorder and major depressive disorder. Journal of Psychiatric Research. 2011;**45**:54-59. DOI: 10.1016/j.jpsychires.2010.05.001

[6] Eschenko ND, editor. Biochemistry of Psychiatric and Neurological Diseases. Selected Sections. St Petersburg, Publishing House of St Petersburg State University; 2004. 204 p

[7] Jenkins TA, Harte MK, Stenson G, Reynolds GP. Neonatal lipopolysaccharide induces pathological changes in parvalbumin immunoreactivity in the hippocampus of the rat. Behavioural Brain Research. 2009;**205**:355-359. DOI: 10.1016/j.bbr.2009.07.014

[8] Mura G, Petretto DR, Bhat KM, Carta MG. Schizophrenia: From epidemiology to rehabilitation. Clinical Practice & Epidemiology in Mental Health. 2012;**8**:52-66. DOI: 10.2174/1745017901208010052

[9] Lieberman JA, Kinon FJ, Loebel AD. Dopaminergic mechanisms in idiopathic and drug-induced psychoses. Schizophrenia Bulletin. 1990;**16**:97-110

[10] Waziri R, Baruah S. A hyperglycinergic rat model for the pathogenesis of schizophrenia: Preliminary findings. Schizophrenia Research. 1999;**37**:205-215

[11] Konradi C, Heckers S. Molecular aspects of glutamate dysregulation: Implications for schizophrenia and its treatment. Pharmacology & Therapeutics. 2003;**97**:153-179

[12] Boksha I. Specific Metabolism of Glutamate in Schizophrenia. LAP Saarbrucken, Germany: Lambert Academic Publishing; 2012. p. 196

[13] Wood SJ, Yücel M, Pantelis C, Berk M. Neurobiology of schizophrenia spectrum disorders: The role of oxidative stress. Annals of the Academy of Medicine, Singapore. 2009;**38**:396-401

[14] Yao JK, Reddy R. Oxidative stress in schizophrenia: Pathogenetic and therapeutic implications. Antioxidants & Redox Signaling. 2011;**15**:1999-2002

[15] Prilipko LL, Lederman RR. Lipid peroxidation processes as a factor in modification of membrane proteins of nerve cells in schizophrenia. Vestnik Rossiĭskoĭ Akademii Meditsinskikh Nauk. 1982;**1**:33-36

[16] Ryazantseva NV, Novitsky VV, Agarkov AP, Stepovaya EA, editors. Pathology of Cell Membranes in Schizophrenia. Tomsk: Publishing House of Tomsk State University; 2004. p. 122

[17] Kliushnik TP, Siriachenko TM, Sarmanova ZV, Otman IN, Dupin AM, Sokolov RE. Changes of the level of serum antibodies to neuroantigens in patients with schizophrenia during the treatment. Zhurnal nevrologii i psikhiatrii imeni S.S. Korsakova (Moscow). 2008;**108**:61-64

[18] Deakin J, Lennox BR, Zandi MS. Antibodies to the N-methyl-D-aspartate receptor and other synaptic proteins in psychosis. Biological Psychiatry. 2014;**75**:284-291. DOI: 10.1016/j.biopsych.2013.07.018

[19] Steiner J, Schiltz K, Bernstein HG, Bogerts B. Antineuronal antibodies against neurotransmitter receptors and synaptic proteins in schizophrenia: Current knowledge and clinical implications. CNS Drugs. 2015;**29**:197-206. DOI: 10.1007/s40263-015-0233-3

[20] Levite MJ. Glutamate receptor antibodies in neurological diseases. Neural Transom (Vienna). 2014;**121**:1029-1075. DOI: 10.1007/s00702-014-1193-3

[21] Torrey EF, Yolken RH. The schizophrenia–rheumatoid arthritis connection: Infectious, immune, or both? Brain, Behavior, and Immunity. 2001;**15**:401-410. DOI: 10.1006/brbi.2001.0649

[22] Othman SS, Kadir KA, Hassan J, Hong GK, Singh BB, Raman N. High prevalence of thyroid function test abnormalities in chronic schizophrenia. Australian & New Zealand Journal of Psychiatry. 1994;**28**:620-624. DOI: 10.3109/00048679409080785

[23] Hardoy MC, Cadeddu M, Serra A, Moro MF, Mura G, Mellino G, Bhat KM, Altoé G, Usai P, Piga M, Carta MG. A pattern of cerebral perfusion anomalies between major depressive disorder and Hashimoto thyroiditis. BMC Psychiatry. 2011;**11**:148. DOI: 10.1186/1471-244X-11-148

[24] Pollak TA, Beck K, Irani SR, Howes OD, David AS, McGuire PK. Autoantibodies to central nervous system neuronal surface antigens: Psychiatric symptoms and psychopharmacological implications. Psychopharmacology. 2016;**233**:1605-1621. DOI: 10.1007/s00213-015-4156-y

[25] Owen MJ, Sawa A, Mortensen PB. Schizophrenia. Lancet. 2016;**388**:86-97. DOI: 10.1016/S0140-6736(15)01121-6

[26] Schmitt A, Leonardi-Essmann F, Durrenberger PF, Parlapani E, Schneider-Axmann T, Spanagel R, Arzberger T, Kretzschmar H, Herrera-Marschitz M, Gruber O, Reynolds R, Falkai P, Gebicke-Haerter PJ. Regulation of immune-modulatory genes in left superior temporal cortex of schizophrenia patients: A genome-wide microarray study. The World Journal of Biological Psychiatry. 2011;**12**:201-215. DOI: 10.3109/15622975.2010.530690

[27] Kavanagh DH, Tansey KE, O'Donovan MC, Owen MJ. Schizophrenia genetics: Emerging themes for a complex disorder. Molecular Psychiatry. 2014;**20**:72-76. DOI: 10.1038/mp.2014.148

[28] Miller BH, Wahlestedt C. MicroRNA dysregulation in psychiatric disease. Brain Research. 2010;**1338**:89-99. DOI: 10.1016/j.brainres.2010.03.035

[29] Sun XY, Lu J, Zhang L, Song HT, Zhao L, Fan HM, Zhong AF, Niu W, Guo ZM, Dai YH, Chen C, Ding YF, Zhang LY. Aberrant microRNA expression in peripheral plasma and

mononuclear cells as specific blood-based biomarkers in schizophrenia patients. Journal of Clinical Neuroscience. 2015;**22**:570-574. DOI: 10.1016/j.jocn.2014.08.018

[30] Shi W, Du J, Qi Y, Liang G, Wang T, Li S, Xie S, Zeshan B, Xiao Z. Aberrant expression of serum miRNAs in schizophrenia. Journal of Psychiatric Research. 2012;**46**:198-204. DOI: 10.1016/j.jpsychires.2011.09.010

[31] Lai CY, SL Y, Hsieh MH, Chen CH, Chen HY, Wen CC, Huang YH, Hsiao PC, Hsiao CK, Liu CM, Yang PC, Hwu HG, Chen WJ. MicroRNA expression aberration as potential peripheral blood biomarkers for schizophrenia. PLoS One. 2011;**6**:e21635. DOI: 10.1371/journal.pone.0021635

[32] Perkins DO, Jeffries CD, Jarskog LF, Thomson JM, Woods K, Newman MA, Parker JS, Jin J, Hammond SM. MicroRNA expression in the prefrontal cortex of individuals with schizophrenia and schizoaffective disorder. Genome Biology. 2007;**8**:R27. DOI: 10.1186/gb-2007-8-2-r27

[33] Moreau MP, Bruse SE, David-Rus R, Buyske S, Brzustowicz LM. Altered microRNA expression profiles in postmortem brain samples from individuals with schizophrenia and bipolar disorder. Biological Psychiatry. 2011;**69**:188-193. DOI: 10.1016/j.biopsych.2010.09.039

[34] Ripke S, O'Dushlaine C, Chambert K, Moran JL, Kähler AK, et al. Genome-wide association analysis identifies 13 new risk loci for schizophrenia. Nature Genetics. 2013;**45**:1150-1159. DOI: 10.1038/ng.2742

[35] Schizophrenia Psychiatric Genome-Wide Association Study (GWAS) Consortium. Genome-wide association study identifies five new schizophrenia loci. Nature Genetics. 2011;**43**:969-976. DOI: 10.1038/ng.940

[36] Hauberg ME, Holm-Nielsen MH, Mattheisen M, Askou AL, Grove J, Børglum AD, Corydon TJ. Schizophrenia risk variants affecting microRNA function and site-specific regulation of NT5C2 by miR-206. European Neuropsychopharmacology. 2016;**26**:1522-1526. DOI: 10.1016/j.euroneuro.2016.06.014

[37] Yin J, Lin J, Luo X, Chen Y, Li Z, Ma G, Li K. miR-137: A new player in schizophrenia. International Journal of Molecular Sciences. 2014;**15**:3262-3271. DOI: 10.3390/ijms15023262

[38] Olde Loohuis NF, Ba W, Stoerchel PH, Kos A, Jager A, Schratt G, Martens GJ, van Bokhoven H, Nadif Kasri N, Aschrafi A. MicroRNA-137 controls AMPA-receptor-mediated transmission and mGluR-dependent LTD. Cell Reports. 2015;**11**:1876-1884. DOI: 10.1016/j.celrep.2015.05.040

[39] Siegert S, Seo J, Kwon EJ, Rudenko A, Cho S, Wang W, Flood Z, Martorell AJ, Ericsson M, Mungenast AE, Tsai LH. The schizophrenia risk gene product miR-137 alters presynaptic plasticity. Nature Neuroscience. 2015;**18**:1008-1016. DOI: 10.1038/nn.4023

[40] Topol A, Zhu S, Hartley BJ, English J, Hauberg ME, Tran N, Rittenhouse CA, Simone A, Ruderfer DM, Johnson J, Readhead B, Hadas Y, Gochman PA, Wang YC, Shah H, Cagney G,

Rapoport J, Gage FH, Dudley JT, Sklar P, Mattheisen M, Cotter D, Fang G, Brennand KJ. Dysregulation of miRNA-9 in a subset of schizophrenia patient-derived neural progenitor cells. Cell Reports. 2016;**15**:1024-1036. DOI: 10.1016/j.celrep.2016.03.090

[41] Murai K, Sun G, Ye P, Tian E, Yang S, Cui Q, Sun G, Trinh D, Sun O, Hong T, Wen Z, Kalkum M, Riggs AD, Song H, Ming G, Shi Y. The TLX-miR-219 cascade regulates neural stem cell proliferation in neurodevelopment and schizophrenia iPSC model. Nature Communications. 2016;**7**:10965. DOI: 10.1038/ncomms10965

[42] Lahti AC, Weiler MA, Tamara M, Parwani A, Tamminga CA. Effects of ketamine in normal and schizophrenic volunteers. Neuropsychopharmacology. 2001;**25**:455-467. DOI: 10.1016/S0893-133X(01)00243-3

[43] Strous RD, Shoenfeld Y. Schizophrenia, autoimmunity and immune system dysregulation: A comprehensive model updated and revisited. Journal of Autoimmunity. 2006; **27**:71-80. DOI: 10.1016/j.jaut.2006.07.006

[44] Bergink V, Gibney SM, Drexhage HA. Autoimmunity, inflammation, and psychosis: A search for peripheral markers. Biological Psychiatry. 2014;**75**:324-331. DOI: 10.1016/j.biopsych.2013.09.037

[45] Lerner RA, Tramontano A. Antibodies as enzymes. Trends in Biochemical Sciences. 1987;**12**:427-430. DOI: 10.1016/0968-0004(87)90208-8

[46] Schultz PG, Lerner RA. From molecular diversity to catalysis: Lessons from the immune system. Science. 1995;**269**:1835-1842

[47] Keinan E, editor. Catalytic Antibodies. Weinheim: Wiley-VCH Verlag GmbH and Co; 2005. p. 586

[48] Nevinsky GA, Kanyshkova TG, Buneva VN. Natural catalytic antibodies (abzymes) in normalcy and pathology. Biochemistry (Moscow). 2000;**65**:1245-1255

[49] Nevinsky GA, Buneva VN. Human catalytic RNA- and DNA-hydrolyzing antibodies. Journal of Immunology. 2002;**269**:235-249

[50] Nevinsky GA, Favorova OO, Buneva VN. Natural catalytic antibodies – New characters in the protein repertoire. In: Golemis E, editor. Protein-Protein Interactions; a Molecular Cloning Manual. New York, Cold Spring Harbor: Spring Harbor Lab. Press; 2002. pp. 532-534

[51] Nevinsky GA, Buneva VN. Catalytic antibodies in healthy humans and patients with autoimmune and viral diseases. Journal of Cellular and Molecular Medicine. 2003;**7**:265-276. DOI: 10.1111/j.1582-4934.2003.tb00227.x

[52] Nevinsky GA, Buneva VN. Natural catalytic antibodies-abzymes. In: Keinan E, editor. Catalytic Antibodies. Weinheim: Wiley-VCH Verlag GmbH and Co; 2005. p. 505-569. DOI: 10.1002/3527603662.ch19

[53] Nevinsky GA. Natural catalytic antibodies in norm and in autoimmune diseases. In: Brenner KJ, editor. Autoimmune Diseases: Symptoms, Diagnosis and Treatment. New York, USA: Nova Science Publishers; 2010. pp. 1-107

[54] Nevinsky GA. Natural catalytic antibodies in norm and in HIV-infected patients. In: Kasenga FH, editor. Understanding HIV/AIDS Management and Care—Pandemic Approaches the 21st Century. Rijeka, Croatia: InTech; 2011. pp. 151-192

[55] Nevinsky GA. Autoimmune processes in multiple sclerosis: Production of harmful catalytic antibodies associated with significant changes in the hematopoietic stem cell differentiation and proliferation. In: Conzalez-Quevedo A, editor. Multiple Sclerosis. Rijeka, Croatia: InTech; 2016. pp. 100-147

[56] Nevinsky GA. Catalytic antibodies in norm and systemic lupus Erythematosus. In: Khan WA, editor. Lupus. Rijeka, Croatia: InTech; 2017. pp. 41-101. DOI: 10.5772/67790

[57] Shoenfeld Y, Ben-Yehuda O, Messinger Y, Bentwitch Z, Rauch J, Isenberg DI, Gadoth NG. Autoimmune diseases other than lupus share common anti-DNA idiotypes. Immunology Letters. 1988;**17**:285-291. DOI: 10.1016/0165-2478(88)90043-0

[58] Blanco F, Kalsi J, Isenberg DA. Analysis of antibodies to RNA in patients with systemic lupus erythematosus and other autoimmune rheumatic diseases. Clinical and Experimental Immunology. 1991;**86**(1):66-70. DOI: 10.1111/j.1365-2249.1991.tb05775.x

[59] Sato T, Uchiumi T, Arakawa M, Kominami R. Serological association of lupus autoantibodies to a limited functional domain of 28S ribosomal RNA and to the ribosomal proteins bound to the domain. Clinical and Experimental Immunology. 1994;**98**:35-39. DOI: 10.1111/j.1365-2249.1994.tb06603.x

[60] Hirokawa K, Takasaki Y, Takeuchi K, Kaneda K, Ikeda K, Hashimoto H. Anti-TS1-RNA: Characterization of novel antibodies against sequence-specific RNA by random RNA selection in patients with Sjögren's syndrome. The Journal of Rheumatology. 2002; **29**:931-937

[61] Ikeda K, Takasaki Y, Hirokawa K, Takeuchi K, Hashimoto H. Clinical significance of antibodies to TS1-RNA in patients with mixed connective tissue disease. The Journal of Rheumatology. 2003;**30**:998-1005

[62] Founel S, Muller S. Antinucleosome antibodies and T-cell response in systemic lupus erythematosus. Annals of Internal Medicine (Paris). 2002;**153**:513-519

[63] Andryushkova AA, Kuznetsova IA, Buneva VN, Toporkova LB, Sakhno LV, Tikhonova MA, Chernykh ER, Orlovskaya IA, Nevinsky GA. Formation of different abzymes in autoimmune-prone MRL-lpr/lpr mice is associated with changes in colony formation of haematopoietic progenitors. Journal of Cellular and Molecular Medicine. 2007;**11**:531-551. DOI: 10.1111/j.1582-4934.2007.00048.x

[64] Andryushkova AA, Kuznetsova IA, Orlovskaya IA, Buneva VN, Nevinsky GA. Antibodies with amylase activity from the sera of autoimmune-prone MRL/MpJ-lpr mice. FEBS Letters. 2006;**580**:5089-5095

[65] Andryushkova AS, Kuznetsova IA, Orlovskaya IA, Buneva VN, Nevinsky GA. Nucleotide- hydrolyzing antibodies from the sera of autoimmune-prone MRL-lpr/lpr mice. International Immunology. 2009;**21**:935-945

[66] Doronin VB, Parkhomenko TA, Korablev A, Toporkova LB, Lopatnikova JA, Alshevskaja AA, Sennikov SV, Buneva VN, Budde T, Meuth SG, Orlovskaya IA, Popova NA, Nevinsky GA. Changes in different parameters, lymphocyte proliferation and hematopoietic progenitor colony formation in EAE mice treated with myelin oligodendrocyte glycoprotein. Journal of Cellular and Molecular Medicine. 2016;**20**:81-94. DOI: 10.1111/jcmm.12704

[67] Doronin VB, Korablev A, Toporkova LB, Aulova KS, Buneva VN, Budde T, Meuth SG, Orlovskaya IA, Popova NA, Nevinsky GA. Changes in several disease parameters including Abzymes and hematopoietic progenitor colony formation in brain inflammation and demyelination. Journal of Neurology and Neurological Disorders. 2017;**3**:302

[68] AAulova KS, Toporkova LB, Lopatnikova JA, Alshevskaya AA, Sennikov SV, Buneva VN, Budde T, Meuth SG, Popova NA, Orlovskaya IA, Nevinsky GA. Changes in haematopoietic progenitor colony differentiation and proliferation and the production of different abzymes in EAE mice treated with DNA. Journal of Cellular and Molecular Medicine. 2017;**12**:3795-3809

[69] Buneva VN, Nevinsky GA. Exceptional multiplicity of catalytic antibodies with different catalytic activities in the blood of patients with autoimmune and viral diseases. Molekulyarnaya Biologiya (Moscow). 2017;**51**:969-984

[70] Sinohara H, Matsuura K. Does catalytic activity of Bence-Jones proteins contribute to the pathogenesis of multiple myeloma? Applied Biochemistry and Biotechnology. 2000;**83**:85-94

[71] Kozyr AV, Kolesnikov AV, Aleksandrova ES, Sashchenko LP, Gnuchev NV, Favorov PV, Kotelnikov MA, Iakhnina EI, Astsaturov IA, Prokaeva TB, Alekberova ZS, Suchkov SV, Gabibov AG. Autoantibodies to nuclear antigens: Correlation between cytotoxicity and DNA-hydrolyzing activity. Applied Biochemistry and Biotechnology. 1998;**75**:45-61

[72] Andrievskaya OA, Buneva VN, Naumov VA, Nevinsky GA. Catalytic heterogenity of polyclonal RNA-hydrolyzing IgM from sera of patients with lupus erythematosus. Medical Science Monitor. 2000;**6**:460-470. DOI: 10.12659/MSCR.894649

[73] Andrievskaya OA, Buneva VN, Baranovskii AG, Gal'vita AV, Benzo ES, Naumov VA, Nevinsky GA. Catalytic diversity of polyclonal RNA-hydrolyzing IgG antibodies from the sera of patients with systemic lupus erythematosus. Immunology Letters. 2002;**81**:191-198. DOI: 10.1016/S0165-2478(02)00006-8

[74] Baranovskii AG, Kanyshkova TG, Mogelnitskii AS, Naumov VA, Buneva VN, Gusev EI, Boiko AN, Zargarova TA, Favorova OO, Nevinsky GA. Polyclonal antibodies from blood and cerebrospinal fluid of patients with multiple sclerosis effectively hydrolyze DNA and RNA. Biochemistry (Mosc). 1998;**63**:1239-1248

[75] Bezuglova AM, Konenkova LP, Doronin BM, Buneva VN, Nevinsky GA. Affinity and catalytic heterogeneity and metal-dependence of polyclonal myelin basic protein-hydrolyzing IgGs from sera of patients with systemic lupus erythematosus. Journal of Molecular Recognition. 2011;**24**:960-974. DOI: 10.1002/jmr.1143

[76] Bezuglova AM, Konenkova LP, Buneva VN, Nevinsky GA. IgGs containing light chains of the λ-and κ-type and of all subclasses (IgG1–IgG4) from the sera of patients with systemic lupus erythematosus hydrolyze myelin basic protein. International Immunology. 2012;**24**:759-770. DOI: 10.1093/intimm/dxs071

[77] Bezuglova AM, Dmitrenok PS, Konenkova LP, Buneva VN, Nevinsky GA. Multiple sites of the cleavage of 17- and 19-mer encephalytogenic oligopeptides corresponding to human myelin basic protein (MBP) by specific anti-MBP antibodies from patients with systemic lupus erythematosus. Peptides. 2012;**37**:69-78. DOI: 10.1016/j.peptides.2012.07.003

[78] Timofeeva AM, Dmitrenok PS, Konenkova LP, Buneva VN, Nevinsky GA. Multiple sites of the cleavage of 21- and 25-mer encephalytogenic oligopeptides corresponding to human myelin basic protein (MBP) by specific anti-MBP antibodies from patients with systemic lupus erythematosus. PLoS One. 2013;**8**:e51600. DOI: 10.1371/journal.pone.0051600

[79] Polosukhina DI, Kanyshkova TG, Doronin BM, Tyshkevich OB, Buneva VN, Boiko AN, Gusev EI, Favorova OO, Nevinsky GA. Hydrolysis of myelin basic protein by polyclonal catalytic IgGs from the sera of patients with multiple sclerosis. Journal of Cellular and Molecular Medicine. 2004;**8**:359-368. DOI: 10.1111/j.1582-4934.2004.tb00325.x

[80] Polosukhina DI, Buneva VN, Doronin BM, Tyshkevich OB, Boiko AN, Gusev EI, Favorova OO, Nevinsky GA. Metal-dependent hydrolysis of myelin basic protein by IgGs from the sera of patients with multiple sclerosis. Immunology Letters. 2006;**103**:75-81. DOI: 10.1016/j.imlet.2005.10.018

[81] Legostaeva GA, Polosukhina DI, Bezuglova AM, Doronin BM, Buneva VN, Nevinsky GA. Affinity and catalytic heterogeneity of polyclonal myelin basic protein-hydrolyzing IgGs from sera of patients with multiple sclerosis. Journal of Cellular and Molecular Medicine. 2010;**14**:699-709. DOI: 10.1111/j.1582-4934.2009.00738.x

[82] Ponomarenko NA, Durova OM, Vorobiev II, Belogurov AA, Kurkova IN, Petrenko AG, Telegin GB, Suchkov SV, Kiselev SL, Lagarkova MA, Govorun VM, Serebryakova MV, Avalle B, Tornatore P, Karavanov A, Morse HC 3rd, Thomas D, Friboulet A, Gabibov AG. Autoantibodies to myelin basic protein catalyze site-specific degradation of their antigen. Proceedings of the National Academy of Sciences of the United States of America. 2006;**103**:281-286

[83] Ermakov EA, Smirnova LP, Parkhomenko TA, Dmitrenok PS, Krotenko NM, Fattakhov NS, Bokhan NA, Semke AV, Ivanova SA, Buneva VN, Nevinsky GA. DNA-hydrolysing activity of IgG antibodies from the sera of patients with schizophrenia. Open Biology. 2015;**5**:150064. DOI: 10.1098/rsob.150064. PMID:26382278

[84] Nevinsky GA, Buneva VN. Autoantibodies and natural catalytic antibodies in health, multiple sclerosis, and some other diseases. Advances in Neuroimmune Biology. 2012; **3**:157-182

[85] Paul S, Volle DJ, Beach CM, Johnson DR, Powell MJ, Massey RJ. Catalytic hydrolysis of vasoactive intestinal peptide by human autoantibody. Science. 1989;**244**:1158-1162

[86] Gololobov GV, Chernova EA, Schourov DV, Smirnov IV, Kudelina IA, Gabibov AG. Cleavage of supercoiled plasmid DNA by autoantibody fab fragment: Application of the flow linear dichroism technique. Proceedings of the National Academy of Sciences of the United States of America. 1995;**92**:254-257

[87] Vlassov A, Florentz C, Helm M, Naumov V, Buneva V, Nevinsky G, Giegé R. Characterization and selectivity of catalytic antibodies from human serum with RNase activity. Nucleic Acids Research. 1998;**26**:5243-5250. DOI: 10.1093/nar/26.23.5243

[88] Vlasov AV, Baranovskii AG, Kanyshkova TG, Prints AV, Zabara VG, Naumov VA, Breusov AA, Giege R, Buneva VN, Nevinskii GA. Substrate specificity of serum DNA- and RNA-hydrolyzing antibodies of patients with polyarthritis and autoimmune thyroiditis. Molekulyarnaya Biologiya (Moscow). 1998;**32**:559-569

[89] Vlassov AV, Helm M, Florentz C, Naumov V, Breusov AA, Buneva VN, Giege R, Nevinsky GA. Variability of substrate specificity of serum antibodies obtained from patients with different autoimmune and viral deseases in reaction of tRNA hydrolysis. Russian Journal of Immunology. 1999;**4**:25-32

[90] Vlasov AV, Helm M, Naumov VA, Breusov AA, Buneva VN, Florentz C, Giege R, Nevinskii GA. Features of tRNA hydrolysis by autoantibodies from blood serum of patients with certain autoimmune and virus diseases. Molekulyarnaya Biologiya (Moscow). 1999;**33**:866-872

[91] Ermakov EA, Ivanova SA, Buneva VN, Nevinsky GA. RNA- and microRNA-hydrolyzing IgG antibodies from blood of patients with schizophrenia. Biochemistry (Moscow). 2018 in press

[92] Krasnorutskii MA, Buneva VN, Nevinsky GA. Antibodies against DNA hydrolyze DNA and RNA. Biochemistry (Moscow). 2008;**73**:1547-1560 ISSN 0006-2979

[93] Krasnorutskii MA, Buneva VN, Nevinsky GA. Antibodies against RNA hydrolyze RNA and DNA. Journal of Molecular Recognition. 2008;**21**:338-347. DOI: 10.1002/jmr.906

[94] Krasnorutskii MA, Buneva VN, Nevinsky GA. Immunization of rabbits with DNase I produces polyclonal antibodies with DNase and RNase activities. Journal of Molecular Recognition. 2008;**21**:233-242. DOI: 10.1002/jmr.890

[95] Krasnorutskii MA, Buneva VN, Anti-RNase NGA. Antibodies against pancreatic ribonuclease a hydrolyze RNA and DNA. International Immunology. 2008;**20**:1031-1040. DOI: 10.1093/intimm/dxn061

[96] Krasnorutskii MA, Buneva VN, Nevinsky GA. Immunization of rabbits with DNase II leads to formation of polyclonal antibodies with DNase and RNase activities. International Immunology. 2009;**21**:349-360. DOI: 10.1093/intimm/dxp004

[97] Andrievskaia OA, Kanyshkova TG, Iamkovoi VI, Buneva VN, Nevinskii GA. Monoclonal antibodies to DNA hydrolyze RNA better than DNA. Doklady Akademii Nauk (Russian). 1997;**355**:401-403

[98] Terryberry W, Thor G, Peter JB. Autoantibodies in neurodegenerative diseases: Antigen-specific frequencies and intrathecal analysis. Neurobiology of Aging. 1998;**19**:205-216

[99] Reindl M, Linington C, Brehm U, Egg R, Dilitz E, Deisenhammer F, Poewe W, Berger T. Antibodies against the myelin oligodendrocyte glycoprotein and the myelin basic protein in multiple sclerosis and other neurological diseases: A comparative study. Brain. 1999;**122**:2047-2056

[100] Parshukova DA, Smirnova LP, Buneva VN, Semke AV, Ivanova SA. Proteolytic hydrolysis of myelin basic protein by IgGs during long-term treatment of schizophrenia. European Neuropsychopharmacology. 2015;**25**(S2):S272-S273. DOI: 10.1016/S0924-977X(15)30317-5

[101] Parshukova DA, Smirnova LP, Ermakov EA, Bokhan NA, Semke AV, Ivanova SA, Buneva VN, Nevinsky GA. Autoimmunity and immune system dysregulation in schizophrenia: IgGs from sera of patients hydrolyze myelin basic protein.

[102] Fersht A. Enzyme Structure and Mechanism. 2nd ed. W. H. Freeman, Co: N.Y; 1984. p. 475

[103] Ames BN. Dietary carcinogens and anticarcinogens. Oxygen radicals and degenerative diseases. Science. 1983;**221**:1256-1264

[104] Sies H, editor. Oxidative Stress: Oxidants and Antioxidants. N.Y: Academic Press; 1991. p. 650

[105] Cutler RG. Antioxidants and aging. The American Journal of Clinical Nutrition. 1991; **53**:373S-379S

[106] Beckman KB, Ames BN. The free radical theory of aging matures. Physiological Reviews. 1998;**78**:547-581

[107] Feuers RJ, Weindruch R, Hart RW. Caloric restriction, aging, and antioxidant enzymes. Mutation Research. 1993;**295**:191-200

[108] Morkovkin VM, Kartelishev AV. Pathochemistry of Schizophrenia (Pathogenetic, Diagnostic and Prognostic Aspects). Moscow: Medicine; 1988. pp. 1-256

[109] Krotenko NV, Smirnova LP, Loginov VN, Gorbatsevich LA, Ivanova SA. Comparative activity of antioxidant enzymes in erythrocytes of patients with schizophrenia and multiple sclerosis. Actual Probl Psychiat Narcol (Tomsk, Russia). 2007;**13**:108-110

[110] Gilgun-Sherki Y, Melamed E, Offen D. The role of oxidative stress in the pathogenesis of multiple sclerosis: The need for effective antioxidant therapy. Journal of Neurology. 2004;**251**:261-268

[111] Koch M, Mostert J, Arutjunyan AV, Stepanov M, Teelken M, Heersema D, De Keyser J. Plasma lipid peroxidation and progression of disability in multiple sclerosis. European Journal of Neurology. 2007;**14**:529-533

[112] Smirnova LP, Krotenko NV, Krotenko NM, Loginov VN, Dukhan MV, Ivanova SA, Maltseva YL. Activity of antioxidant enzymes in erythrocytes of patients with mental and neurological disorders. Siberian Herald Psychiatry and Addiction Psychiatry (Tomsk, Russia). 2008;**1**:133-135

[113] Ivanova SA, Shchigoreva Yu G, Boiko AS, Semke AV, Uzbekov MG, Bokhan NA. Glucose-6-phosphate dehydrogenase and catalase activities in erythrocytes of schizophrenic patients under pharmacotherapy with traditional antipsychotics. Neurochemical Journal (Moscow). 2014;**8**:66-70

[114] Smirnova LP, Krotenko NV, Grishko EV, Alifarova VM, Ivanova SA. The state of the antioxidant system during therapy of patients with multiple sclerosis. Biochemistry, Supplement (Moscow). Series B: Biomedical Chemistry. 2011;**5**:76-80

[115] Mates JM, Perez-Gomez C, Nunez de Castro I. Antioxidant enzymes and human diseases. Clinical Biochemistry. 1999;**32**:595-603

[116] Mates JM, Sanchez-Jimenez F. Antioxidant enzymes and their implications in pathophysiologic processes. Frontiers in Bioscience. 1999;**4**:D339-D345

[117] Frei B, Stoker R, Ames BN. Antioxidant defenses and lipid peroxidation in human blood plasma. Proceedings of the National Academy of Sciences of the United States of America. 1988;**85**:9748-9752

[118] Zenkov NK, Lankin VZ, Men'shikova EB. Oxidative Stress. Biochemical and Pathophysiological Aspects. Moscow: MAIK, Nauka/Interperiodica; 2001. pp. 3-343

[119] Shcheglova TV, Tolmacheva AS, Ovchinnikova LP, Sinitsyna OI, Vasilenko NL, Buneva VN, Nevinsky GA. Superoxide dismutase, catalase, peroxidase and peroxide-independent oxidoreductase activities of IgG antibodies from the blood of Wistar rats. Russian Journal of Immunology (Moscow). 2011;**5**:11-20

[120] Tolmacheva AS, Blinova EA, Ermakov EA, Buneva VN, Vasilenko NL, Nevinsky GA. IgG abzymes with peroxidase and oxidoreductase activities from the sera of healthy humans. Journal of Molecular Recognition. 2015;**28**:565-580. DOI: 10.1002/jmr.2474

[121] Tolmacheva AS, Zaksas NP, Buneva VN, Vasilenko NL, Nevinsky GA. Oxidoreductase activities of polyclonal IgGs from the sera of Wistar rats are better activated by combinations of different metal ions. Journal of Molecular Recognition. 2009;**22**:26-37. DOI: 10.1002/jmr.923

[122] Ermakov EA, Smirnova LP, Bokhan NA, Semke AV, Ivanova SA, Buneva VN, Nevinsky GA. Catalase activity of IgG antibodies from the sera of healthy donors and patients with schizophrenia. PLoS One. 2017;**12**:e0183867. DOI: 10.1371/journal.pone.0183867

[123] Polosukhina DI, Buneva VN, Doronin BM, Tyshkevich OB, Boiko AN, Gusev EI, Favorova OO, Nevinsky GA. Hydrolysis of myelin basic protein by IgM and IgA antibodies from the sera of patients with multiple sclerosis. Medical Science Monitor. 2005;**11**:BR266-BR272

[124] Burbaeva GS, Turishcheva MS, Vorobyeva EA, Savushkina OK, Tereshkina EB, Boksha IS. Diversity of glutamate dehydrogenase in human brain. Progress in Neuro-Psychopharmacology & Biological Psychiatry. 2002;**26**:427-435. DOI: 10.1016/S0278-5846(01)00273-1

[125] Kostrikina IA, Buneva VN, Nevinsky GA. Systemic lupus erythematosus: Molecular cloning of fourteen recombinant DNase monoclonal kappa light chains with different

catalytic properties. Biochimica et Biophysica Acta. 2014;**1840**:1725-1737. DOI: 10.1016/j.bbagen.2014.01.027

[126] Botvinovskaya AV, Kostrikina IA, Buneva VN, Nevinsky GA. Systemic lupus erythematosus: Molecular cloning of several recombinant DNase monoclonal kappa light chains with different catalytic properties. Journal of Molecular Recognition. 2013;**26**:450-460. DOI: 10.1002/jmr.2286

[127] Timofeeva AM, Buneva VN, Nevinsky GA. Systemic lupus erythematosus: Molecular cloning and analysis of 22 individual recombinant monoclonal kappa light chains specifically hydrolyzing human myelin basic protein. Journal of Molecular Recognition. 2015;**28**:614-627. DOI: 10.1002/jmr.2476

[128] Timofeeva AM, Ivanisenko NV, Buneva VN, Nevinsky GA. Systemic lupus erythematosus: Molecular cloning and analysis of recombinant monoclonal kappa light chain NGTA2-Me-pro-ChTr possessing two different activities-trypsin-like and metalloprotease. International Immunology. 2015;**27**:633-645. DOI: 10.1093/intimm/dxv042

[129] Timofeeva AM, Buneva VN, Nevinsky GA. Systemic lupus erythematosus: Molecular cloning and analysis of recombinant monoclonal kappa light chain NGTA1-Me-pro with two metalloprotease active centers. Molecular BioSystems. 2016;**12**:3556-3566

[130] Hifumi E, Matsumoto S, Nakashima H, Itonaga S, Arakawa M, Katayama Y, Kato R, Uda T. A novel method of preparing the monoform structure of catalytic antibody light chain. The FASEB Journal. 2016;**30**:895-908. DOI: 10.1096/fj.15-276394

[131] Hifumi E, Taguchi H, Kato R, Uda T. Role of the constant region domain in the structural diversity of human antibody light chains. The FASEB Journal. 2017;**31**:1668-1677. DOI: 10.1096/fj.201600819R

[132] Wentworth AD, Jones LH, Wentworth P Jr, Janda KD, Lerner RA. Antibodies have the intrinsic capacity to destroy antigens. Proceedings of the National Academy of Sciences of the United States of America. 2000;**97**:10930-10935

[133] Wentworth P Jr, Jones LH, Wentworth AD, Zhu X, Larsen NA, Wilson IA, Xu X, Goddard WA 3rd, Janda KD, Eschenmoser A, Lerner RA. Antibody catalysis of the oxidation of water. Science. 2001;**293**:1806-1811

[134] Wentworth P Jr, Nieva J, Takeuchi C, Galve R, Wentworth AD, Dilley RB, DeLaria GA, Savev A, Babior BM, Janda KD, Eschenmoser A, Lerner RA. Evidence for ozone formation in human atherosclerotic arteries. Science. 2003;**302**:1053-1056

[135] Ikhmyangan EN, Vasilenko NL, Buneva VN, Nevinsky GA. IgG antibodies with peroxidase-like activity from the sera of healthy Wistar rats. FEBS Letters. 2005;**579**:3960-3964

[136] Ikhmyangan EN, Vasilenko NL, Buneva VN, Nevinsky GA. Metal ions-dependent peroxidase and oxidoreductase activities of polyclonal IgGs from the sera of Wistar rats. Journal of Molecular Recognition. 2006;**19**:91-105

[137] Ikhmyangan EN, Vasilenko NL, Sinitsina OI, Buneva VN, Nevinsky GA. Substrate specificity of rat sera IgG antibodies with peroxidase and oxidoreductase activities. Journal of Molecular Recognition. 2006;**19**:432-440

[138] Tolmacheva AS, Vasilenko NL, Zaksas NP, Sinitsina OI, Buneva VN, Nevinsky GA. Immunoglobulins a from the blood of healthy Wistar rats oxidize amines. Russian Journal of Immunology (Moscow). 2009;**3**:39-48

[139] Poser CM, Paty DW, Scheinberg L. New diagnostic criteria for multiple sclerosis: Guidelines for research protocols. Annals of Neurology. 1983;**13**:227-231

[140] Kurtzke JF. Rating neurological impairment in multiple sclerosis: An expanded disability scale (EDSS). Neurology. 1983;**33**:1444-1452

[141] Williamson RA, Burgoon MP, Owens GP, Ghausi O, Leclerc E, Firme L, Carlson S, Corboy J, Parren PW, Sanna PP, Gilden DH, Burton DR. Anti-DNA antibodies are a major component of the intrathecal B cell response in multiple sclerosis. Proceedings of the National Academy of Sciences of the United States of America. 2001;**98**:1793-1798

[142] Shuster AM, Gololobov GV, Kvashuk OA, Bogomolova AE, Smirnov IV, Gabibov AG. DNA hydrolyzing autoantibodies. Science. 1992;**256**:665-667

[143] Buneva VN, Andrievskaia OA, Romannikova IV, Gololobov GV, Iadav RP, Iamkovoi VI, Nevinskii GA. Interaction of catalytically active antibodies with oligoribonucleotides. Molekulyarnaya Biologiya (Moscow). 1994;**28**:738-743

[144] Nevinsky GA, Breusov AA, Baranovskii AG, Prints AV, Kanyshkova TG, Galvita AV, Naumov VA, Buneva VN. Effect of different drugs on the level of DNA-hydrolyzing polyclonal IgG antibodies in sera of patients with Hashimoto's thyroiditis and nontoxic nodal goiter. Medical Science Monitor. 2001;**7**:201-211

[145] Baranovskii AG, Ershova NA, Buneva VN, Kanyshkova TG, Mogelnitskii AS, Doronin BM, Boiko AN, Gusev EI, Favorova OO, Nevinsky GA. Catalytic heterogeneity of polyclonal DNA-hydrolyzing antibodies from the sera of patients with multiple sclerosis. Immunology Letters. 2001;**76**:163-167

[146] Baranovskii AG, Buneva VN, Doronin BM, Nevinsky GA. Immunoglobulins from blood of patients with multiple sclerosis like catalytic heterogeneous nucleases. Russian Journal of Immunology (Moscow). 2008;**2**:405-419

[147] Parkhomenko TA, Buneva VN, Tyshkevich OB, Generalov II, Doronin BM, Nevinsky GA. DNA-hydrolyzing activity of IgG antibodies from the sera of patients with tick-borne encephalitis. Biochimie. 2010;**92**:545-554. DOI: 10.1016/j.biochi.2010.01.022

[148] Odintsova ES, Kharitonova MA, Baranovskii AG, Sizyakina LP, Buneva VN, Nevinsky GA. DNA-hydrolyzing IgG antibodies from the blood of patients with acquired immune deficiency syndrome. Molekulyarnaya Biologiya (Moscow). 2006;**40**:770-777

[149] Parkhomenko TA, Doronin VB, Castellazzi M, Padroni M, Pastore M, Buneva VN, Granieri E, Nevinsky GA. Comparison of DNA-hydrolyzing antibodies from the

cerebrospinal fluid and serum of patients with multiple sclerosis. PLoS One. 2014;**9**: e93001. DOI: 10.1371/journal.pone.0093001

[150] Doronin VB, Parkhomenko TA, Castellazzi M, Padroni M, Pastore M, Buneva VN, Granieri E, Nevinsky GA. Comparison of antibodies hydrolyzing myelin basic protein from the cerebrospinal fluid and serum of patients with multiple sclerosis. PLoS One. 2014;**9**:e107807. DOI: 10.1371/journal.pone.0107807

[151] Doronin VB, Parkhomenko TA, Castellazzi M, Cesnik E, Buneva VN, Granieri E, Nevinsky GA. Comparison of antibodies with amylase activity from cerebrospinal fluid and serum of patients with multiple sclerosis. PLoS One. 2016;**11**:e0154688. DOI: 10.1371/journal.pone.0154688

[152] O'Connor KC, Bar-Or A, Hafler DA. Neuroimmunology of multiple sclerosis. Journal of Clinical Immunology. 2001;**21**:81-92

# Permissions

All chapters in this book were first published in PD, by InTech Open; hereby published with permission under the Creative Commons Attribution License or equivalent. Every chapter published in this book has been scrutinized by our experts. Their significance has been extensively debated. The topics covered herein carry significant findings which will fuel the growth of the discipline. They may even be implemented as practical applications or may be referred to as a beginning point for another development.

The contributors of this book come from diverse backgrounds, making this book a truly international effort. This book will bring forth new frontiers with its revolutionizing research information and detailed analysis of the nascent developments around the world.

We would like to thank all the contributing authors for lending their expertise to make the book truly unique. They have played a crucial role in the development of this book. Without their invaluable contributions this book wouldn't have been possible. They have made vital efforts to compile up to date information on the varied aspects of this subject to make this book a valuable addition to the collection of many professionals and students.

This book was conceptualized with the vision of imparting up-to-date information and advanced data in this field. To ensure the same, a matchless editorial board was set up. Every individual on the board went through rigorous rounds of assessment to prove their worth. After which they invested a large part of their time researching and compiling the most relevant data for our readers.

The editorial board has been involved in producing this book since its inception. They have spent rigorous hours researching and exploring the diverse topics which have resulted in the successful publishing of this book. They have passed on their knowledge of decades through this book. To expedite this challenging task, the publisher supported the team at every step. A small team of assistant editors was also appointed to further simplify the editing procedure and attain best results for the readers.

Apart from the editorial board, the designing team has also invested a significant amount of their time in understanding the subject and creating the most relevant covers. They scrutinized every image to scout for the most suitable representation of the subject and create an appropriate cover for the book.

The publishing team has been an ardent support to the editorial, designing and production team. Their endless efforts to recruit the best for this project, has resulted in the accomplishment of this book. They are a veteran in the field of academics and their pool of knowledge is as vast as their experience in printing. Their expertise and guidance has proved useful at every step. Their uncompromising quality standards have made this book an exceptional effort. Their encouragement from time to time has been an inspiration for everyone.

The publisher and the editorial board hope that this book will prove to be a valuable piece of knowledge for researchers, students, practitioners and scholars across the globe.

# List of Contributors

**Agota Barabassy, Balázs Szatmári, István Laszlovszky and György Németh**
Gedeon Richter Plc., Budapest, Hungary

**Ahmet Emre Sargın**
Department of Psychology, Uskudar University, Istanbul, Turkey

**Kadir Özdel**
Dışkapı Yıldırım Beyazıt Training and Research Hospital, Ankara, Turkey

**Mehmet Hakan Türkçapar**
Department of Psychology, Hasan Kalyoncu University, Gaziantep, Turkey

**Siew Yim Loh**
Faculty of Medicine, University of Malaya, Kuala Lumpur, Malaysia

**Cătălina Angela Cri-an**
Department of Neurosciences, Discipline of Psychiatry and Pediatric Psychiatry, Iuliu Hațieganu University of Medicine and Pharmacy, Cluj-Napoca, Romania Psychiatric Clinic I, Emergency County Hospital, Cluj-Napoca, Romania

**Susan Weiner**
Private Residence, North Potomac, MD, USA

**Anca Dobrean**
Department of Clinical Psychology and Psychotherapy, Babeş-Bolyai University, Cluj- Napoca, Romania

**Costina-Ruxandra Păsărelu**
Doctoral School Evidence-Based Assessment and Psychological Interventions, Babeş-Bolyai University, Cluj-Napoca, Romania

**Ariel Cariaga-Martinez and Raúl Alelú-Paz**
Laboratory for Neuroscience of Mental Disorders Elena Pessino, Madrid, Spain

**Delia M. Podea, Aurora I. Sabau and Karol J. Wild**
"Vasile Goldis" Western University of Arad, County ClinicalEmergency Hospital of Arad, Psychiatry Department, Arad, Romania

**Esmaeil Shahsavand Ananloo**
Department of Genomic Psychiatry and Behavioral Genomics (DGPBG), Roozbeh Hospital, School of Medicine, Tehran University of Medical Sciences (TUMS), Tehran, Iran

**Tomas Sverak**
Department of Psychiatry, Masaryk University and University Hospital Brno, Czech Republic Central European Institute of Technology (CEITEC MU), Masaryk University, Brno, Czech Republic

**Pavla Linhartova, Adam Fiala and Tomas Kasparek**
Department of Psychiatry, Masaryk University and University Hospital Brno, Czech Republic

**Valentina N. Buneva, Evgeny A. Ermakov and Georgy A. Nevinsky**
Institute of Chemical Biology and Fundamental Medicine of Siberian Division of Russian Academy of Sciences, Novosibirsk, Russia

# Index

www.ingramcontent.com/pod-product-compliance
Lightning Source LLC
LaVergne TN
LVHW060550210926
848485LV00005B/1288